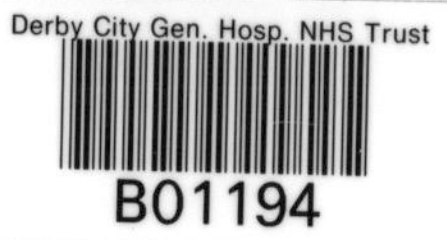

Blackstone's Guide to the

HUMAN FERTILISATION AND EMBRYOLOGY ACT 1990

Abortion and Embryo Research
The New Law

Blackstone's Guide to the

HUMAN FERTILISATION AND EMBRYOLOGY ACT 1990

Abortion and Embryo Research
The New Law

Derek Morgan BA
Senior Fellow in Health Care Law, University College Swansea

and

Robert G Lee LLB
Director of Education, Wilde Sapte, Solicitors, London

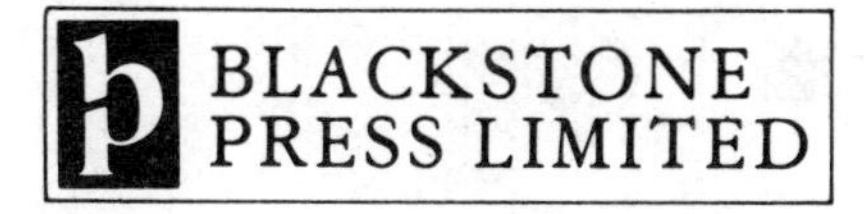

First published in Great Britain 1991 by Blackstone Press Limited,
9-15 Aldine Street, London W12 8AW. Telephone 081-740 1173

ISBN: 1 85431 105 0

British Library Cataloguing in Publication Data
A CIP catalogue record for this book is available from the British Library

Typeset by Style Photosetting Ltd, Mayfield, East Sussex
Printed by Loader Jackson Printers, Arlesey, Bedfordshire

Contents

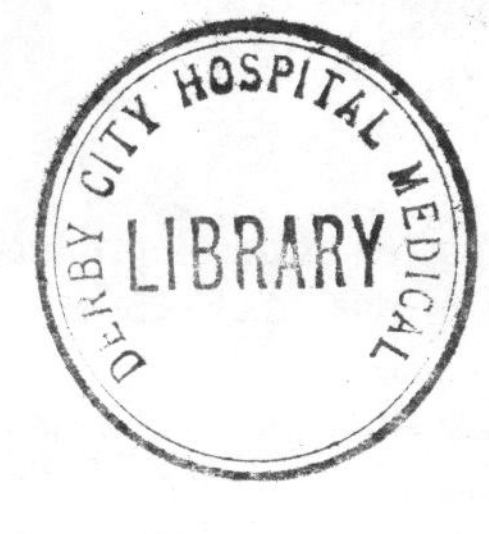

Preface

[This] is a turning point in medical research and in the destiny of mankind. Nothing like this Bill has previously been placed before Parliament.

Lord Houghton, House of Lords, Official Report, 20 March 1990, Col. 244.

Introducing the Human Fertilisation and Embryology Bill to the House of Commons the then Secretary of State for Health, Kenneth Clarke said that this was probably the single most important piece of legislation which a government had brought forward in the last 20 years. It deals with matters which lie at the heart of the people that we say we are, and those which we aspire to become.

In this introductory commentary to the Act we have tried to make the substance of the legislation comprehensible against the background philosophical, ethical, scientific and political debates which have framed its arrival on the statute book.

We have only pared the surface of the rich seam of literature which assisted conception and reproductive technology has generated. Our intellectual debts to that literature are clear. In producing this book we have drawn heavily and in various ways on the goodwill and support, intellectual and material of a number of colleagues and friends. Over a long period of time, Celia Wells, Frances Price, Brian Wynne and Peter Braude have been counsellors and guides to our understanding of this area and our translation of that into this book. Celia Wells has read and commented on the whole manuscript and we have benefited enormously from her advice; Gillian Douglas read and made improvements to every chapter. In addition, Peter Alldridge, Richard Bryden, Veronica English, Don Evans, Jennifer Gunning, Katherine O'Donovan and Frances Price have read and commented upon various chapters or sections. That we did not always heed their advice exonerates them from any responsibility for what follows. Anne Lee prepared the drawings and the figures for Chapter 1; Michelle Bennett enabled us to keep in touch with one another; we are indebted to each of them for those particular contributions. We would also like to thank the Interim Licensing Authority and the Royal College of Obstetricians and Gynaecologists for giving us permission to reproduce material.

Heather Saward and Alistair MacQueen at Blackstone Press were persuaded to accept this book onto their list in April 1990. Their editorial and production contribution to it has been outstanding, and we are delighted to be able to acknowledge this.

Derek Morgan
Robert Lee

List of Abbreviations

BMA	British Medical Association
CMO	Chief Medical Officer
HUFEA	Human Fertilisation and Embryology Authority
ILA	Interim Licensing Authority
LBR	Live Birth Rate
OPCS	Office of Population Censuses and Surveys
PMR	Perinatal Mortality Rate
RCOG	Royal College of Obstetricians and Gynaecologists
VLA	Voluntary Licensing Authority

Glossary

AID: Artificial insemination (of a woman) using donated gametes or a mixture of donor and husband's sperm. Now more commonly referred to as donor insemination (qv) to avoid confusion with AIDS.

AIH: Artificial insemination (of a woman) using husband's sperm.

AIP: Artificial insemination (of a woman) using her partner's sperm.

Alpha foetoprotein: a plasma protein characteristic of the foetus, found in the amniotic fluid (qv) and in small quantities in maternal serum. The level of AFP in maternal blood can be used to screen for neural tube defects and in conjunction with HCG (qv) levels to estimate the risk for Down's syndrome in the foetus.

Amniocentesis: a procedure, usually carried out between 14 and 18 weeks of pregnancy, in which about 20 millilitres of the amniotic fluid is withdrawn through a needle inserted through the abdomen and the uterine wall into the amniotic sac in which the foetus is developing. The fluid and the foetal cells it contains may be tested for genetic disease in the foetus.

Amnion: the inner membrane forming the sac in which the embryo (qv) develops.

Amniotic fluid: the fluid filling the cavity between the embryo and the amnion. Secreted initially by the amnion, it is later supplemented by foetal urine.

Blastocyst: the hollow ball of cells (qv) resulting from cleavage (qv) of the zygote (qv) which implants (qv) in the lining of the uterine cavity before gastrulation (qv).

Cell: the basic unit of all living organisms. Complex organisms such as humans are composed of somatic (body) cells and germ line (reproductive) cells.

Chimera: an individual consisting of cells or tissues of diverse genetic constitution.

Chorion: the outer membrane tissue of the primitive placenta which surrounds the embryo (qv), amnion (qv) and yolk sac.

Chorionic villi: microscopic finger-like fronds of chorionic tissue.

Chorion villus sampling (CVS): a procedure usually effected between 8 and 12 weeks of pregnancy, by which a small amount of the chorionic villi is biopsied for genetic analysis.

Chromosome: a threadlike structure of DNA (qv) and associated proteins found coiled tightly together in the cell nucleus (qv) which carries genetic information in the form of genes (qv). In humans each somatic cell (qv) contains 46 chromosomes — 23 pairs; one of each chromosome in the pair is of maternal and one of paternal origin. Of these 22 are matching pairs and one pair determines sex (XX = female, XY = male).

Cleavage: the stage of cell division between fertilisation and the development of cell differentiation to form the blastocyst (qv).

Cloning: the production of two or more genetically identical individuals by nucleus substitution (qv; 'fusion cloning') or by mechanical division of a cleaving zygote (qv) to yield identical cells each of which can form a new individual ('embryo division' (qv)); rendered a criminal offence under HUFE Act s. 3(3)(d).

Corona radiata: the innermost layer of cells (qv) of the cumulus mass (qv) which surrounds the egg.

Cumulus mass: (cumulus oophorus) the 'cloud' of nurse cells from within the follicle shell surrounding the egg.

Cryopreservation: the protective storage, usually in liquid nitrogen at − 196C, of gametes or embryos. A practice to be regulated under Human Fertilisation and Embryology Act 1990, ss. 14(1)(c), (3), (4) and sch. 2, para. 2, which provides that embryos may not be stored for longer than 5 years and gametes for not longer than 10 years. Women's eggs obtained following superovulation (qv) may also be cryopreserved. The long term effects of freezing are unknown.

DIPI: direct intraperitoneal sperm insemination, involves the injection of washed sperm through the top of the vagina into that part of the peritoneal cavity (known as the Pouch of Douglas) in the vicinity of the fallopian tubes (qv).

DNA: deoxyribonucleic acid, the major constituent of the chromosomes (qv), and the hereditary material of most living organisms.

Donor insemination: the fertilisation of a woman's egg without sexual intercourse. Semen, either fresh or previously frozen, is placed into the cervix usually by a third party using a syringe; a treatment used to establish a pregnancy for a woman whose husband has no or very few sperm.

Ectogenesis: the complete development of an embryo (qv) outside the body.

Egg donation: process where a fertile woman donates an egg to be fertilised *in vitro* (qv) with the semen of the partner of a woman who is infertile.

Embryo: the product of human conception, often understood to cover the period from fertilisation to the end of the eighth week of pregnancy, during which time all the main organs are formed. Pre-embryo is sometimes used to cover the first fourteen days' development after fertilisation. Around this point the 'primitive streak' (qv) develops.

Embryo biopsy: the removal and culture of one or two cells (qv) from an embryo (qv) still *in vitro* (qv) to determine their genetic make-up, in order to detect defects which may result in the birth of severely handicapped babies.

Embryo division: the splitting of an *in vitro* (qv) embryo (qv) at an early stage when each section may continue development. This may produce multiple copies of the single original embryo, and may be considered a form of cloning — fission cloning.

Embryo (or ovum) transfer: the process of transferring a fertilised egg in the course of IVF (qv) or GIFT (qv) procedures, where following development *in vitro* for two or three days, or after flushing from a woman's uterus by lavage (qv; at 5 days), an early embryo is placed in the uterus of an infertile woman in order to try and achieve implantation and pregnancy.

Embryonic disc: a two-tiered disc of cells which derives from the inner cell mass of the blastocyst (qv) and from which the embryo (qv) will grow.

Exsanguination: depriving the body of blood, usually through bleeding.

Fallopian tubes: the organs which carry an egg from the ovary to the womb.

Fertilisation: the fusing together of the maternal and paternal genetic material from the sperm and the egg. The process of fertilisation is commonly regarded as beginning with the passage of sperm through the cumulus oophorus (qv) and ending at syngamy (qv).

Foetus: in humans, the developing embryo from about eight weeks on until birth, when organogenesis is complete and recognisable human features have been established.

Follicle: a fluid-filled cavity containing cystic space which develops in the ovary in which the oocyte develops and is nourished. The oocyte is released surrounded by the cumulus mass when the follicle ruptures at ovulation.

Fundus: the top (cranial) part of the womb (qv) above the point of entry of the fallopian tubes (qv).

Gametes: the reproductive cells (qv), sperm and egg, which fuse to form a zygote (qv). Each human gamete contains a basic set of 23 chromosomes (qv) — a haploid set; on fusion of egg and sperm a full (diploid) set of 46 chromosomes results. All other (somatic) cells in the body contain 46 chromosomes in their nuclei (qv).

Gastrulation: the stage during which the primitive embryonic cells reorganize to form the germ layers (qv).

Gene: the unit of inheritance; that element of DNA (qv) in which the amino-acid sequence of a protein is encoded. Everyone inherits two copies of each gene. A dominantly inherited genetic disease occurs when only one copy of the gene is sufficient to produce the disease, e.g. Huntington's chorea; a recessively inherited disease only occurs if both copies of the defective gene are present, e.g. Tay-Sachs' disease, Sickle cell disease.

Genome: the basic set of genes (qv) in the chromosomes (qv) in any cell (qv) organism or species. Humans have a genome of 23 chromosomes.

Germ layers: the three main layers of cells at gastrulation (qv) stage of development, from which various tissues and organs of the body are formed.

GIFT: gamete intra-fallopian transfer; a process by which an egg or eggs are transferred with sperm into the woman's fallopian tubes (qv) so that fertilisation can occur *in vivo*.

Human chorionic gonadotrophin: (HCG) a protein hormone normally secreted by the chorionic villi (qv) of the placenta. Its presence in the maternal blood or urine indicates pregnancy. It is also used therapeutically as a single injection to stimulate luteinising hormone required for the maturation of the oocytes (qv) before ovulation or asperation.

Human menopausal gonadotrophin: a mixture of the two polypeptide hormones, follicle stimulating hormone and luteinising hormone. Prepared from the urine of menopausal women, it is used to stimulate oocyte (qv) development in the ovary (qv) as part of superovulation.

Implantation: the process whereby the embryo (qv) becomes burrowed in the lining of the uterus (qv); for the purposes of the Human Fertilisation and Embryology Act 1990, s. 2(3) a woman is not to be treated as carrying a child until the embryo (qv) has implanted.

Inner cell mass: (or basal cell mass), a clump of cells growing within and to one side of the blastocyst (qv) from which the embryo (qv) develops.

In vitro: literally, in glass. More commonly to represent the test-tube of popular imagery or more generally, the laboratory.

IUI: inter-uterine insemination, AID with superovulation; a woman is given drugs in order to stimulate superovulation and a sperm sample is then injected into the uterine cavity using a fine catheter through the neck of the womb, beyond the cervix and into the uterine cavity.

IVC: intra-vaginal culture, a method whereby sperm and aspirated oocytes are incubated together in a container held in a woman's vagina in order to effect fertilisation *in vitro* without the need for complex laboratory facilities. After 2 days any cleaving embryos are transferred to the woman's uterus.

IVF: *in vitro* (qv) fertilisation (qv), a 'treatment service' within HUFE Act s. 2(1), in which a woman's egg is fertilised by mixing with sperm outside the body in a petri dish (the 'test-tube').

Karyotype: the chromosomal make-up of cells of an individual; the microscopic appearance of a set of chromosomes, including their number, shape and size.

Laparoscopy: examination of the pelvic or other abdominal organs with a fibreoptic telescope inserted surgically below the navel. During laparoscopy, suction applied to the needle can be used in the recovery of eggs from follicles (qv) in the ovary.

Lavage: the removal of a fertilised egg or cleavage stage embryo from the womb (qv) before implantation (qv) by washing out the uterine cavity.

Meiosis: (reduction division) the process by which a diploid cell nucleus divides into four nuclei each with half the number of chromosomes of the parent nucleus; the process necessary for the formation of haploid gametes (qv).

Morula: the ball of cells which forms at about 3-4 days after insemination of the egg resulting from cleavage of the fertilised ovum.

Nucleus: the part of the cell (qv) which contains the genetic material DNA (qv); it is separated from the other cell contents by a nuclear membrane.

Nucleus substitution: the substitution of the nucleus of an ovum by the nucleus of a somatic cell (qv).

Oocyte: a female cell (qv) that has entered meiosis (qv).

Ovary: the female reproductive organ in which oocytes are produced from pre-existing germ cells.

Ovulation: the release of an egg from a follicle (qv) in the ovary (qv).

Ovum: egg; female gamete (qv).

Phenotype: the physical characteristics of an organism, determined by the genotype and the environment.

POST: peritoneal oocyte and sperm transfer, a procedure which involves the collection of eggs from a woman's ovary (qv) and their transfer with sperm directly into the peritoneal cavity — the cavity of the abdomen where the fallopian tubes and the uterus are situated. Not suitable where a woman's fallopian tubes (qv) are blocked or missing.

Primitive streak: a groove which develops in the embryonic disc (qv) about 14–15 days after fertilisation, into which a third layer of cells, the upper ectoderm layer, invaginates the disc to form the three germ layers. The primitive streak is taken to be the first sign that an embryo will develop; if the primitive streak does not form, embryonic development does not progress and there will be no foetus (qv). The legal significance of this is established in the Human Fertilisation and Embryology Act 1990, ss. 11(1)(c) and 3(3); the moral significance remains contested.

Pro-nucleus: a small round structure(s) seen within the egg after fertilisation which contain the haploid sets of chromosomes (genetic material of each gamete (qv)) surrounded by a membrane. A normal fertilised egg should contain 2 pro-nuclei, one from the egg and one from the sperm.

Recombinant DNA: one of the processes, also known as 'genetic engineering' where DNA (qv) from one organism is introduced into the DNA of another.

Selective reduction: the procedure in which one or more normal foetuses in a multiple pregnancy resulting from assisted conception are destroyed. Clinical guidance now suggests that no more than three or very occasionally four eggs or embryos should be transferred to the womb, thus reducing the incidence of high multiple pregnancy (see RCOG Guidelines, 'Guidelines on Assisted Reproduction Involving Superovulation', August 1990). The foetuses destroyed are usually those closest to the fundus of the uterus. The procedure may be hazardous to the remaining foetus(es), as miscarriage of them results in about 1:50 cases.

Sperm: a mature male germ cell, produced in the testicles.

Superovulation: the medical stimulation of the ovary (qv) with hormones to induce the production of multiple egg-containing follicles in a single menstrual cycle. A number of different regimes are used to induce superovulation; recruitment of follicles being obtained through the administration of pituitary gonadotrophins (CFSH and LH) or oestrogen analogues. An injection of LCG is given at the end of this treatment to induce superovulation so that egg collection may be timed correctly. LCG may also be given as support after embryo transfer. Risks include ovarian hyperstimulation syndrome or the formation of ovarian cysts.

Syngamy: the coming together of the pronucleii at the conclusion of the process of fertilisation (qv). Pairing of the maternal and paternal haploid sets (qv) of chromosomes (qv) is followed by division of the fertilised egg into two cells.

Transvaginal Aspiration: a method of egg recovery in which a needle is inserted through the top of the vagina into the ovary lying in the peritoneal cavity (qv).

Trisomy: having three chromosomes (qv) of one type instead of the normal two (e.g., trisomy 21, responsible for Down's syndrome; trisomy 18, responsible for Edward's syndrome (qv)).

Transvaginal oocyte recovery: now most commonly used for IVF (qv), where the woman's bladder is empty and a needle is passed through the vagina under ultrasound guidance in order to recover eggs.

TUDOR: transvesical ultrasound directed oocyte recovery, an alternative to laparoscopic or transvaginal egg recovery, in which a woman empties her bladder and then fills it with saline solution, and then a needle for recovering the eggs is inserted through her abdomen and bladder and towards the ovary (qv).

Ultrasound: high frequency sound waves that can be focused and the reflected energy used to image tissues, organs or structures within the body.

Ultrasound-guided aspiration: A non-surgical method for egg retrieval where ultrasound images are used to guide the path of the needle into the follicle.

Uterus: the womb; the female organ in which the foetus grows during pregnancy.

ZIFT: zygote intra-fallopian transfer; where eggs fertilised *in vitro* are transferred to the fallopian tubes (qv) at the zygote (pronuclear) stage (1 day); cf. GIFT for unfertilised eggs.

Zona pellucida: the transparent membrane or shell which surrounds the oocyte.

Zygote: the cell (qv) formed by the union of sperm and egg.

Chapter 1
Introduction: Law, Morals and Assisted Conception

The relationship between law and scientific investigation, and between law and fundamental moral principles is always open for debate and examination. Within the 49 sections of the Human Fertilisation and Embryology Act are some of the most difficult, most intractable and fundamental moral questions of which any society becomes seized. What has characterised the twentieth century more clearly than any preceding is that we have assumed the power to cause death on a hitherto unimagined scale and, increasingly, to take scientific control of life itself (Jonathan Glover, *Fertility and The Family: The Glover Report on Reproductive Technologies to the European Commission* ((1989), Fourth Estate, p. 1)).

The Human Fertilisation and Embryology Act represents a marshalling of arguments after nearly two decades of scientific research and ethical and philosophical debate. It would be idle to suppose that the form in which the Act is framed will represent anything more than a temporary statement on the morality of the issues under examination. As with abortion, the questions involved are of such importance to the moral health of society that the process of debate and decision will be constant. Perhaps that is much as it should be. Believing that such fundamental moral and legal issues can be 'solved' betrays a misunderstanding of what moral disagreement is about, as much as it does about the political process of legislating life or regulating reproduction. This is probably only just the starting point.

The result, for the time being, is the creation of a statutory licensing authority with responsibility to review and licence the provision of certain treatments for infertility, and to licence and supervise scientific experiments on early human embryos, or pre-embryos as some would call them. If a committee had been charged to manufacture a name for this statutory licensing authority which could not be the subject of an easy acronym, it might be thought that the Human Fertilisation and Embryology Authority was a pretty good shot. In the absence of any other obvious candidate we refer throughout the text to this body as HUFEA or 'the Authority.' In addition, the Act sets out to reform the lawful grounds of access to abortion. In that respect, it makes the most fundamental changes to abortion law since 1967; it recasts it in a way which was almost inconceivable at the outset of Parliamentary debate.

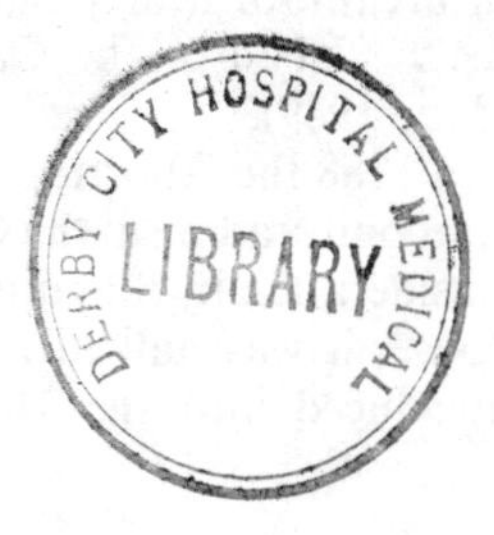

The moral skirmishes which followed publication of the Warnock Report in 1984 suggested that the debates on and eventual resolution of the questions involved would provoke bitter Parliamentary battles and even more intensive public lobbying (Cmnd 9314, *Report of the Committee of Inquiry into Fertilisation and Embryology,* subsequently republished with an introduction by Mary Warnock as *A Question of Life* ((1985), Oxford, Basil Blackwell). The original report was debated in the House of Commons in November 1984 (see House of Commons, Official Report 23 November 1984 cols. 528-43 and 547-90). That gave an early indication of the nature of the debate which had been joined. This was emphasised by the debates which accompanied the unsuccessful private members' Bills introduced by MPs Enoch Powell, Ken Hargreaves (twice) and Alistair Burt in 1985, 1986 and 1987. These Unborn Children (Protection) Bills failed to gain Parliamentary majorities. They would have made it an offence to create, store or use a human embryo for any purpose other than to assist a specified woman to become pregnant. In each case, a registered medical practitioner would have had to apply in writing to the Secretary of State for consent to the fertilisation of a human ovum *in vitro*. That authority would only have been forthcoming if the Secretary of State was satisfied as to:

(i) the arrangements made for the procedure;
(ii) the competence and experience of the medical and other personnel to be involved; and
(iii) the suitability of the premises where the procedure would have been carried out.

In tandem with these debates were continued, and again unsuccessful, attempts to amend the Abortion Act 1967. In the 23 years since its enactment — and the 1967 Act was the seventh backbench attempt to introduce some grounds for lawful abortion — and down to reform in the present Act no fewer than 15 attempts were made through private members' legislation to secure reforms to the 1967 Act. In that time medical opinion and medical technology moved forward, and it became possible, although with poor chances of success and poor prognosis, to salvage premature babies born as little as 24 or 25 weeks after conception (see *Medical Care of the Newborn in England and Wales,* (1989), Royal College of Physicians of London, for a review of current practice). Allied with a number of disturbing reports of abortions which appeared to have produced a live birth, pressure for reform of the Act became, literally, irresistible. One case led not only to a coroner's inquest, but also a Parliamentary debate. This concerned reports that an abortus of about 21 weeks had been deposited in a kidney dish at the side of a ward, where it had made apparent attempts to struggle for breath for nearly three hours before being disposed of by a nursing officer (see the debate on the 'Carlisle Baby case', House of Commons, Official Report, 8 June 1989).

In 1988 the Abortion (Amendment) Bill sponsored by David Alton received its second reading in the Commons by 296 votes to 251, and spent 30 hours under consideration by Standing Committee. When the Bill returned to the floor of the House, it was 'talked out' on Report. An Abortion (Amendment) Bill 1989, introduced into the House of Lords by Lord Houghton to pre-empt the consideration of abortion law reform in the Human Fertilisation and Embryology Bill sought to reduce the time limit within which abortions could lawfully be performed under the Act in England and Wales from 28 to 24 weeks. This limit has met with widespread medical and legal approval (see, for example, the recommendations of the Lane Committee, *Report on the Workings of the Abortion Act 1967*, Cmnd 5579, 1974, para. 208; and of the Working Party of the Royal College of Obstetricians and Gynaecologists and Others, *Report on Foetal Viability and Clinical Practice*, (1984), pp. 14-15). Disquiet has been expressed, as well, about the operation of a number of the other provisions in the 1967 Act, particularly the 'conscience clause' (s. 4), permitting those medical and nursing staff (see *Royal College of Nursing of the United Kingdom* v *Department of Health and Social Security* [1980] AC 800) who have a conscientious objection to participating in any abortion procedure from being required to do so, unless to save the life of the woman who is seeking the abortion. Such concern led to an investigation by the House of Commons Social Services Committee into the operation of the section (see 'Abortion Act 1967 "Conscience Clause"', Social Services Committee, 10th Report, 1990, HC 123, which recommends extending the operation of the clause to ancillary staff (para. 46) and deleting the present 'burden of proof' requirement, presently on the person claiming a conscientious objection (para. 47). The Report notes the existence of discrimination against those exercising their conscientious objection but confessed the Committee's inability to see an easy way to eradicate it (para. 44)).

But there comes a time when fundamental moral disagreement collides with public and professional demands for certainty or consistency, however illusory these eventually prove to be. The nature and moment of scientific work in the past 25 years has ensured that new questions have been put upon the moral and legal agendas. Moreover, they will not go away. The continued pressure for abortion law reform, which surfaced again in the course of this Bill's passage, exemplifies a simple point. Whatever Parliament has here decided about, say, experimentation or research with human embryos, it would be mistaken to assume that pressure for reform will not immediately be gathered and the debate rejoined. We have, it seems, lifted some veils which can no longer be firmly held back. The Human Fertilisation and Embryology Act is a transitory marker in continued moral reflection.

There is also an important sense in which science has crossed a Rubicon for which there is no return ticket. This is reflected in one of the contributions made by the Labour Party frontbench spokeswoman on health, Harriet Harman, to the Standing Committee debates:

> Human fertilisation and embryology are an area of rapid change and continuous advances in our knowledge. When we came to debate the Bill there were many new issues on the agenda which were not considered by the Warnock Committee because they had not even been thought of just those few years before. It is wrong to suggest that passing a law — which we fully support — that says that in principle research shold be allowed to go ahead within a legislative framework somehow marks the end of the debate. The matter will remain one of public interest and also of controversy (Official Report, Standing Committee B, 8 May 1990, col. 49).

Assisted reproduction has introduced a new vocabulary to, and challenged old philosophies of, families and family law. It has also demanded a new literacy of lawyers, lay people and legislators. (We have included some of the more common terms likely to be encountered in the Glossary.) While the past 40 years has seen the meltdown of the nuclear family and its surrounding myths and ideologies, — in less than ten years half of all children born in the United Kingdom will be brought up outside the 'conventional' family — new demons, chimeras and spirits have been summoned to haunt the new families which technological and personal upheavals have introduced. This has been accompanied by the rise of the 'want' society; one in which it has become fashionable to seek the fulfilment of wants and to accept far less readily, if at all, that some desires cannot, should not, or even must not be satisfied or satiated.

There is a sense in which children are an example of this, and assisted conception part of the response, which includes also adoption, surrogacy, and the sale or stealing of children and newborns, sometimes on an international scale. This, in its turn, has fed the arguments of clinicians who service those wants to seek the widest possible freedom. The Human Fertilisation and Embryology Act brought before Parliament the issues surveyed by the Warnock Committee Report published in 1984. The moral turbulence has centred on embryos, particularly on embryos created outside the body, and especially on research with such embryos. It has swept through the legislative process, and is reflected in the way in which the Act has been drafted, interpreted and debated inside and outside Parliament. The limited way in which the licensing authority may be able to discharge its supervisory role owes much to the perceptions of problems created by the Warnock Report. The Act is a Warnock Act. This is true not only in its following the report of the Warnock Committee, but also in the more important sense that the science in question is that of 1984, updated in an ad hoc and piecemeal way. The Act represents a limited attempt to capture or to understand the exponential technological leaps since then. In that important sense, Warnock is not only the benchmark but the workbench of the present legislation.

Types of Philosophical Argument

Followers of previous political debates in this area will not be surprised to find that much of the moral argument has centered on 'personhood', with contributors looking for an absolute point at which something becomes a person. The unspoken assumption is that the way in which we decide on the dividing line, the criteria, is where the morally important work is to be done. There is no shortage of candidates here; moral philosophers, religious leaders, pressure groups and scientific contributors have canvassed conception, nidation, the beginning of the primitive streak, or of the neural streak, quickening, viability and birth at which someone becomes a 'person' or entitled to receive the respect owed to a person. Nor does the argument end there. Some commentators have suggested that what matters is an ability to sense and value life, so that birth as such presents no logical stopping point at which the debates about personhood must end — or begin. It follows that the argument actually surrounds adequate notions of what it is to be a person.

There are alternative approaches to this question, which start from and bring an entirely different perspective. One reverses the 'criterial' approach, and holds that it is only possible to find out what a person is by using morality to find out how a person might arrive out of that. It suggests that we cannot define morality outside, by reference to external criteria, which can then be applied to tell us what our moral position is (or should be). This position holds that otherwise there is nothing that morality can tell us, or anything that human agency can achieve (i.e., there is nothing to distinguish between morality and law). This suggests that there will inevitably be disagreement because we are not looking for one criterion, for a definition of a person. Indeed, it suggests that there is no morally correct position to arrive at; there is no right moral answer. Who or what is a person depends not on a conclusion reached — through applying some criteria — but on a conviction shown.

There is a third type of position, close to the one which Warnock herself appears to have held, which posits that there is no absolute point at which a person arrives and has moral status, no absolute point at which a person 'materialises', but that a person emerges as a gradually present moral entity and one which is possessed of more and more rights as a juridical person. If we then want to make particular legal or political decisions, we do have to select a point or a series of points. This, although it does not presently represent the status of UK law, is, we suspect, the one to which it is moving. At present, English law holds that a foetus can possess different rights as it moves towards birth. Indeed, after birth the sorts of rights that it possesses can differ (see e.g., Derek Morgan, 'Letting Severely Handicapped Babies Die Legally' (1989) 53 *Bulletin of the Institute of Medical Ethics* 13-18). Our abortion law, with its present concepts of 'capable of being born alive' and 'viability', or our law on congenital injuries and pre-natal torts, family law disputes commencing prior to birth and now our laws on embryo experimentation, strongly suggest a differential rights approach. At no point do we accord the foetus special status. These different sorts of approach, although not clearly articulated as such, can be identified as approaches taken during the moral and political debates in the lead up to this particular legislation.

Law and Morals

There is, of course, a further complicated relationship. It is that between morality and law. Once we have discussed the ethics or morality of a particular issue, it does not then follow necessarily that this has to be translated into legal language. That will depend on what we see to be the relationship, if any, between law and morals. Questions about whether an activity is right or wrong, morally innocuous or repugnant, and the arguments supporting those views, belong to moral philosophy. We have identified above only three of the many possible approaches which can be brought to bear in this analysis. The question of whether we should then have laws governing any particular issue, and what shape and rationale those laws might take, belong to legal and political philosophy. There is no necessary, simple connection to be made between the rightness, wrongness or moral indifference to an act or practice, and the propriety or desirability of having a law which requires, permits or forbids it. Of course, we may have a position which holds, for example, that any conduct which is morally repugnant should be and is unlawful. Similarly, we may hold that because conduct is prohibited by legal fiat endorsed with sanction — whether criminal or civil — it is therefore a moral imperative not to break that law. We could hold this latter position simply because we felt that whatever was unlawful was necessarily immoral, or because, whatever our judgment of the morality of the particular law, we placed a particular moral primacy on obeying the law, even if we find it to be morally repugnant.

We can put this another way. That there is no general direct connection between law and morality can be tested straightforwardly. One may consider that an act may be wrong, and wrong only because it is against the law; then there would be a direct connection between the morality and legality of an act. But generally we do not believe that to be the case. We look for some background, justifying moral reason for the law to be the way it is. Debate in legal philosophy then turns on whether morals and law should be coextensive and coterminous, or whether there should be, in the Wolfenden Committee's memorable phrase, some acts which are 'not the law's business':

> Unless a deliberate attempt is to be made by society, acting through the agency of the law, to equate the sphere of crime with that of sin, there must remain a realm of private morality and immorality which is, in brief and crude terms, not the law's business (Wolfenden Report, Report of the Committee on Homosexual Offences and Prostitution, Cmnd 247, 1957 para. 257).

While it seems to follow from this that the scope of moral debate need pay no necessary attention to law, the question for lawyers has been the extent to which the law is or should or indeed can be coterminous with moral positions, and if so, with which one(s).

A traditional starting point for lawyers and political philosophers has been the statement by the nineteenth century thinker John Stuart Mill that:

> The only purpose for which power can be rightfully exercised over any member of a civilised community against his will is to prevent harm to others. His own good, either physical or moral is not a sufficient warrant (*On Liberty*)

We do not want to dwell here on the difficulties to which this dictum has given rise; what is harm?, who counts as others?, must force be used to prevent harm to others, or is this merely a necessary condition?, and what is wrong with the parentalist intervention of others to prevent one causing harm to oneself? In other words, is Mill correct that the state must always misperceive the individual's interests, or be untimely in its intervention? But the responses to the Wolfenden Report, which recalls Mill's harm principle, illustrate some of the fundamental differences in contemporary thought about the relationship between law and morals.

We need to dwell here briefly on the role of the public/private distinction which commended itself to Wolfenden. It does need to be observed, however, that Mill was not himself the author of the distinction. Rather, Mill argued that for something to be brought within the moral sphere it had to involve definite harm to some assignable other. The issue of public regulation arose from that. For Mill, there was no 'bolt-hole' labelled 'private' into which one could escape and claim immunity from public regulation. Insofar as Wolfenden appears to suggest that there is, the public/private spheres of morality have to be traced back to some other source, of which Machiavelli in *The Prince* is an early example. For Mill, it was appropriate to argue whether the public sanction of the law was more or less appropriate than some less formal mechanism, but this did not depend on a supposed distinction between private and public conduct. Anything that fell within the moral realm properly understood, in that it involved harm to another, was amenable to public regulation. (This important clarification is executed by Alan Ryan in his essay 'John Stuart Mill and the Art of Living' (1963) *The Listener*, 21 October 1968).

One of the core questions posed by a respondent to Wolfenden, Patrick Devlin, was whether Wolfenden was correct in assuming and stating that society does not have the right to pass judgment on all matters of morals (Devlin, *The Enforcement of Morals* ((1965), Oxford). Are morals a matter, and exclusively a matter, for private judgment, or is there a public morality? Herbert Hart, in responding to Devlin, recharacterised the questions which Devlin had asked:

> Is the fact that certain conduct is by common standards immoral sufficient to justify making that conduct punishable by law? Is it morally permissible to enforce morality as such? (H. L. A. Hart, *Laws, Liberty & Morality* (1968), Oxford).

Devlin's response to these questions was broadly yes, Hart's no. In an important respect, Hart and Devlin were in agreement. Both believed that if one can establish an identifiable harm to society, then the proper ground for intervention is established. Where they disagreed was on whether morality constitutes a seamless web from which is spun a common, shared morality.

For Devlin, this was a constitutive part of what a society was, such that equating sin and crime was what defined law. Devlin's view is that what makes a society is precisely its shared morality and that creating a society without common agreement on good and evil is doomed to failure. The same would apply to a society in which the common agreement evaporates. The use of law to enforce such agreement is as justifiable as its use to ensure the well-being of anything else that is essential to the existence of that society. Devlin believed, however, that law should be used only in some cases. He suggested four principles of restraint in the extent to which it should be used to enforce even that commonly shared notion of good and evil:

(i) that only what is beyond the limits of tolerance — and this means a real feeling of revulsion and not mere dislike — should be punished by law;
(ii) the extent of tolerance of departures from moral standards will vary over generations;
(iii) as far as possible privacy should be protected;
(iv) the law is concerned with a minimum and not a maximum standard of behaviour.

Hart's response evolves from Mill's harm principle. While he includes harm to oneself, which Mill would have disavowed, Hart argued that recognition of individual liberty as a value involves,

> as a minimum, acceptance of the principle that the individual may do what he wants, even if others are distressed when they learn what it is that he does unless, of course, there are other good grounds for forbidding it.

Hart criticised Devlin's approach as 'legal moralism'; he charged that on Devlin's own account it *assumes* a congruity between law and morality (rather than substantiating it). But more than that, he argued that it is difficult for Devlin to distinguish between a change in morality and a subversion of it. For Hart, Devlin was locked into an unchanging morality in which any change was discernible only as a subversion of morality. This seems a particularly important exchange when put in the context of, say, abortion or embryo research.

A third approach to this question of the relationship between law and morality has been suggested by Rosalind Hursthouse. As she points out, the confusion of questions about morality and legislation is particularly common in arguments about abortion (and we would add embryo research, although for different reasons). As she elaborates, one reason for the confusion is the oppositional tactics taken in debate:

> Many people, particularly women, do think there is something wrong about having an abortion, that it is not a morally innocuous matter, but also think that the current abortion laws are if anything too restrictive, and find it difficult to articulate their position on the morality of abortion without apparently betraying the feminist campaign concerning legislation (*Beginning Lives,* (1987), Basil Blackwell, p. 15).

There are many echoes of this in the radical and the liberal feminist writings on abortion (Cp., for example, Adrienne Rich, *Of Woman Born,* (1976, p. 273-4) Caroline Whitbeck, 'The Moral Implications of Regarding Women as People', in W. Bondelson et. al., (eds.), *Abortion and the Status of the Fetus* ((1984), Reidel, pp. 247-72). This enables us to suggest different approaches to, say, abortion and embryo research, which recognise their ambiguity, as well as their complexity.

Stances on Abortion and Embryo Research

Hursthouse is one writer who has addressed the confusions between questions of law, morality and legislation. She has argued that once the distinction between the questions of law and morality is separated out it becomes possible to identify four different positions on abortion. We suggest that this analysis might conveniently be applied to the arguments surrounding embryo research and the other contents of the Human Fertilisation and Embryology Act 1990.

Morality of abortion	*Laws on abortion*	*Position*
Wrong	Restrictive	Conservative
Innocuous	Restrictive	'Totalitarian'
Innocuous	Liberal	Liberal/Radical
Wrong	Liberal	Liberal/Moderate

(Rosalind Hursthouse, *Beginning Lives,* (1987) Basil Blackwell, p. 15)

The first position is the familiar one in which legislation about morality is based on a conservative moral view. This view is perhaps the most easily identifiable in the Parliamentary debates which have accompanied criticism of the reform implemented in the Abortion Act 1967, and is represented in the Parliamentary debates on the 1990 Act by MPs such as Bernard Braine, Ann Widdecombe, David Alton and in the House of Lords the Duke of Norfolk.

The two liberal views are an innovative and challenging position introduced by Hursthouse. It is much more difficult, whether in the abstract or in the context of Parliamentary speeches and votes, to identify which of the alternative positions an individual holds. An alternative way of describing the positions might be the liberal/moderate as the 'lesser of two evils', where the death of the foetus (or destruction of the embryo) is compared with and transcended by the rights or interests of the individual woman (or society generally). This may be contrasted with the liberal/radical position, where it is the moral insignificance of abortion which facilitates the approach. In the embryo research debates, it is perhaps easier to distinguish those who believe that embryo research does not involve anything of moral worth (the pre-human embryo) and those who hold that it does attract moral worth (the human pre-embryo). For those of the latter position, the value which attaches to the embryo is not sufficient to outweigh the benefits which may be derived from research in terms of infertility treatments; the alleviation of suffering to future generations caused by the existence of genetically inherited diseases or chromosomal disorders; the search for improved methods of contraception or the better understanding of the causes of infertility and miscarriage.

Those who argue that the embryo and the foetus is not a person, or does not have personhood or is not a human being, hold that abortion (and hence embryo research) are morally innocuous. For them, abortion is no different from the removal of cancerous tissue or an appendix. Hence, the desirability of liberal abortion laws does not depend on the present lack of safe and effective birth control or the plight of a woman overburdened with children or with a child who is likely to suffer from a serious physical or mental handicap. It depends only on the argument that men and women should have the same access as to appendectomies or cancer treatments.

If, however, abortion is not morally innocuous, then there is a problem for those who believe that women should be allowed access to lawful abortion facilities on a straightforward basis. It is important for the Liberal/Radical to consider, concerning morality, what sort of wrong they believe abortion to be, and concerning legislation, whether it is the sort of moral wrong over which the state may or should exercise formal control. If, as conservatives believe, abortion is a form of homicide, no morally responsible person should be able to proceed without legal repercussion. If abortion, though not as wrong as homicide, is still nevertheless morally compromised, there remains the problem of whether a woman should be given access to lawful abortion services (to do a wrong or inflict a harm, as Devlin might put it).

If an act is morally compromised, it is not obvious that a right to do it should be enshrined in and protected by law. This does not say that liberal legislation cannot be justified by those who think abortion is morally wrong. Their appeal, however, will lie beyond 'the right to choose':

the 'fashionable and liberal' way of regarding abortion as a morally innocuous event is dangerous because of its tendency to harm women, a tendency which makes it almost as anti-feminist as that of the anti-abortion campaigners (Mira Dana, quoted in Hursthouse, op.cit., p. 24. This seems a purposive recall of the arguments of Rich, supra.)

What is Infertility and What are its Causes?

This immediately provokes the question of whether infertility is an illness or a disease which should be treated. For some, infertility is a 'disease' just as any other; like cancer it is about pathological physiology and it shares with cancer the pathology of cells having 'gone wrong.' The 'plight' of 'the infertile' has thus been seen as legitimating the time, technology and resources expended on it (we return to this comparison in our discussion of the regulation of treatment services, infra, Chapter 5). For others, infertility is a grief, not a disease, and is something sent to burden those unable to conceive.

There are a number of points which are pertinent here. First, fertility is closely allied to the general position of women and men in society, and infertility is as much a social construct as a biological fact; the facts of infertility are loaded with the values of society. Secondly, expenditure on the 'disease' of infertility represents costs foregone elsewhere. The value of assisted conception technology to the wider community has not been extensively debated (but see infra, Wagner and St Clair and respondents, discussed at pp. 120–22). In a world where there is little shortage of people or children, although not all of them may be of the 'approved' colour or able bodied and minded, it is legitimate to ask whether resources should be committed to infertility work at all. Such concerns prompted one MP, Sir Michael McNair-Wilson to observe during Parliamentary debates that:

> . . . in a world that is suffering from overpopulation and that is still afflicted with so many curable illnesses, can the medical profession justify the huge expenditure of vast resources on the more esoteric aspects of medicine, when that money could buy immediate and more easily achievable relief for so many? (House of Commons, Official Report 23 April 1990, col. 89).

Of course, it is possible to challenge both the assumptions which lie behind this sort of observation and the conclusion to which it is made to give rise. So, on the one hand, the 'myth' of overpopulation has been questioned (see Susan George, *How the Other Half Dies,* (1982)) as something more simply understood as a failure to distribute resources equitably. On the other hand, it may be just foolish to think that by hostaging people with fertility problems to their 'fate' that the population policies of the globe will thereby be resolved. There seems to be an extraordinary argument that by penalising those with infertility the sins of omission in the political processes of the world will be absolved. It is nonetheless the case that infertility treatments remain costly and their success rates low, it is undoubtedly necessary to guard against the production of high expectations and the increased grief which a failure (often repeated failure) of those expectations often engenders.

Reproduction has come to occupy an increasingly prominent role in the theatre of the personal. It has moved downstage, from being seen as a minor bit part of personhood, to be cast as one of the essential characteristics of its successful production and realisation. Issues such as childbirth, child-rearing and child care are thus more easily identifiable as raising core questions of social justice. Hence, although there is no area of health care practice where resources are committed with infinite guarantee, the decision about how resources are allocated to infertility treatments cannot be made on the basis of salving our conscience about misallocations which we make elsewhere. Family life, howsoever that is constructed, construed or conceived, continues to exert an important and a powerful hold over issues of personal identity, reproduction and responsibility. (For an overview of the different approaches to the place and power of the family see Diana Gittins, *The Family in Question* ((1985), Macmillan), and D H J Morgan, *The Family, Politics and Social Theory* ((1985), Routledge). For two radically different perspectives compare Michelle Barrett and Mary McIntosh, *The Anti-Social Family* ((1982), Verso) with *Council of Europe, Parliamentary Assembly, Report on Family Policy,* (Doc. 5870, 5 April 1988) and House of Lords, Official Report 29 November 1989, cols. 425-94, debate on Motion — The Family).

Estimates vary of the incidence of infertility, but most agreed figures suggest that at least one in ten couples are affected at some stage in their lives. In Britain this would mean something like 50,000 new cases of infertility each year. But one detailed study in 1985 of one single District Health Authority estimated that at least one in six couples need specialist help at some time in their lives because of an average infertility of two and a half years (M G R Hull, 'Population Study of Causes, Treatment and Outcome in Infertility' *British Medical Journal* 14 December 1985; cf. the summary of the 'Dobson Report'; D Mathieson, 'Infertility Services in the NHS: What's Going On': a report prepared for Frank Dobson MP, House of Commons, in Lesley Doyal's essay, 'Infertility — A Life Sentence: Women and the National Health Service' in Michelle Stanworth (ed.), *Reproductive Technologies: Gender, Motherhood and Medicine* ((1987), Polity Press, pp. 174-90), arguing that the problems of infertility services are not unique and that they reflect the broader failure of the NHS to meet women's needs and expectations. Doyal elsewhere suggests that infertility services reflect the general insensitivity and sexism apparent in the inadequate health care provision for women, see Lesley Doyal, 'Women and the National Health Service: The Carers and the Careless', in E Lewin and V Olesen, (eds.), *Women, Health and Healing* ((1985), Tavistock).

Whatever conclusion is reached on this point, further disputatious points arise. Suppose, for example, that we agree that resources should indeed be devoted to infertility treatments. The first question which then arises is whether all types of infertility should be viewed in the same way? IVF, for example, was originally used for inoperably blocked fallopian tubes. In Denmark, which has a restrictive approach, it is largely confined to such treatment. (See 'Laws on the Establishment of an Ethical Council and the Regulation of Certain forms of Bioethical Research' (English translation reproduced in Jan Stepan (ed.), *International Survey of Laws on Assisted Procreation,* ((1990), Zurich, Schulthess Polygraphischer Verlag), pp. 104-105).) In the United Kingdom, however, it is also indicated in endometriosis, ovulation disorders, anti-sperm antibodies and male infertilities, many of which, it is argued, are socially or environmentally caused.

Secondly, should non-clinical criteria be employed as a way of rationing access to the scarce resource which treatment services represent? For example, the Warnock Committee averred that:

> To judge from the evidence, many believe that the interests of the child dictate that it should be born into a home where there is a loving, stable, heterosexual relationship and that, therefore, the deliberate creation of a child for a woman who is not a partner in such a relationship is morally wrong . . . we believe that as a general rule it is better for children to be born into a two-parent family, with both father and mother, although we recognise that it is impossible to predict with any certainty how lasting such a relationship will be (Warnock Report para. 2.11, and see paras. 4.16 and 5.10).

In other words, the Committee felt more comfortable with the idea of a child born into a home where the uncertainty of its parents' commitment to one another was mediated by the different genders of those whom it assumed would be the child's primary carers. These assumptions have not gone unchallenged, although they appear to have been smuggled into the Act as a way of rationing or restricting access to treatment services. (We return to this point in our discussion of 'Access to Treatment Services' in Chapter 5.)

It is an aspiration of many of those who work in the field that the 'treatment' or care of those with infertility should be but the first practical application of embryo research and IVF work. The additional benefits of a contraceptive vaccine, the resolution of causes of miscarriage, and the detection of genetic and chromosomal abnormalities in pre-implantation embryos or early foetuses remain the longer-term goals of this branch of research.

A third area which needs comment is that such 'infertility treatments' as there are are not freely available to all who would wish to use them. Most services are available only in private clinics, and hence to those who can pay the fees which the clinics charge. Throughout the present Parliamentary debates the lack of available treatment services on the NHS was referred to as 'a tax on the infertile'. And even for those women or couples who can afford access, for whom assisted conception technologies and techniques open up a realm of choice about childlessness, the success is limited.

The costs of infertility treatments, the practices which clinics adopt and procedures which they offer vary enormously. And there are wide regional variations in the availability of treatments. Oxford Regional Health Authority has 18.8 clinics for each million women aged 15-44. North Western RHA has one clinic for 863,000 women. Of 121 health authorities surveyed in a report by the Labour Party's health spokeswoman Harriet Harman, the average is 8.5 clinics per million women (*Trying for a Baby: A Report on the Inadequacy of NHS Infertility Services*, (1990), p. 4). The waiting time for an appointment is up to 10 weeks in one third of the District Health Authorities, 10-20 weeks in 58% and more than 20 weeks in 9% of the authorities. It is exceptional for an authority to provide what would be regarded as a comprehensive infertility service which would include: dedicated infertility clinics; ultrasound scanning; rapid radioimmune assay (a diagnostic test); micro-surgery; and on a regional basis, access to *in vitro* fertilisation and AID services.

A particular feature which the report notes is that scant literature or information is available about services. Little formal advice is given to GPs, although most health authorities rely on GPs being 'fully aware of the services available.' One of the specific duties of HUFEA (under s. 8(b)) will be to publicise the services provided to the public by the Authority or provided in pursuance of licences. An amendment in Commons' Committee which would have required HUFEA to publish and circulate to all GPs information about treatment services available in every Regional Health Authority; to report annually to the NHS Training Authority on the adequacy of counselling services and to have advised the Secretary of State on the nature and extent of any unmet demand for the provision of treatment services governed by the Act was defeated.

As we shall see, s. 16(1) enables HUFEA to levy a fee from any applicant for a licence. Fees are expected to meet two-thirds of HUFEA's operating costs, with the Government budgeting for the cost of setting up the HUFEA at £138,000 for 1990/91, £232,000 for 1991/92 and £159,000 for 1992/93, with broadly equivalent sums in future years. One of the estimates based on these costs is that the licence fee may be somewhere between £40-50,000 per annum, out of a total budget of some £2ml for large centres. For academic or NHS departments' clinics, where they are not able to pass on the costs to patients, the implications were thought to be serious. Under s. 16(7) it is open to HUFEA to set different fees for different types of clinic, or fees may be limited to the levels of work undertaken by each centre. The Government does not intend to fund HUFEA fully from public finances, and perhaps a substantial part of the operating revenue will come form charges levied from clinics and collected ultimately from women or couples undergoing infertility treatments. One of the perceived dangers of these costs is that it will make it important, if not imperative, for other income to be brought into centres to cover these costs by offering, for example, unlicensed GIFT treatments.

On the question of whether this lack of central funding was discriminating against those who used infertility services, the 'tax on the infertile' as it was several times called, Baroness Faithful in the House of Lords put the Government's position: 'money available in this area is open to abuse' (House of Lords, Official Report 6 March 1990, col. 1109), although she did not go on to specify the Government's worries. The Medical Research Council figure for the costs of IVF treatment has put the cost, including salaries, materials and drugs, at £1,587 per successful pregnancy (sometimes referred to as each clinical pregnancy). The Midland Fertility Services Unit believes the cost per live birth (not pregnancy) to be about £8,000, while the King's College estimate puts the cost per treatment cycle at £1,200. Treatment costs vary widely from clinic to clinic. Only two Centres, University Hospital of Wales in Cardiff and St Mary's Hospital in Manchester, provide assisted conception facilities on the NHS. There are 23 centres which are wholly private and 17 which receive either partial funding from the NHS or make use of some NHS facilities but charge the patient for the cost of the treatment. The ILA comment, once again, that funding for this type of treatment under the NHS 'remains grossly inadequate' (*ILA Fifth Report*, (1990), p. 12).

This observation is concurred with in the Harman Report, presented to Parliament in April 1990. It notes that definitions of infertility are not static and that variable definitions do not help in planning the necessary provision of treatment services. However, in contrast with the ILA's estimate that 275,000 couples in the United Kingdom could benefit from IVF treatment, the Report's responses yield an estimate that only 50,000 initial referrals are made per year to infertility clinics. The Report comments:

> Whilst fertility services remain regarded as a luxury which cannot be afforded in a cash-starved NHS, the advances of modern science are available only to a limited few. And the knowledge that such services are available leads many couples to mortgaging their home and their future to pay for fertility treatment (p. 3).

There is a wide range of professional, demographic and socio-political factors which may affect the construction of the results obtained about the 'success rates' from any given clinic following its provision of infertility services. This can vary according to a clinic's decision to treat only a certain number or type of infertility cases each year; the age structure of the client population; the professional skill and expertise of the clinicians, and so on. These points need to be appreciated in studying the most recent figures published by the ILA showing the rates of treatment outcome (particularly pregnancy and live births) per treatment cycle.

TABLE II

IVF Data 1988

(a) Treatment

	Patients	*Treatment Cycles*	*Egg Collections*	*Pre-embryo Transfers*
Large Centres (6)*	3,858	5,621	4,738	3,687
Medium Centres (19)	3,377	4,466	3,457	2,597
Small Centres (10)	280	402	319	269
Total	7,515	10,489	8,514	6,553

(b) Outcome†

	Pregnancies	*Abortions*	*Ectopics*	*Live Births*	*Perinatal Deaths*
Large Centres (6)	806	169	39	545	15
Medium Centres (19)	511	84	28	388	11
Small Centres (10)	37	11	2	23	0
Total	1,354	264‡	69	956	26§

* The figures in parentheses are the numbers of centres included in the returns.
† 55 cases lost to follow-up (4·1 per cent of all pregnancies).
‡ Includes 36 cases of late abortion (> 12 weeks gestation).
§ Perinatal mortality rate is 26·4 (PMR (E+W) in 1988 was 8·7).

TABLE III

GIFT Data 1988

(a) Treatment

	Patients	*Treatment Cycles*	*Egg Collections*	*Gamete Replacements*
IVF Centres (25)	2,438	2,891	2,347	2,517
Non-IVF Centres (18)	402	501	371	382
Total	2,840	3,392	2,718	2,899

(b) Outcome

	Pregnancies	*Pregnancy/ Patient Treated %*	*Pregnancy/ treatment cycle %**
IVF Centres (25)	628	25·7	21·7
Non-IVF Centres (18)	79	19·6	15·7
Total	707	24·9	20·8

* There is a significant difference (p = ·0025) between the outcome for IVF and non-IVF centres.

TABLE IV

Mean IVF Pregnancy and Live Birth Rates 1988

(a) Pregnancy Rates %

	Per Treatment Cycle	*Range*	*Per Egg Collection*	*Range*	*Per Transfer*	*Range*
Large Centres* (6)	14·3	6·1–20·4	17·0	7·0–25·9	21·9	10·3–30·0
Medium Centres (19)	11·4	3·7–24·0	14·8	6·1–31·4	19·7	7·9–32·5
Small Centres (10)	9·2	0·0–15·2	11·6	0·0–20·9	13·8	0·0–24·1

(b) Live Birth Rates %

	Per Treatment Cycle	*Range*	*Per Egg Collection*	*Range*	*Per Transfer*	*Range*
Large Centres (6)	9·7	0·9–16·4	11·5	1·8–20·4	14·8	2·6–22·8
Medium Centres (19)	8·7	1·5–14·6	11·2	3·1–24·4	14·9	5·0–25·7
Small Centres (19)	5.7	0·0–10·9	7·2	0·0–14·9	8·6	0·0–17·2

* The figures in parentheses are the numbers of centres included in the returns.

TABLE V

Crude Pregnancy and Live Birth Rates per Treatment Cycle 1985–1988

All Centres	*1985*	*1986*	*1987**	*1988*
Pregnancy rate %	11·2	9·9	12·5	12·9
Live birth rate %	8·6	8·6	10·1	9·1†

* Excluding one large centre with incomplete data.
† Excluding 55 pregnancies lost to follow-up.

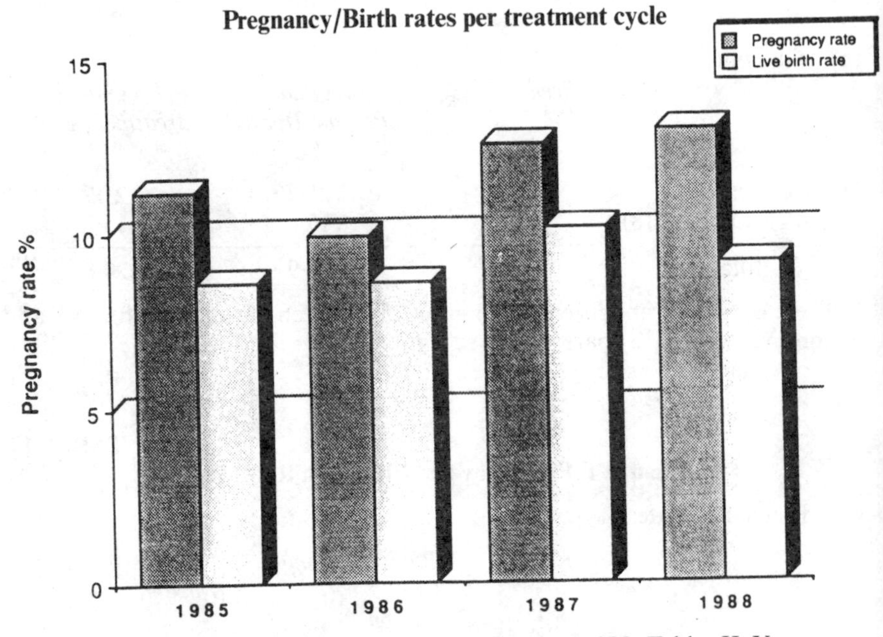

Source: Interim Licensing Authority, Fifth Report, 1990, Tables II–V

Even a brief perusal of Table III gives some interesting data. For all centres there were 956 live births in 10,489 treatment cycles, a less than 1:10 success rate. With 26 perinatal deaths (death in the first 28 days after birth), the perinatal mortality rate was 26.4 per 1,000; the overall PMR in England and Wales for 1988 was 8.7. And while the live birth rates show a significant difference between the large centres (those attempting more than 400 treatment cycles a year) — with a live birth rate of 9.7%; medium centres (attempting 100-400 t.c. p.a.) — with a LBR of 8.7%; and small centres (attempting less than 100 t.c. p.a.) — showing a LBR of only 5.7%; these figures have to be read in light of the caveat which we mentioned above; some large centres, for example, may be very selective in the patients or types of infertility which they will treat; some small centres may take on the 'hopeless cases' rejected by other, perhaps larger clinics.

This leads us into a final, and important point. The experience of infertility may produce anger, grief, resentment, bewilderment and frustration. In short it may produce a 'crisis of infertility', which is said to have an adverse impact on self-esteem, self-image, psychological well-being, marital relationships and sexual satisfaction. Some of these stereotypical pictures have, however, been challenged in recent research. Rachel Cook, John Parsons, Bridget Mason and Susan Golombok interviewed 59 women attending infertility clinics for IVF and AID treatment. The women and their partners (of whom 34 responded) were asked to complete a questionnaire assessing their anxiety, depression, marital functioning, sexual satisfaction and strategies for coping with infertility ('Emotional, Marital and Sexual Functioning in Patients Embarking upon IVF and AID Treatment for Infertility', (1989) 7 *Journal of Reproductive and Infant Psychology* 87-93). While the researchers discovered that both men and women experienced high levels of anxiety, they did not find that they experienced depression, nor that there was a significant level of problems in marital and sexual functioning. Dividing those patients into high and low distress groups, the researchers concluded that those patients who were more anxious and/or depressed were more likely to engage in avoidance-coping strategies, but that this bore no relation with marital or sexual functioning. Cook et.al. conclude that:

> It is perhaps not surprising that infertility patients show high levels of anxiety given the stressful nature of the treatment, especially IVF. Depression, on the other hand, is more often associated with loss, and perhaps depression is more likely to occur after unsuccessful treatment. In fact, it appears . . . that infertility patients embarking upon treatment are particularly optimistic about the likelihood of becoming pregnant and having a baby (at p. 92, citations omitted).

In view of this last observation, it may be imperative for the counselling to which patients are to be directed (see s. 13(6), infra Chapter 5) to apprise patients of the results which they are likely to meet, and for the counselling to be available throughout the treatment cycle programme, and even afterwards.

In addition, as Naomi Pfeffer has argued, the adequacies of these stereotypical assessments may be challenged in a different way. Desperation, she has argued, is only one of a potential range of emotions which 'the infertile' do, or may be expected to, manifest. Not all such emotions are negative and desperation may result not from the condition of infertility but from 'the insensitive and humiliating treatment sometimes received at the hands of medical and other authorities' (Naomi Pfeffer, 'Artificial Insemination, *In Vitro* Fertilisation and the Stigma of Infertility' in Michelle Stanworth, (ed.), *Reproductive Technologies: Gender, Motherhood and Medicine* ((1987), Oxford, Polity Press, p. 81)). This point is echoed by Robert Edelmann and Susan Golombok who observe that 'differences in anxiety between [those whose infertility is] unexplained and organic groups may be a result of the investigative procedures and the uncertain diagnosis rather than a cause of infertility' ('Stress and Reproductive Failure' (1989) 7 *Journal of Reproductive and Infant Psychology* 79-86, at p. 80). Pffefer concludes with an important metawand which should be remembered when talking of the 'plight of the infertile':

> The decision to embark on parenthood, to undertake a major change in social status, antedates the attempt to conceive, particularly today when more

effective means of fertility control are available. This decision is the result of processes that are shaped by social and historical forces, the impact of which are shared by the fertile and infertile alike; there is nothing peculiar about the motivation for parenthood of those who later find themselves infertile (op. cit., at p. 83).

Concerns with Infertility

Medical advance has identified more and more potential causes of infertility, and the group of patients whose fertility cannot be attributed to any anatomical, physiological or pathological cause and whose infertility is 'unexplained', now rarely exceeds 18% of 'infertility patients'. (See Edelmann and Golombok, op.cit., p. 79.) Some of the causes are iatrogenic, arising from contraception, drugs, abortion, surgery or invasive diagnostic procedures. Other causes are environmental — including a wide range of factors such as alcohol, poor nutrition, stress and background toxins — although more research is needed to identify securely causal relationships. Infertility can also arise from physiological factors: undescended testes, endometriosis (the presence of endometriotic tissue — normal uterine lining — in abnormal locations, such as the fallopian tubes, ovaries or peritoneal cavity), lack of sperm motility and so on. It does seem correct to observe that there is a concern with infertility that is unparalleled in earlier times (although we could not make the same observation with respect to fertility). We want here to suggest tentatively four reasons why that might be so.

First, there do seem to be more individuals or couples presenting with primary infertility. This may in part arise out of changing patterns of family planning, including delayed childbearing, careers, chosen childlessness and changing choices. For many (especially women) in the late 1960s and 1970s, while reproductive choices were changing alongside slow and gradual economic and employment liberation, they tended towards the redefiniton of *chosen* childlessness. Coupled with this, the changing patterns of family unit and the increased acceptance of the dissolubility of them, led to changing patterns of relationship and family units. The combined effects of this is that many, especially women, found their reproductive choices changing. This led to an abandonment of earlier choices about reproduction and childlessness, with a consequent desire to become pregnant later in their reproductive lives, and/or a desire to have children in a number of sequential partnerships. This produces a desire to remain (re)productive for longer. Hence childbirth became for some more condensed, through choice, and attendant on apparent improvements in reliable contraceptive options.

Secondly, it would seem that an increasing number of couples with primary infertility are seeking treatment. The importance of assistance may grow as fewer newborn babies are available for adoption. This arises from a combination of contraception, abortion and slow but growing acceptance of single women keeping children born to them rather than their being adopted, either with the active support and encouragement of the state through social welfare programmes, or at least not in the face of open state-sanctioned hostility. Greater toleration of illegitimacy has been reflected in legislative changes aimed at removing the remaining vestiges of stigma and the adverse consequences of illegitimacy. Heightened expectations concerning the way in which we can assert control over our lives may lead to a reluctance or refusal to accept an involuntarily childless state. This may be especially true with rising incomes, so that a higher percentage of infertile couples can afford to make their voice loudly heard and expect to be listened to.

Medical advance provides a third reason, as an increasing number of physicians offer more sophisticated techniques of diagnosis and treatment. The birth and evolution of the technology of assisted reproduction has been rapid, but even relatively low-tech. methods, such as surrogacy, have become more prominent. (For a review of the growth and development of assisted conception technologies see Edward Yoxen, *Unnatural Selection: Coming to Terms with the New Genetics,* ((1986) Heinemann.) On the other hand, it has to be said that demand for infertility treatment far outstrips supply. Estimates vary, but it seems that between 1 in 10 and 1 in 8 of all couples is established as the best estimate of the numbers of those who will experience infertility at some stage in their reproductive lives.

Finally, we cannot ignore the role of the media in reflecting shades of opinion not simply upon issues of infertility, but also on questions of family and sex. We have seen a strong promotion of 'family' values on a political plane, firmly underpinned by the media. In the summer of 1990, 'The Family' became firmly entrenched in the political battles between major political parties. Coverage of questions of infertility by the media has ranged from stories of high technology pioneers on the frontiers of science to stories of grandmothers having babies for their daughters and daughters having children for their mothers; from the human misery of those who have been 'trying for a baby' for years to fears of a 'Brave New World' mentality to accompany the technology. This media attention has reflected and been reflected in public interest and attitudes.

In an important review of public attitudes, Stephen Harding has gauged the changes gradually taking place with respect to assisted conception and abortion (see Stephen Harding, 'Trends in Permissiveness' in Roger Jowell, Sharon Witherspoon and Lindsay Brook, (eds.), *British Social Attitudes,* 5th Report pp. 38-42). Comparing cross-nationally, and over a range of personal sexual issues, the British emerge as close to the West European average; more censorious than the Danes, French and Dutch, less so than the Irish (North and South), Italians and Spanish.

Compared with the responses in 1985, Harding concludes that there is generally far greater disquiet where donated gametes are concerned, whether AI or IVF, than with any form of assisted conception using only the couple's own gametes. There is little change in the widespread acceptance of AIH and *in vitro* fertilisation using the husband's sperm, but where the problem of infertility is addressed by someone outside the immediate family, respondents are generally far less sympathetic, and are becoming less so. Where AIH is concerned, 90% of respondents in 1985 thought it should be allowed by law; 89% in 1987. Whereas embryos created *in vitro* involving the husband's gametes attracted 83% support in 1985, that had risen to 87% in 1987. But when the issue of AID was raised, only 53% in 1985 and 50% in 1987 thought the law should permit it.

With respect to abortion, Harding notes that 'the results paint an unequivocal picture' (p.41). Despite the various attempts at legislative reform, public support

Attitudes to Artificial Fertility Measures (A216) by sex, age within sex and religion

SHOULD THE LAW ALLOW A MARRIED COUPLE TO USE THE FOLLOWING METHODS?	TOTAL	SEX		AGE WITHIN SEX						RELIGION			
		Male	Female	MALE			FEMALE			Roman Catholic	C of E/ Anglican	Other Christian	(No religion)
				18-34	35-54	55+	18-34	35-54	55+				
Artificial insemination: husband as donor	%	%	%	%	%	%	%	%	%	%	%	%	%
Allowed by law	89	89	89	90	93	82	96	92	78	82	88	87	93
Not allowed by law	9	10	7	9	6	16	3	6	13	15	9	11	5
Other/Don't know	2	1	4	*	1	2	1	2	9	3	4	2	2
Artificial insemination: anonymous donor													
Allowed by law	50	53	47	64	57	36	61	49	27	40	46	45	58
Not allowed by law	47	45	48	34	41	61	38	47	62	56	49	52	39
Other/Don't know	4	2	5	1	2	3	1	4	11	4	5	3	3
'Test-tube' embryo implanted													
Allowed by law	85	84	86	90	87	75	93	90	73	78	84	84	89
Not allowed by law	12	13	10	9	10	22	6	7	19	17	12	15	8
Other/Don't know	3	2	4	1	3	3	1	4	8	5	5	2	2
'Surrogate mother': without payment													
Allowed by law	36	41	31	49	42	32	33	37	19	24	33	31	43
Not allowed by law	61	57	65	49	56	65	66	59	70	73	63	66	55
Other/Don't know	4	2	5	2	2	3	1	4	10	3	5	3	2
'Surrogate mother': paid													
Allowed by law	23	29	17	35	29	22	20	20	9	16	20	20	27
Not allowed by law	74	69	79	63	69	75	79	77	81	81	76	78	70
Other/Don't know	3	2	5	2	1	2	2	3	10	3	5	2	2
BASE: A RESPONDENTS													
Weighted	*1243*	*587*	*636*	*195*	*213*	*179*	*217*	*241*	*196*	*124*	*441*	*220*	*441*
Unweighted	*1281*	*600*	*680*	*184*	*225*	*191*	*215*	*252*	*211*	*124*	*463*	*228*	*445*

Source: *British Social Attitudes*, Fifth Report, p. 48.

Circumstances in which abortion should be legalised (A215) by sex, age within sex, religion and marital status

SHOULD THE LAW ALLOW AN ABORTION IN EACH CASE?	TOTAL	SEX		AGE WITHIN SEX						RELIGION				MARITAL STATUS		
		Male	Female	MALE			FEMALE			Roman Catholic	C of E/ Anglican	Other Christian	(No religion)	Married now	Separated/ divorced/ widowed	Never married
				18-34	35-54	55+	18-34	35-54	55+							
	%	%	%	%	%	%	%	%	%	%	%	%	%	%	%	%
The woman decides on her own she does not wish to have the child	54	54	54	62	49	53	57	57	45	34	55	49	61	53	50	59
The couple agree they do not wish to have the child	59	63	55	71	60	59	63	57	43	38	57	55	67	58	50	66
The woman is not married and does not wish to marry the man	56	57	55	62	55	56	60	58	47	32	56	54	64	56	52	58
The couple cannot afford any more children	58	61	54	59	62	61	59	54	50	37	57	53	66	59	53	54
There is a strong chance of a defect in the baby	89	88	90	90	87	88	94	91	85	68	92	92	91	91	85	85
The woman's health is seriously endangered by the pregnancy	94	94	93	95	95	91	97	95	88	78	95	94	97	95	90	92
The woman becomes pregnant as a result of rape	93	94	93	95	94	92	97	92	90	79	94	93	97	94	88	93
BASE: A RESPONDENTS																
Weighted	*1243*	*587*	*656*	*195*	*213*	*179*	*217*	*241*	*196*	*124*	*441*	*320*	*441*	*887*	*140*	*217*
Unweighted	*1281*	*600*	*680*	*184*	*225*	*191*	*215*	*252*	*211*	*124*	*463*	*228*	*445*	*905*	*165*	*210*

Source: *British Social Attitudes*, Fifth Report, p. 49.

for lawful abortion in all circumstances has increased significantly among demographic groups over the four-year period. Even among Catholic respondents, traditionally thought to be the most hostile to abortion, 79% now favour abortion in the case of rape and 78% when the mother's health is endangered. Agreement that foetal abnormality should be grounds for abortion has also grown dramatically in this group, from 51% in 1983 to 68% in 1987. Harding remarks that the trend towards more liberal attitudes to abortion stands out from trends on other sexual issues. One reason could be that abortion has come to be seen more as a matter of women's rights than of sexual morality. On the other hand it can be seen that the largest part of the shift towards more liberal views about abortion, particularly for reasons of preference, took place between 1983 and 1985 (the dates of the two previous BSA Reports).

Why Legislate?

We may now move on to ask why the Human Fertilisation and Embryology Act 1990 was introduced. Here, we are concerned to investigate why there has been a growing concern with questions of fertility and infertility; we are not so immediately concerned with the question of why we choose now as the time to legislate. In this section, we also examine in outline the main provisions of the Act.

In introducing the legislation to the House of Commons, the then Secretary of State for Health, Kenneth Clarke, declared:

> The Human Fertilisation and Embryology Bill is, in my opinion, one of the most significant measures to be brought forward by a Government in the last 20 years. It is a complex and sensitive Bill that deals with matters that are fundamental to the well-being of our society. It proposes a new and detailed system of statutory regulation of certain types of infertility treatment. If the House agrees with the view taken in another place, that regulation would extend to research involving human embryos (House of Commons, Official Report, 2 April 1990, col. 915).

Commenting in the earlier House of Lords debate, Lord Houghton had said that the Bill:

> is a turning point in medical research and in the destiny of mankind. Nothing like this Bill has previously been placed before Parliament (House of Lords, Official Report, 20 March 1990, col. 244).

John Hannam MP perhaps captured most succinctly the thinking behind the need for legislative intervention. He argued that legislation was necessary to regulate research on embryos, to protect the integrity of reproductive medicine, and to protect scientists and clinicians from legal action and sanction. In addition, some people feared unregulated embryo research, being prepared to support work in specific areas such as infertility and genetic disease, but uneasy at the thought of reproductive technology taking more sinister directions such as genetic interference with the embryo.

Of the fundamental moral issues involved, such as embryo research and abortion, the legislation and the accompanying debates had much to say. But the Act also introduces fundamental and wide-ranging reforms into the burgeoning scientific and commercial worlds of assisted conception. We cannot here provide an historical survey of the main developments (see Yoxen, op.cit., especially Chapters 2-4). It will suffice to say that the development of such varied techniques as artificial insemination by donor (AID), *in vitro* fertilisation (IVF), gamete intrafallopian transfer (GIFT) and embryo transfer (ET), the main forms of assisted conception with which we shall be here concerned, have become commonplace news items in the last decade, and also big business. And while assisted conception practices have a lengthy pedigree, with AID and surrogacy being practised on an unknowably wide scale, the involvement of health care professionals in counselling and treating the growing incidences of infertility has introduced a new dimension. The public commitment of science and technology, some of it cutting edge technology, to questions at the very frontiers of human life itself, have disclosed fears and hopes, anguish and aspirations, which have involved a quantum leap in our imaginations and our languages.

These assisted conception techniques bring with them as many philosophical, moral and legal problems as the more obvious cases of embryo research and abortion. And, while they have not commanded the news coverage, the resolution of these issues into Parliamentary debates and the resulting legislation illustrates the enormous range which this Act addresses. It introduces statutory control of a new form of clinical practice; it brings to the forefront of attention questions as to the provision of and payment for assisted conception services. The Government's refusal to commit more resources to the area was repeatedly criticised. In parallel with this, these new reproductive techniques have been developed at a time of resurgence in expression of feminist thought and values. Importantly among the issues which this has disclosed has been the centrality of the views of women. And in the assisted conception debate, the way in which their interests, desires, plans and goals are accounted for, discounted, factored in or out, have assumed a major importance. But the conclusions to which this leads various commentators are not uniform, other than perhaps in the view that where such issues fundamentally affect the life, well-being, health and emotions of women, men should take a back seat. This was most forcefully expressed during the Parliamentary debates by Teresa Gorman, a backbench Conservative MP, usually noted for her strong commitment to market individualism. In the debate on abortion law reform she interjected with this analysis of the arguments of those who sought to reduce the time limits, or the grounds on which access to lawful abortion could be obtained:

> Although superficially we are talking about medicine, science and when, where and whether we should stop abortion, emotions and deep passions bubble up from underneath. . . . Those motives form one of the deepest, most misogynous strands in human society. For centuries theologians have equated sex with sin and celibacy with grace. They have regarded women as little more than flower pots in which future generations of children, preferably boy children, are reared. . . . I hope that the majority of my colleagues, perforce mainly male, who do not have to bear the responsibility of an unwanted birth and pregnancy

> and who do not have to make such decisions, will not have the temerity, arrogance, inhumanity and insensitivity to make those decisions for women (House of Commons, Official Report 24 April 1990, cols. 230-32).

Although vigorously opposed by some women MPs, this view echoes a common strand of feminist thought and philosophy; where decisions affecting women, and their reproductive health and interests are concerned, it is the individual woman herself who should have the right, and hence the responsibility, of making such fundamental decisions about the morality of what she does.

Not all of those who participated in debates were whole heartedly in favour of assisted conception at all. For example, Alan Amos, (House of Commons, Official Report 23 April 1990, col. 106) argued that:

> IVF is inefficient, expensive, time-consuming and dangerous for women. It can lead to cysts, coagulation, strokes, heart problems, ovarian cancer and many other problems.

And, objecting to the legislation in the House of Lords debate on Report, Lord Kennet complained that the Bill had been forced through in ignorance. He said that in three important respects the legislation had been pioneered without full consideration. Parliament knew little or nothing of the prevalence, causes and nature of infertility. Although the Office of Population Censuses and Surveys was now to be charged with responsibility for collecting that data, it did not presently exist.

Secondly, he felt that the possible drawbacks of IVF and Embryo Transfer had not been canvassed. Finally, the whole question of the cost of infertility treatments had not been disclosed. The figures which have been published, suggest a *marginal cost* for pregnancy achieved (not baby successfully born) as a result of a treatment service at the NHS clinic at Hammersmith Hospital in London at £16,000. This included salary costs, drugs and materials, but not any overheads. A figure of £25,000 was suggested by Wagner and St Clair in a study published in *The Lancet* in October 1989, but a comparison of the two figures has not been made (we return to this argument, infra, Chapter 5). Indeed, the true costs of each pregnancy and successful birth would also have to include: an apportioned share for each healthy baby of the accumulated research costs; similarly for the cost of special post-natal care, whether in the clinic or at home; of the extra care needed for the higher incidence of multiple births following ovarian stimulation, IVF or GIFT; the extra costs of care associated with the production of more children with genetic abnormalities which may later materialise. A cause for disquiet which was not properly explored during the debates is that higher order pregnancies are attended with major risks of morbidity and mortality. The risk of stillbirth is six times higher than for a singleton pregnancy, for example, and the risk of death in the infant's first year is nearly ten times greater. The rate of death below the age of one is 8.5 per 1,000 for singletons. With twins this rises to 44.7 per 1,000, and for triplet and other higher order births the rate is 92.5 per 1,000. A similar discontinuity is evident in the risk of stillbirths, where the figures per 1,000 are respectively 5.0, 18.3 and

32.9 (see OPCS, *Mortality Statistics* (for 1986), series DG3; we return to deal with these points in Chapter 5).

In addition, there would need to be some account taken of the usually hidden emotional costs of infertility treatments borne by the couple undergoing treatment services. These would include the emotional, physical and psychological costs of dealing with, and perhaps accepting the inability to have a child; the sexual, social and genetic costs and, for some families, the financial costs of caring for children, sometimes several children with slight to severe handicap and disability as a result of the treatment. Two particular examples of these costs were highlighted during the passage of the Bill.

The first concerned the experiences of Helen Pusey (*New Statesman* 19 May 1990). Helen Pusey suffered temporary blindness, kidney failure and pleurisy at the end of her quadrupule GIFT pregnancy waiting for an emergency caesarean. Two of the Pusey quads died, one twenty minutes after birth the other at five months; the two 'surviving' have multiple handicaps. It has emerged that she was not told, let alone counselled, about the possibilities of multiple birth following GIFT, until a few moments before going to theatre for the operation.

A second example was highlighted by *The Mail on Sunday* on June 10 1990. It concerns the trauma experienced by Marie Charlesworth undergoing treatment at the Perth Memorial Hospital in Western Australia. Following the transfer to her of four eggs, each successfully implanted and began to develop. Marie Charlesworth asked the clinicians to terminate three of the embryos, but they refused. By the time of birth, Marie had decided to part with two or three of the eventual children. Fourteen months later, that intention has been effected, and the three boys to whom she gave birth have been adopted by a family in the West Australian state. She and her husband felt unable to cope with the emotional traumas of what were essentially 'unwanted' multiple births, even though the West Australian Government had offered financial assistance to deal with such an unexpectedly large family.

Finally, the Act seeks to regulate embryo research. In what began (at least until abortion was added to its provisions) as the most controversial part of the legislation, the Bill was introduced with two possible variants of the embryo research clause. The eventual shape of the legislation would depend on the vote taken upon whether a permissive or restrictive line was taken on the question of research. In the event, on a free vote, the permissive line received support, but with a 30% vote against. It was a complaint thereafter that the Standing Committee considering the Bill contained only two out of its 18 members who were specifically and publicly committed to a 'pro-life' view.

It is thought that about 5,000 embryos are presently used for research purposes each year in the UK (see Michael McNair-Wilson MP, House of Commons, Official Report 20 June 1990, col. 964, quoting figures reportedly from Oxford University). There are a number of reasons, even once it is decided that research on embryos should be permitted, why the law might wish to regulate that research. Warnock stated that 'the human embryo per se has no legal status' (para. 11.16). This remains broadly the case following the passage of the Act, as we explain later in this chapter (see, infra, p. 82 et seq.). Nonetheless, surrounding questions of how, why, where and when research on embryos may be pursued need to be addressed.

For example, should we permit research only on 'spare' embryos created in the course of treatment services? This position was adopted by Lord Jackobovits in the House of Lords, in an amendment which was defeated (House of Lords, Official Report 6 March 1990, col. 1059; and lost again in the Commons, see House of Commons, Official Report June 20 1990, col. 998). Jackobovits argued that it was surely repugnant to create human life solely for the purpose of destroying it in embryo experiments. He sought also to introduce an amendment to sch. 2 to the Act (which sets out a list of purposes for which embryo research may be permitted) in order to exclude 'eugenic or frivolous' motives. Here, he argued that embryo research, for example, to satisfy a preference for sons, or smaller humans who would reduce the payload of spaceships, should be addressed and arrested before it got under way. Similarly, he wished to prohibit the use of embryos for research into contraceptives, which was described by Jackobovits as an insufficiently urgent purpose.

The listing of such amendments illustrates the difficulties in drawing boundaries around the margins of embryo research even once a decision, in principle, is taken by majority to allow it. In the debates, there were four schools of thought on embryo research:

(i) those for whom any research was acceptable and permissible;
(ii) those who did not want research at all;
(iii) those who did not want any form of destructive research but who were prepared to countenance therapeutic research for the benefit of each embryo;
(iv) those who wanted research to be permitted if at all only on spare embryos created in the course of providing treatment services and which would otherwise be allowed to perish / condemned to die if not implanted.

This final stance addresses Jackobovits' point. *In vitro* fertilisation usually produces surplus embryos which cannot be transferred to the woman's uterus. Only one clinic, at the Jessop Hospital for Women in Sheffield, does not use ovarian hyperstimulation to assist in the production of multiple eggs. The argument, then, that they may be used in beneficial research is that this does them no additional injury. Opponents of creation only for the purpose of research were fearful of the development of 'embryo farms' (see Frank Field, House of Commons, Official Report, 20 June 1990, col. 936). Such fears, doubtless felt most strongly, dictated that the law could no longer remain silent on the questions of whether, how, why, where and when embryo research could be undertaken.

The 1990 Act — An Overview

The statutory scheme has been introduced to ensure that these sensitive issues of moral and legal complexity are dealt with in a clear framework. It seeks to balance what are the sometimes conflicting interests of the involuntarily childless and the children of the reproduction revolution. Similarly, it seeks to mediate between the families who may benefit from research into the causes of genetically inherited disease or chromosomal abnormalities (who may suffer from what has been called 'reproductive blight'), and the human embryo or foetus. In all cases, the broader social, moral and philosophical interests which disclose fundamentally different ways of conceiving of the world and the ways in which it may be inhabited are brought into conflict. In short, the Act is one important manifestation of who we are and who we say we want to become; the question which it raises is 'who to be or not to be?'

In short, the Act has three fundamental objectives:

(1) to provide a statutory framework for the control and supervision of research involving human embryos;
(2) to provide for the licensing of certain types of assisted conception practice, namely those which involve the creation of a human embryo outside the body, or partly inside and partly outside, and any treatment service which involves the use of donated gametes (egg and sperm) or donated embryos;
(3) to effect changes to the Abortion Act 1967.

Each may be briefly surveyed.

Certain infertility treatments ('treatment services') will be permitted only under licence from a new statutory body, the Human Fertilisation and Embryology Authority (HUFEA). This body will have the authority to issue three, and only three, types of licence: a treatment licence, a research licence and a storage licence. A treatment licence or a storage licence may be issued only for a maximum period of five years, after which a re-application must be made. A research licence is valid only for a maximum of three years.

A treatment licence may authorise one or more of the following: bringing about the creation of embryos *in vitro;* keeping embryos; using gametes; testing the condition of the embryo for replacement; placing an embryo into a woman; using a 'hamster test' to determine the potency and normality of human sperm; and other practices which may later be specified by the Authority. Hence, a licence will be necessary for IVF, AID (if treatment services are offered), Donor GIFT, Egg Donation and IVC. The Government do not intend that a licence should be necessary where fertilisation takes place within a woman's body using her egg(s) and her husband's sperm (AIH) or, where they are unmarried, her partner's sperm (AIP). AIH, AIP and non-donor GIFT are outwith the licensing requirements (this is the intention; whether it had been achieved in respect of GIFT is something which we examine, infra., Chapter 5).

A storage licence will permit the storage of gametes or embryos, or both.

A research licence will permit the creation of embryos *in vitro,* and their use for specified projects of research. The research (or experimentation; the choice of terms is apt to reflect in part one's moral judgment) must be directed towards one or more of a defined number of aims and only where HUFEA is satisfied that the research is necessary or desirable. These aims are:

(i) the promotion of advances in the treatment of infertility;
(ii) increasing knowledge about the causes of congenital disease;
(iii) increasing knowledge about the causes of miscarriages;
(iv) developing more effective techniques of contraception;
(v) developing methods for detecting the presence or absence of gene or chromosome abnormalities before implantation of an embryo.

In respect of abortion, the Act makes some fundamental changes to the Abortion Act 1967. For the first time a specific time limit is written into legislation. In England and Wales, the time limit within which most lawful abortions must now be performed is 24 weeks. There are, however, three new grounds on which abortion is available at any time up to birth. In Scotland, where the common law and not statute (the Infant Life (Preservation) Act 1929) applied in relation to child destruction, it was previously thought by some commentators that lawful abortion could be performed at any time up to birth. Effectively, however, most abortions in Scotland were performed broadly in line with the position in England and Wales. The 1990 Act now introduces this new statutory time limit into that jurisdiction as well. Amendments made to the Bill at the Report stage in the House of Commons, 21 June 1990, removed Northern Ireland from the scope of the new abortion provisions, and saw the attempts to amend the Bill to make access to abortion more straightforward defeated. Also defeated was an attempt to reintroduce time limits in respect of abortion on the grounds of foetal handicap and the health of the woman.

There are other examples of the statutory control of medical treatment, such as abortion, female circumscision, human organ donation, treatments for detained patients under the Mental Health Act 1983, but in none of these is the treatment regulated. In this respect HUFEA is a first.

There are some ancillary aspects of assisted conception, each of which raises ethical and legal problems of some nicety or complexity which have not been addressed in the Act. The major one of these is the statutory regulation of GIFT — gamete intrafallopian transfer — and whether or how it should be subject to statutory regulation. After a great deal of pressure, the Government remained unmoved on the inclusion of GIFT but conceded an amendment on Report which clarified the ability of HUFEA to seek to bring the procedure under review by way of regulations. The consequences of this manoeuvre are discussed below in Chapter 4. The following matters, which are not included in the Act, give rise to their own difficulties.

1. The Act nowhere deals with the special position of minors and gamete donation. It is presumably left to the common law, or to any guidance which HUFEA is minded to offer in the Code. There may be good reason to distinguish between the donation of sperm and the donation of eggs, particularly in relation to minors. While the general direction of the Act is to discourage unthinking donations of any kind, it might have been appropriate to address the question of whether the donation of eggs or sperm should be undertaken by a young woman or man under some specified age at all. A specific exception could perhaps have been considered in the course of therapeutic surgery, such as an hysterectomy. Under the common law, *Gillick* v *West Norfolk and Wisbech Health Authority* [1985] 3 All ER 402 provides that a minor may validly consent to medical treatment without parental involvement when he or she has acquired sufficient intellectual and emotional maturity and understanding to be capable of making up her or his own mind on the matter requiring decision. The Family Law Reform Act 1969, s. 8 provides that a minor of the age of 16 may give an effective consent to surgical, medical or dental treatment as valid as if he or she were of the age of majority (18). With a person under that age, it is clear applying *Gillick*

that there may be some minors sufficiently mature to be capable of going beyond understanding the nature of the donation, to an appreciation of what it involves. A doctor would have to be satisfied that a minor appreciated any moral and emotional questions involved, and any health risks associated with the donation, before concluding that the minor had the requisite capacity to consent. It is unfortunate that for the avoidance of doubt a clear policy preference was not announced by the legislature, but the counselling provision of s. 13(6) might be relied upon to produce some safeguards.

2. The Act does not indicate whether or how a review of a decision to refuse licensed treatment services to a woman or a couple may be brought. This could arise in two ways. First, through any medical or other necessary personnel invoking the conscience clause ground of s. 38. Secondly, on the s. 13(5) 'welfare of the child' ground. In *R* v *Ethical Committee of St Mary's Hospital (Manchester) ex parte Harriot* [1988] 1 FLR 512, a woman who had formerly worked as a prostitute believed that she was excluded from continuing treatment services once the clinic discovered her history. She challenged the decision of the Centre to exclude her. She also challenged the advice of the Local Ethical Review Committee (established in accordance with DHSS Circular HSC IS 153) which had concurred with the clinic that in withdrawing the services in these circumstances it was acting perfectly correctly. Schiemann J dismissed her claim. However, he held that while the LERC was not under a duty to investigate her case before giving its advice, and was merely an informal body whose function was to provide a forum for professional discussion, the court could nonetheless review the policy of an Ethics Committee. Holding that the committee could be subject to judicial review, he suggested that it was incumbent upon a committee to give lawful advice. Thus, it could not advise to exclude all Jewish or Black applicants, for example. Nor could it reach a decision which no reasonable committee could have reached. And, without argument on the point, the judge accepted a submission from counsel that it would be lawful for a clinic to adopt the sort of criteria which are used to assess the suitability of a couple or occasionally a single person for adoption purposes.

A question which discloses similar difficulties about access has arisen before the courts in France. Alain Parpalaix was warned that the treatment he was about to undergo for cancer of the testicles might cause sterility. He deposited sperm before the treatment with CECOS — Centre d'Etude et de Conservation du Sperme. He later married Corrine Richard, the woman with whom he had been living. Following his death, she sought the court's assistance in forcing CECOS to deliver to her his sperm. In *Parpalaix* v *CECOS et Federation Francaise des Centres d'Etude et de Conservation du Sperme,* (unreported) the court ordered that CECOS should hand over Parpalaix's sperm to his widow, as it had tacitly approved Parpalaix's intention; it had not, for example, specifically warned that it would refuse to hand over the sperm. Further, the court decided that there being no legislation or regulation which prevented the request being met, and that since one of the aims of marriage was procreation, nothing in natural law prohibited the transfer.

These reasons provide a useful template for the development of HUFEA's or individual licensed centres' approaches to questions of conscience or etiquette under the Act. The framework of the consents schedule of the Act — sch. 3 — makes it clear that the wishes of the donators or genitors are the fulcrum upon which the ethical scales are to be weighed. Clarification would, however, have been beneficial. As the Act stands, it is not clear to what extent a licensing committee may take into account a centre's policy on access to infertility treatment when deciding licensing issues.

3. The Act does not presently state whether there is to be a limit on the number of donations which any individual donor may make, whether of sperm or of eggs. Warnock would have limited the number of children which could be born from any one donor to ten. It was thought that it would be too difficult to enforce such a limit, presumably of either donations or resulting children, and hence undesirable for it to be provided in the Act. And, additionally, it was resisted as representing an intrusion into clinical practice which could not be justified. No explicit connection was made between the two reasons. However, this point will be dealt with in the Code of Practice to be drawn up under s. 25.

4. The Act provides, in s. 28(2), (5), that in determining the status of any child born to a married woman, the consent of her husband shall be presumed, and shall thereby determine fatherhood, unless he is able to show that he is not the father of the child. The section does not go on to specify whether anybody else with a legitimate interest may have standing to rebut the presumption and show that he is not the father of the child. This heralds a wider set of unspoken values concerning the nature of the relationships for which assisted conception may be appropriate.

5. The difficult question of circumstances in which a doctor may be under an obligation to a third party to break the usual duty of confidence owed to a patient is given added force in respect of assisted conception. The type of question which might arise here is whether a doctor or other health care worker who discovers a genetic disease in a donor's child is placed under a duty to report that fact to the donor and any other person whose health may be affected. We cannot deal extensively with that question here, but based on *Tarasoff* v *Regents of the University of California* 131 Cal. Rptr. 14 (1976) and *W* v *Egdell* [1989] 1 All ER 1089 (CA) we would suggest the emergence of a positive duty to warn, which may have enormous implications in respect of genetic screening and donor disease (see further, Robert Lee 'Medical Confidentiality: A Confidence Trick' in Linda Clarke, (ed.), *Confidentiality and Law* ((1990) Lloyds). The implications of genetic mapping and genetic screening are rapidly assuming such importance that legislation may soon be necessary to deal with moral and ethical questions as large as those addressed here. The Government has asked Sir Cecil Clothier QC, a former Parliamentary Ombudsman and former member of the ILA to chair a committee to examine some of the ethical and legal problems which will arise in the area of genetic mapping, and this committee is expected to report in 1991 or 1992.

6. Is donation of gametes and embryos the supply of goods or provision of services? Or both? The importance of this question arises if it is argued that an action against a donor or a clinic could lie not just with respect to negligence in respect of defective gametes, but also under the strict liability regime of the

Consumer Protection Act 1987 for defective products. Body products, such as blood or sperm, once separated from the body and in the control of someone are capable of being owned (*R* v *Welsh* [1974] Road Traffic Reports 478, *R* v *Rothery* [1976] Road Traffic Reports 550). But whether sperm, eggs or fertilised ovum are 'products' for the purposes of the 1987 Act is not settled. The American courts in the early 1970s began to hold that blood was a product for the purposes of tortious liability, often to be reversed by the legislature declaring it to be a service incident to treatment. However, some courts have responded by distinguishing between the supply of blood from a commercial blood bank and from a hospital. Where the supply is the primary objective of the commercial concern and only an incidental concern of the service provided by the hospital, a blood bank has been found liable in contract for the supply of defective blood (see *Cunningham* v *MacNeal Memorial Hospital* 266 N E 2d 897 (Ill 1970) and *Belle Bonfils Memorial Blood Bank* v *Hansen* 579 P 2d 1158 (Colo 1978). The point has not yet arisen in the United Kingdom, but a related, potentially far more controversial, issue arises in asking whether the embryo is a person or a chattel. Lord Hailsham pleaded in debate that:

> It is wrong to try to define a human embryo in terms of established legal definitions which are plainly inapplicable to human embryos. Why must an embryo be one or the other? Why cannot it be just an embryo? (House of Lords, Official Report 6 February 1990, col. 751).

In the USA, in *Del Zio* v *Presbyterian Hospital* 74 Civ 3588 (SD, NY, 1976) the US District Court for the Southern District of California appeared to treat the embryo as though it were a chattel, whereas in the first instance Tennessee case of *Davis* v *Davis* (1989) (reversed on other grounds on appeal, see Tennessee Court of Appeals (1990)), the embryo was clearly understood to be a person. The legal importance of these questions (their philosophical and moral importance we take to be self-evident, see our discussion of 'philosophical approaches', supra, pp. 4–5) can be seen again in the pending US case, *York* v *Jones,* where a couple who wish to transfer from Virginia to California frozen embryos are attempting to discover whether this amounts to inter-state commerce and what consequences follow. In Europe such questions as to whether we are dealing with the free movement of goods under Articles 30-36 of the Treaty of Rome, or the free movement of persons arise. Does a frozen embryo need a passport, or immigration papers or an import/export licence? In the Act the embryo is nowhere given a status either as a chattel or as a person. Warnock observed (para.10. 11) that:

> Until now the law has never had to consider the existence of embryos outside the mother's uterus. The existence of such embryos raises potentially difficult problems as to ownership. The concept of ownership of human embryos seems to us to be undesirable. We recommend that legislation be enacted to ensure that there is no right of ownership in a human embryo.

And yet as Kennedy and Grubb remark, Warnock gives to the couple who have stored an embryo rights to use and dispose of it (paras. 10.11 and 12); rights of sale of gametes and embryos where licensed (13.13); and limited circumstances where drug testing may be carried out on embryos created specifically for that purpose (para. 12.5). In light of this they pointedly ask:

> What special status does an embryo have if it may be the object of research during the first fourteen days of gestation and thereafter destroyed? What is ownership if it is not the right to control, including to dispose of by sale, or otherwise? (Ian Kennedy and Andrew Grubb, *Medical Law: Text and Materials* ((1989), Butterworths p. 682).

It seems consistent with the approach taken in the Act, especially if the arguments as to toti-potentility of the cells up to the appearance of the primitive streak are accepted, that only after that time does the legal category of person even begin to emerge (we discuss this point in Chapter 3, which examines embryo research). This is not to say that it is then possessed of legal personality. Indeed it seems from *R* v *Tait* [1989] 3 All ER 613 that a five-month-old foetus is not a person for the purposes of the Offences Against the Person Act 1861. A fortiori, then, an embryo before that time will not be. It is indeed consistent with this scheme to regard the pre-embryo, sperm and eggs as more like property than anything else, although we may refuse to recognise a full sense of property in relation to them, in the sense that we may regard them as something to which obligations and responsibilities are owed, but which cannot be owned in the full sense of the ownership of other chattels.

Thus, it is not possible straightforwardly to say whether an embryo can be stolen, bequeathed, kidnapped or perhaps most controversially, patented. Certainly, in respect of genetically engineered plants and animals, the United States and the United Kingdom and European countries have allowed patenting and genetically engineered mice, known as an 'oncomouse', are available for sale in the United States. And if a cryopreservation facility were destroyed in a fire, would a claim on the Centre's insurance policy which limited claims to loss or damage to property include the embryos held in storage? Or not?

Finally it is unclear what effect frozen embryos or gametes will have on the rule against perpetuities and whether a testator will be able to bind property by relation to the birth of a child from a fertilised ovum in cryopreservation. The question is whether what Leach has called a posthumous child 'en ventre sa frigidaire' is a 'life in being' for the purposes of the rule? (W Barton Leach, 'Perpetuities in the Atomic Age' (1962) 48 *American Bar Association Journal* 942, at p.942). If A dies and leaves his property 'to all my children', does this include or exclude frozen embryos which may not be implanted for twenty or thirty years? (but cf. s. 14(1)(c) and (4) specifying a present statutory limit of five years for embryos and s. 14(1)(c) and (3) a limit of ten years for gametes).

These, and no doubt a variety of other questions, as yet unframed, will face us in the future. The very application of such a bewildering array of common law concepts to the ever growing possibilities which embryology throws up makes out an excellent case for Parliamentary consideration and statutory regulation. That the Human Fertilisation and Embryology Act is incomplete does not mean that it is unwelcome. But it will not be the last word on the subject.

Chapter 2
Abortion

The Politics of Abortion

Reform of the abortion law in England, Wales and Scotland has long been on the political agenda. The Abortion Act 1967 does not extend to Northern Ireland, where the statutory defences which that Act introduced do not apply. An attempt to amend the Bill in order to extend the operation of the 1967 reforms was defeated at Report stage in the Commons by 267 votes to 131. The last time that the now defunct Northern Ireland Assembly had voted on the issue in 1984, a proposal to extend the 1967 Act was defeated by 20 votes to 1. Women travel from Northern Ireland to obtain abortions in England and Wales; in 1988, 1,815 such operations were performed on women from the six counties. However, most of the parliamentarians (all male) from the Province who spoke in the present debates vehemently denounced any attempt to extend the legislation. (House of Commons, Official Report, 21 June 1990, cols. 1134-75; for a review of the practice in the six countries see, *Abortion in Northern Ireland: The Report of an International Tribunal* (1989), Beyond the Pale Publications).

Since a statutory scheme of defences to a charge of abortion — or the procurement of a miscarriage as the offence is still technically described — was introduced to supplement that recognised at common law, there have been continuing calls for a review of the parameters of the legislation and the way which it is used in practice. Criticism of the Abortion Act 1967 has come from those who believe that its limited ambit is overlooked in practice in order to condone what has come to be called 'abortion on demand.' Further, they charge that the effective limit for most lawful abortions (between 24 and 28 weeks) has led to a large number of women from other countries using British abortion facilities as a way of evading their own national legislation on access to abortion services. An allied concern is simply the number of abortions performed; in 1969, there were 54,819 recorded abortion operations; in 1985, the recorded figure was 171,873 and in the most recent available, those for 1989, the figure is reported as 170,500 (Office of Population Censuses and Surveys, *Population Trends 61,* 1990 HMSO). This means that one in five of all pregnancies is ended through a termination.

INTERNATIONAL COMPARISONS OF ABORTION — NOVEMBER 1990

Nation	Law	Indications	Time Limit	Availability	1984 Total (residents only)	Abortion rate # 1984	% before 12 weeks
UK	Abortion Act 1967 (as amended s. 37 Human Fertilisation and Embryology Act)	Risk to life of woman or her mental or physical health. Substantial risk of handicap in child (i) greater risk than that of termination that pregnancy would injure a woman's physical or mental health (ii) termination necessary to prevent grave permanent injury to woman's physical or mental health (iii) continuation of pregnancy involves risk to life of pregnant woman greater than of termination. (iv) immediately necessary to save life of woman	(i) 24 weeks (ii), (iii), (iv) and (v) without limit	In NHS hospital or approved private hospital or nursing home	136,400 (England and Wales) 9,400 (Scotland)	12.8 8.9	84
Australia	State laws apply — mostly based on UK 1861 Act and liberalised by case law	Physical and mental health of woman. Foetal defect. Rape	14 to 28 weeks	Free-standing clinics in NSW and Victoria and in public hospitals. Woman reimbursed by Medicare	54,000	15.2	
Belgium	1990	Abortion available on limited grounds		In some free University Hospitals. Women go outside country, mainly to Holland	N/A	N/A	N/A
Canada	Overturned by Supreme Court January 1988 (*Morgentaler* v *R*)				62,300	10.2	
Denmark	Act No 350, June 1973	On request Medical, genetic, rape or social with permission of committee	12 weeks 2nd trimester	Local hospitals. Women are reimbursed	20,700	18.4	97.5
France	Law 75-17, 1975 Law 79-1204, 1979	On request Risk to woman's life or health. Foetal handicap	12 weeks from LMP No limit	Public hospitals and private clinics 80% reimbursed	177,000	14.9	97

German Federal Republic	Law 15, 1976	Rape or sexual crime, social, psychological reason Medical reasons. Genetic reasons	12 weeks from concep-tion No limit 22 weeks	Free of charge to woman with statutory health insurance	97,900*	7.3	93
Italy	Law 194, 1978	On demand Medical or genetic reasons or rape	Up to 90 days No limit	In state hospitals only. Free of charge	227,400	19.0	
Netherlands	Law 1981 Regulations 1984	Intolerable situation to be determined by woman and her doctor	24 weeks	Public hospitals and free-standing clinics. Women reimbursed	18,700	5.6	89**
Norway	Act 50, June 1975 Law 66, Sec 1-4 June 1978	On request Medical. Genetic, Rape	12 weeks 18 weeks	Free of charge	14,100	15.9	
Spain	Organic Law 9, July 1985	Rape. Genetic reasons. Medical reasons	12 weeks 22 weeks No limit	In public hospitals but mainly in private clinics	N/A	N/A	N/A
Sweden	Abortion Law 595, June 1974 (implemented 1975)	On request. With approval from Nat. Board of Health	18 weeks after 18 weeks	Free of charge in public hospitals	30,800	17.7	95
USA	1973 Supreme Court decision in *Roe* v *Wade* made state laws banning abortion unenforceable. 1989 Supreme Court decision in *Webster* undermined earlier decisions and throws issue back to States	5 states make abortion illegal. Other states, e.g. California and Virginia have liberal laws. Many states prohibit public funding of abortion		Predominantly in private hospitals and clinics	1,515,000	27.4	92

* includes German women obtaining abortions abroad but number at home under reported ** residents and non-residents
# abortions per 1,000 women 15-44 † Rebuttable presumption at 28 weeks gestation

Source: Jennifer Gunning, *Human IVF, Embryo Research, Foetal Tissue for Research and Treatment, and Abortion: International Information* (HMSO (1989), p. 7)

Critics of the present distribution of NHS facilities and their accessibility referred to discrepancies such as a 95% NHS abortion rate in North Devon (where health care professionals operate a unique system of immediate telephone referral from the GP to a consultant such that a woman can obtain an appointment within a day and access to abortion facilities within a week) compared with an NHS abortion rate of 5% in South Birmingham. In 1988, 84% of all abortions were performed before 13 weeks of pregnancy and 14% between 13 and 20 weeks. Only 1.7% of pregnancies were terminated at over 20 weeks, what had become increasingly to be seen as late abortions. However, critics pointed to the 1984 Report of the Royal College of Obstetricians and Gynaecologists on abortion provision which noted that of women applying for termination before 12 weeks one in five were delayed until after the 20th week (*Report on Foetal Viability and Clinical Practice* (1984)). In debate Harriet Harman MP and others sought to limit this delay by providing in an amendment that, up until the 12th week of pregnancy, the authority of only one doctor would be sufficient to allow the woman access to abortion facilities (Official Report, House of Commons, 21 June 1990, col. 1134). This amendment was defeated (by 264 votes to 159), and one which provided for certification of a single doctor if she or he was of the opinion formed in good faith that the pregnancy had not exceeded the 12th week was defeated by 28 votes.

On a European scale, the United Kingdom is far more restrictive in allowing patients sympathetic access to abortion services than many other countries. While amongst the countries of the European Community only Eire and Northern Ireland have no statutory provision for lawful abortion, England and Wales admits of the lowest proportion of abortions below eight weeks and the highest at 13-16 weeks and 17 weeks and over. Limitations on access ensure that however 'liberal' the provisions appear, they may nonetheless be struck down as unconstitutional in the United States as an unwarranted intrusion in the privacy of the woman (see the comment of J K Mason, *Medico-Legal Aspects of Parenthood and Reproduction,* (1990), p. 106).

However, when the abortion rate per thousand women in England and Wales is compared internationally, a more surprising picture emerges. While the rates per 1,000 are lower in The Netherlands, [West] Germany, Canada, Eire and Belgium; they are higher than those for England and Wales in the USA, Sweden, Norway, Italy, France, Denmark, Australia, [East] Germany, Poland, Yugoslavia, USSR, Hungary, Czechoslovakia and Bulgaria. In certain countries, these figures may conceal indifference or hostility to women's health and may proceed from the use of abortion, often performed without anaesthetic, as a form of contraception. Of the higher rate countries, legislative attempts to prohibit lawful abortion have been made recently in Czechoslovakia and Poland. Meanwhile, it is the Netherlands, with one of the more liberal abortion laws, which has one of the lowest rates of abortions, at 5.6 per 1,000 pregnancies. Effective family planning, sex education and welfare provision are commonly cited as the main reasons for such a low rate. And in countries which have very restrictive abortion laws, such as West Germany, it is apparent that many women travel outside the jurisdiction, often to Britain, in order to obtain an abortion.

Despite these varied pressures on abortion services, according to 1988 figures, only 23 abortions were carried out after 24 weeks at NHS hospitals. Government administrative action has ensured that no abortion over 24 weeks is carried out in licensed private clinics at all, and not after 20 weeks unless resuscitation equipment is available. Abortion law reform has become a continuing, evolutionary movement in the domestic legal calendar, but international movements alone are likely to dictate that the reforms of the present Act will not represent the last word on abortion for many years. There will remain pressures, both within the United Kingdom and from the Council of Europe to reform British abortion laws, and to secure some greater degree of harmonisation within, at least, Western Europe. Gunning's research (supra) has revealed the diversity of positions taken within some of the countries of the European Community and of the Commonwealth.

The health reforms of the Abortion Act 1967 seem now almost uncontroversial; in 1965 3,050 women were discharged from hospital with post-abortion sepsis, in 1982 that figure was 390. From 1961-63, 160 women were recorded as dying from abortions; in 1985-87 that figure was 2. However, the moral debate which that reform started has far from abated, indeed the demands for reform limiting access to, or prohibiting abortion have become more vociferous and more impassioned each year. This is in part due to the changes which medical practice are said to have wrought; with the ability to maintain successfully the lives of some severely pre-term neonates with the assistance of sophisticated, expensive technology and dedicated nursing and medical care appearing to lower the age limit of 'viability' of low birth weight or pre-term neonates. Such are the special and particular skills that some of these neonates may be brought to lead lives unaffected by the enormous complications and side effects which advanced prematurity brings (see the review of recent data in this field by Celia Wells and Derek Morgan, 'Medicine, Morals, Money and the Newborn' (1989) *J Social Welfare Law* 57-62, and also House of Commons Official Report, 26 July 1990, Cols. 427-28(W) for more recent figures of pre-term births and birthweights).

Additionally, there has been the 'gravitational pull' exercised by developments in the United States of America, where constant legislative and judicial activity in response to public demands have ensured that the abortion question remains one of the most publically visible of private reproductive choices.(see, e.g. *Webster* v *Reproductive Services* 103 S. Ct. 3040 (1989), extensively reviewed and discussed in the essays collected in 'Perspectives on the Abortion Issue' (1990) 15 (2-3) *Special Issue of American J of Law and Medicine* 153-223). Technological advances inherent in the 'reproduction revolution' itself have brought about apparent irony. This is seen as reflected in the heroic struggle for life of severely pre-term neonates in wards adjacent to those offering abortion services; of couples striving with all their personal, emotional and physical energy to conceive life, while others are portrayed as blithely taking it as part of an alternative contraceptive package necessary in a liberated sexual and reproductive marketplace in which choice and freedom are the hallmarks of a mature and well-oiled sexual paradise. In fact, such popular images and stereotypes are far from the realities of life for many women facing abortion decisions, or indeed for many couples undergoing fertility workups.

As a result, the House of Commons voted on the 23 April 1990 for what appears to be one of the most liberal abortion laws of Western Europe. There are a number of features of the debate which give some indication as to the reasons for the voting. What is striking, however, is that both sides of the abortion divide, the 'pro-birth' and the 'pro-choice' lobbies spectacularly misjudged the Parliamentary mood. In the second reading debate in the House of Commons, for example, it was apparent that the pro-birth lobby were confident of victory; thanking the Government for making time available for the issue to be debated and promising that a conclusive vote in 1990 would lead to the development of harmonious Parliamentary accommodation for some long time. They asserted that if a reduction in time limits were achieved in the Human Fertilisation and Embryology Bill, it would not be necessary or desirable for them to return in the next and successive Parliamentary sessions seeking further reductions. When the Bill came back from Committee to be reported to the House, the mood had changed and the pro-birth lobby were forecasting more Parlimentary effort would be forthcoming to reverse the changes which had been wrought.

Arguments for Change: Pro-birth

In contrast, the pro-choice lobby were initially angered that the long title of the Bill demonstrated the Government's intention to make time available, despaired at the consequences of what they feared would be an 18 or 22 week limit, and railed against the misogynist principles upon which the reforms were premised. The types of argument which were then deployed in the debates can be quickly summarised. For many of those who were anti-abortion, or who wanted to seek a reduction in the scope and availability of abortion, the fundamental starting point was conception itself, in the same way as it had been in the debates over embryo research. Life begins at conception, and no one but God has the authority to end it. There were some prepared to accept that rape, incest and related incidents might disclose grounds for termination:

> The pro-life group readily concedes that there are certain tragic circumstances in which an abortion is justified (House of Commons, Official Report 24 April 1990, col. 216).

However, the main force of their arguments relied upon conception as the beginning of life or variations upon that approach. Why, they asked, if embryo experiments were banned from 14 days onwards, was abortion allowed up to 18, 20, or 28 weeks? If it is proper to defend the life of an unborn child when damaged in the womb by a drug such as Thalidomide, why is it so illogical to defend it against being aborted? Free and easy abortion is in the interests of men because it removes for them the problem of pregnancy; the operation involves the consumption of scarce NHS resources compounded by the incidence of women coming from outside the UK for late abortions. They charged that since the 1967 Act there had been a general decline in respect for the sanctity of life. Additionally, some abortions were carried out on some foetuses who were able, or who were capable of being helped, to sustain life, as in the 'Carlisle baby' case, in which it was reported that an aborted foetus 'lived' in a kidney dish for 3 hours (see Introduction); and that recently a doctor at King's College Hospital London had aborted a foetus in a twinned pregnancy at 27½ weeks for a mild form of handicap.

Seeking to lower time limits, this lobby argued that legislation should work for the future and anticipate further technological development which will enable even less mature foetuses to be kept alive. They asked at what point, if at all, the rights of the unborn child prevailed over those of the woman. And they asked why a prostaglandin injection is given to kill a child if in terminating the pregnancy it has already been deemed to be incapable of life (see the discussion infra of 'capable of being born alive' within the Infant Life (Preservation) Act 1929). Abortions were said to be sought on trivial grounds, such as a hare lip or facial deformity. A consultant plastic surgeon from Guy's Hospital, London, whose work includes performing plastic surgery on foetuses in the womb, wrote to MP Ann Widdecombe believing that in debate she had attacked his practice and the ethical basis of the work which he was doing. As Widdecombe was later to relate, he had written to inform her that not only were abortions on such grounds offered, but that they were routinely offered (House of Commons, Official Report 21 June 1990, col. 1188). This led to an unsuccessful attempt to provide, as an alternative to time-limiting such abortions, that doctors in carrying out abortion on the ground of foetal handicap should be required to specify on the abortion form the nature of the handicap justifying the termination. This vote was tied at 197-197 and the Speaker exercised his casting vote to leave the Bill as reported from Committee (see House of Commons, Official Report 21 June 1990, col. 1217-19).

As the unborn child at 18 weeks is complete in organs and sensitive to touch and sound, the foetus can feel pain and the sensory neurones are more sensitive than those of an adult or a newborn. David Alton MP argued that abortion is always the greater of two evils; the argument of choice cannot be accepted as it amounts to choosing to take another's life; 'I believe that that is a modern heresy,' he said (House of Commons, Official Report 24 April 1990, col. 223). This was allied with an appeal that as we are each 'God's handiwork' and that there is a unique plan for each of us in our lives, that uniqueness entails that we cannot be seen as expendable raw material. Finally, the pro-birth proponents argued that back street abortions had been on the decline before the 1967 Act and late abortions were conducted solely for profit; in 1984 over 60% of late abortions were performed by just 11 private clinics.

Arguments for Continuity: Pro-choice

Those who argued in favour of retention or even extension of the current provision pointed out that since Sweden had introduced abortion on demand up to 18 weeks, 95% of all terminations had been carried out before 13 weeks of pregnancy. In addition, they argued for a retention of the upper time limits because of a fear of a return by women to back street abortions, and the time delay in obtaining medical diagnoses. They asserted the woman's right to choose, and emphasised the need to respect her judgment about the disability of any resulting child — her child. Very immature births, it was said, gave rise to brain and other damage which meant the consumption of very high technological resources in the NHS; this striving to keep alive foetuses which had been aborted (as an amendment moved by Baroness Cox to the Commons' amendment would have provided, see House of Lords, Official Report, 18 October 1990, cols.

1043–86) would have been repugnant and self-defeating. The four-week 'grace period' in calculating correctly the date of the last menstrual period, meant in fact that an 18-week limit would reduce the availability of abortions after 14 weeks (the 1984 RCOG survey suggested that only 3% of its members would favour an 18-week limit); and that arguments designed to cut time limits were in fact disguised arguments to do away with all abortions. They pointed to the disappearance of sex education and contraceptive advice services, and the reduction of local authority resources in family planning services (in April 1990 it was reported that a third of authorities were cutting such services) and reports of four week delays in confirming pregnancy testing, which all led to fears about the provision of safe, effective, compassionate abortion services. Prohibiting abortions in the late period — between 24 and 28 weeks — would deny to a very small but important number of women and young girls (23 in 1988) abortions which they desperately need. These would include: cases where late detection of severe foetal abnormality makes any late abortion especially distressing; young women who become pregnant without realising or knowing it and who are frightened and unsupported; women in the menopause with irregular periods who became pregnant without realising it; and those who suffer because of the irregularity of NHS provision.

Change, Continuity and Interests

There are two senses in which the reforms achieved represent a response to medical interests. First, the British Medical Association and the RCOG and other medical bodies and interest groups were in favour of a reduction of the availability of lawful abortion to 24 weeks. This was decisive for many MPs. But secondly, the day before the abortion vote, MPs had voted to allow embryo research ('destructive embryo research' as its opponents called it) up to 14 days after the beginning of the process of fertilisation. One of the main reasons why they had permitted this was because of medical advances which have made the detection and tentative treatment of genetic disease and chromosomal disorder much more readily available. They were mindful that when it came to the implementation of these technological advances, i.e. abortion of affected foetuses, they were talking about the elimination of the problem through the elimination of the patient. This they felt much securer in accepting if strong medical grounds could be adduced in support.

Against that background it is possible to conclude that the UK has now a much more explictly based eugenic abortion policy than before 1990, not just in the sense that abortion on the ground of foetal handicap is to be more readily available, after 28 weeks (see below), but also because it was apparent that the most clearly favoured Parliamentary ground for abortion was the genetic handicap ground. The 'woman's right to choose' argument — advocated by some of those who spoke in debate — held little persuasive force overall, but on this narrow, limited point, it was decisive.

The debate over the abortion limits had been given added impetus by the introduction into the House of Lords of an Abortion (Amendment) Bill 1989 by Lord Houghton, and the judgment of Brooke J in a civil law claim for damages, *Rance* v *Mid Downs Health Authority* (1990) 140 NLJ 325; *The Independent,* 13

February 1990. The Houghton Bill had sought to reduce the time limit for a lawful abortion to 24 weeks. And in judgment in *Rance,* Brooke J had held that 'capable of being born alive' in the Infant Life (Preservation) Act 1929 meant the 'capacity to survive for a few minutes unaided' (see below). We turn now to consider the nature and shape of the reforms which the 1990 Act have produced, and to restate the law of abortion as it stands in the United Kingdom following the passage of the first statutory reform of abortion in nearly a quarter of a century.

The Law of Abortion: The 1861 Act and the 1929 Act

There is much dispute about the attitude of the common law to abortion, whether performed pre- or post-quickening. We cannot review that dispute here (for an introduction see John Keown's *Abortion, Doctors and the Law,* ((1988), Cambridge University Press), but a brief historical sketch will assist in understanding the present reforms.

In an Act of 1803, Lord Ellenborough's Act, Parliament provided that the abortion of a quick foetus (one which has shown the first recognisable movements *in utero,* usually about the 16th to 18th week of pregnancy) was to be a capital offence. In addition, smaller penalties were provided for abortion before quickening. In 1837, the distinction between pre- and post-quickening abortions was dropped, and the capital punishment was removed by an Act on which the Offences Against the Person Act 1861 is modelled. Thus, since 1803 Parliament has laid out prohibited areas of conduct in respect of the developing foetus, and has sanctioned abortion only where the life of the mother was at risk.

The law which establishes the offence commonly referred to as 'abortion' remains as stated in the 1861 Act. Section 58 provides that:

> Every woman, being with child, who, with intent to procure her own miscarriage, shall unlawfully administer to herself any poison or other noxious thing, or shall unlawfully use any instrument or other means whatsoever with the like intent and whosoever, with intent to procure the miscarriage of any woman, whether she be or not with child, shall unlawfully administer to her or cause to be taken by her any poison or other noxious thing, or shall unlawfully use any instrument or other means whatsoever with the like intent, shall be guilty of an offence, and being convicted thereof shall be liable to imprisonment.

That section was buttressed by s. 59 which provides:

> Whosoever shall unlawfully supply or procure any poison or other noxious thing, or any instrument or thing whatsoever, knowing that the same is intended to be unlawfully used or employed with intent to procure the miscarriage of any woman, whether she be or not be with child, shall be guilty of an offence, and being convicted thereof shall be liable to imprisonment for a term not exceeding five years.

That legislation was supplemented in 1929 by the Infant Life (Preservation) Act which had two functions. It attempted to close a perceived lacuna in the protection which the 1861 Act gave to the developing foetus. This followed from the common law distinction between the status of a foetus and of a child born alive. In *R* v *Poulton* (1832) 5 C & P 329, Littledale J had directed a jury that 'with respect to birth, the being born must mean that the whole body is brought into the world; it is not sufficient that the child respires in the progress of birth.' It followed from this, that the killing of a child in the process of birth was not the procurement of a miscarriage nor murder or manslaughter of a child born alive, because the child was not yet a 'reasonable creature in being' as required by the law of homicide. This lacuna had been exploited, for example, in a trial and acquittal at the Liverpool Assizes in June 1928 where Talbot J in charging the Grand Jury had observed that:

> the law upon this matter is unsatisfactory and it is right that every appropriate opportunity should be taken to call public attention to it. It is a felony to procure abortion and it is murder to take the life of a child when it is fully born, but to take the life of a child while it is being born and before it is fully born is no offence whatever (cited in Brightman Committee Report, Select Committee of the House of Lords on the Infant Life (Preservation) Bill HL 50, para. 8. And see the consideration of a similar point in S B Atkinson, 'Life, Birth and Live-Birth' (1904) 20 *Law Quarterly Review* 157).

The following session, Parliament considered, but failed to pass, a Child Destruction Bill 1928, which was the immediate precursor to the Infant Life (Preservation) Act 1929.

In addition, as Mason points out, this Act was designed to legalise the operation of craniotomy — the crushing of an impacted foetal head which inevitably causes foetal death — which was widely practised before caesarian section became commonplace and safer for the woman. (*Medico-Legal Aspects of Reproduction and Parenthood,* (1990), Dartmouth p. 101).

Section 1 of the Infant Life (Preservation) Act created the offence of 'child destruction', punishable with life imprisonment. That section provides:

> (1) Subject as hereinafter in this subsection provided, any person who, with intent to destroy the life of a child capable of being born alive, by any wilful act causes a child to die before it has an existence independent of its mother, shall be guilty of a felony, to wit, of child destruction, and shall be liable on conviction thereof on indictment to penal servitude for life:
>
> Provided that no person shall be found guilty of an offence under this section unless it is proved that the act which caused the death of the child was not done in good faith for the purpose only of preserving the life of the mother.
>
> (2) For the purposes of this Act, evidence that a woman had at any material time been pregnant for a period of twenty-eight weeks or more shall be prima facie proof that she was at that time pregnant of a child capable of being born alive.

Parliament thus closed the loophole by adopting the concept of a child 'born alive' and extended it back to any child *in utereo* which was 'capable of being born alive', up to the moment when it was in fact born alive. In other words, the phrase adopted by Parliament in 1929 extended to cover not only the process of birth, but also that period when the foetus capable of being born alive was still in its mother's womb. The policy of the Act when introduced in 1929 had been to fill a lacuna in the legislation through which, since 1803, Parliament had regulated women's access to abortion services. In 1929 Parliament declared the policy of the law to be that the taking of a potential human life at a stage of gestation where it was capable of independent existence, but before it had that existence independent of its mother, was unlawful, unless the mother's life was in danger. It is unclear from the face of the statute whether the 28th week there referred to is the 'real' 28th week or the 'medical' count, which would make it the 26th week. This point is noted by Glanville Williams (*Textbook of Criminal Law,* (1983) Sweet & Maxwell, 2nd ed., p. 291 n. 1). He suggests that the medical practice of counting pregnancy as commencing from the beginning of the woman's last period before conception, rather than the possible occurence of conception which is about two weeks thereafter in the middle of the menstrual cycle, would mean that the week there referred to would be the 'medical' week, when the woman was likely to have been pregnant for about 26 weeks. He argues that the 'actual' 28 weeks should be taken to have been intended here, as, in favour of the defendant on a charge, being the latest date on which a pregnancy could have commenced.

It is important to note that the 28 week prima facie presumption of a child 'capable of being born alive' is merely that; it could be displaced by evidence to the contrary. These provisions were left intact by the Abortion Act 1967; s. 5(1) of the 1967 Act saved the provisions of the Infant Life (Preservation) Act 1929 which it described as 'protecting the life of the viable foetus'. What the 1967 Act did do was to protect a registered medical practitioner and a pregnant woman in certain specified circumstances from committing the offence of 'procuring a miscarriage' under the 1861 Act. What the 1967 Act did *not* do (quite the opposite) was to introduce any protection in respect of killing a 'child capable of being born alive'. Hence, there was great importance attached to knowing which foetuses were protected by that Act.

In Scotland, where the 1929 Act does not apply, child destruction is a crime at common law, but because no time limit has ever appeared in statute, there has been said to be a much greater degree of flexibility, and in theory abortions have been available up to term. However, in practice a notional limit of 28 weeks has been adhered to by most authorities and medical practitioners there, and even before the introduction of the Abortion Act 1967 controversy in that jurisdiction had been fierce about the limits for lawful abortion. The Lord Advocate had circulated consultants in Scotland with advice that they risked prosecution for carrying out abortions, and this led directly to the inclusion by the newly returned MP David Steel of an extension of his Bill to Scotland. In 1987, there were only two abortions carried out in Scotland after 24 weeks, and in 1988 only one. So, although Scottish law appeared to be more liberal, in fact the 24-week limit was more honoured than breached. The time limits in the 1990 Act now extend explicitly to Scotland.

These laws remained the bedrock of abortion law until 1967. Even a cursory examination of these provisions discloses some of the difficulties of interpretation to which the law was subject. Immediately it is clear that the offence stated in 1861 consists of the unlawful procurement of a miscarriage, but there are three elements which need brief elucidation here.

First, the offence is defined by reference to miscarriage, and is committed by one who unlawfully procures a miscarriage. We shall return to the importance of what constitutes a miscarriage below when we consider the legality of what has come to be called 'selective reduction' of multiple pregnancy.

Secondly, there arises the question of which foetuses are 'capable of being born alive' such that the procurement of their miscarriage would be an offence under the 1929 Act. In an article in *The Lancet,* 10 March 1984, entitled 'Capable of Being born Alive', Dunn and Stirratt from the Bristol Maternity Hospital reviewed their understanding of the legal position under the 1929 Act and added in a footnote; 'at the time of writing two infants of 23 weeks gestation are in our care, one now being 2½ weeks old the other one week old.' The difficulty in this area was that the exception might tend towards the norm. There was, in the Bristol case, no doubt that the baby born 2½ weeks previously was capable not only of being born alive but also of surviving. However, the article did not indicate whether either child survived beyond that time, nor indeed what significance their survival would have had for the interpretation of the law. Indeed, it was not until 20 years after the Abortion Act that the courts were drawn to make a formal ruling on the meaning of 'capable of being born alive' and its relationship with the concept of 'viability' introduced in 1967.

In *C* v *S* [1987] 1 All ER 1230, Lord Donaldson MR said that a child was capable of being born alive if it was capable of independent or assisted breathing if:

> [the foetus] has reached the normal stage of development and . . . is incapable of breathing, it is not in our judgment 'a child capable of being born alive' within the meaning of the 1929 Act (at p. 1241).

Earlier he had said that a foetus of 18-21 weeks gestation, while demonstrating 'real and discernible signs of life' — in that the cardiac muscle is contracting and a primitive circulation developing —

> even if then delivered by hysterectomy, would be incapable ever of breathing *either naturally or with the aid of a ventilator*. It is not a case of the foetus requiring a stimulus or assistance (emphasis added).

This appears to settle that the 1929 Act protects only the 'viable' foetus, and not the wider category of foetuses decribed by the common law as those of live birth; infants, however premature, alive at the moment of birth. As Williams suggests, this accords with the view apparently adopted by Parliament in the Abortion Act 1967 s. 5(1), which refers to the 1929 Act as protecting viable foetuses (*Textbook*, pp. 303-04). The use of the word 'viable' in the Abortion Act s. 5(1) (which saved the operation of the 1929 Act alongside the Abortion Act) has been accepted as shorthand for 'capable of being born alive' and as not effecting any change in the foetuses which were subject of the 1929 Act's protection (per Brooke J in *Rance*, supra). But Lord Donaldson's dicta, that the child must be 'capable of breathing' does not examine the meaning of viability in the sense of describing how long such survival must be in order to have satisfied the requirement of the child possessing the capacity to survive. It substitutes for one formulation, that in the 1929 Act, another — that of capacity to breathe, with or without assistance.

In her first instance judgment in *C* v *S* Heilbron J observed that 'viability . . . embraces not only being born alive but surviving, for however short a time' (p. 1238). She added, however, that:

> 'capable of being born alive' does not have a clear and plain meaning. It is ambiguous. It is a phrase which is capable of different interpretations, and probably for the reason that it is also a medical concept . . . the expertise of doctors may well be required and gratefully received to assist the court (p. 1239; original emphasis).

More recently, Brooke J had to consider the meaning of this phrase in *Rance* v *Mid Downs Health Authority* (supra). Here, parents claimed that a hospital's medical staff had negligently failed to discover a foetal abnormality, and hence deprived the woman of the opportunity of having an abortion. They sought damages for the shock, trauma, distress and pain associated with the subsequent birth and the subsequent cost of bringing up a severely handicapped child. The Health Authority defended the negligence action by arguing that the scan which would have disclosed the abnormality was carried out at 26 weeks. They argued that the foetus would then have been 'capable of being born alive' and hence that an abortion, even if carried out within the period of 28 weeks, would have been unlawful. They contended that it would be contrary to public policy to award damages for the negligent failure to carry out an unlawful act.

In an extensive review of the formulation and operation of the 1929 Act, Brooke J recalled the opinion of the Brightman Committee, the Select Committee of the House of Lords on the Infant Life (Preservation) Bill (1987-8), introduced into the House of Lords in that session (see House of Lords Papers HL50, 1987-88). There the Committee had surveyed a bewildering diversity of views, all held in good faith, by medical practitioners as to the meaning of this phrase. The Committee had observed that:

> as a matter of legal interpretation, this expression probably means capable of being brought into the world alive independently of the mother, for a period however short, even a matter of minutes. The general opinion, however, among the medical profession and other persons concerned with the subject of abortion, is that 'capable of being born alive' means 'viable' in the sense of the capacity to survive for an appreciable period, which witnesses variously describe or wish to see defined as capable of 'sustained independent existence', 'being able to breathe at the time of birth so that long term survival is possible', 'not only the capacity of being born but also viability (i.e. the possiblility of sustaining life)' and 'capable of sustained survival'. The Committee think that the majority of those concerned with this problem of interpretation equate

> 'capable of being born alive' with 'capable of sustained survival' for some period not precisely defined. Even the draftsman of the 1967 Act used the word 'viable' to describe the effect of the 1929 Act in the section 5 proviso. The Committee fully appreciate the common sense of this approach but find difficulty in seeing how directions could be given to a jury with sufficient precision if that approach be correct.

Brooke J found less difficulty with this question of interpretation:

> The difficulty was not with the concept 'capable of being born alive,' but with proving to a jury's satisfaction, without the help of a statutory presumption of information derived from modern technological know-how, that the child in question had those attributes.

He continued that:

> the words 'born alive' are clear, and the meaning of the words 'capable of being born alive' are also clear. . . . [A child is] born alive if, after birth, it exists as a live child, that is to say breathing and living by reason of its breathing through its own lungs alone, without deriving any of its living or power to live by or through any connection with its mother. . . . Once the foetus has reached a state of development in the womb that it is capable, if born, of possessing those attributes, it is capable of being born within the meaning of the 1929 Act.

Brooke J's stress on the child's unaided survival introduces an ambiguity which he had claimed not to discover on the face of s. 1(1) itself. His judgment is open to two interpretations: that to be capable of being born alive a child must be capable of breathing through its own lungs alone without assistance; or alternatively, that the independence which the child must possess is that of its mother and independence of any other assistance, mechanical or otherwise, which may be necessary or available. It is, however, consistent with the dicta of Lord Donaldson in *C* v *S*, (supra), that the breathing must take place other than by or through connection with its mother. That necessary dependence must have been overcome, whether in fact the umbilical link has been broken or not. It is not necessary that the child be able to sustain its lung function without mechanical ventilation. To require otherwise would mean that all the varied circumstances in which neonates might require ventilation would be cases of children who were not capable of being born alive, and failure to attend to them or render medical assistance would not be culpable. Indeed Brooke J went on to consider the submission of counsel for the plaintiffs that 'capable of being born alive' meant viable in the sense of 'being born alive and surviving into old age in the normal way without intensive care or surgical intervention'. This argument was underlined by arguing that, when the Act was passed in 1929, Parliament can only have had in mind the capacity of a neonate to survive naturally and without artificial ventilation or other assistance. This approach would have avoided the uncertainties introduced by having to specify for how long the survival must be to count as a capacity to be born alive. But Brooke J rejected that interpretation; it would, he said, entail the view that Parliament intended that the phrase it had adopted in the 1929 Act was for individual juries to give substance to, with the result that some children in the course of being born would be denied protection because their expectation of life was not assured at the moment of birth.

Finally, the 1861 statute clearly contemplated that there were circumstances in which an abortion could be lawfully performed, even before the Abortion Act 1967 introduced statutory defences to the offence. The grounds for such action were considered in the important case in 1939, *R* v *Bourne* [1939] 1 KB 687. There, Macnaughten J examined the meaning of the word 'unlawfully' in s. 58, in the light of the wording of the 1929 Act. He concluded that:

> the word unlawfully [in s. 58] is not . . . a meaningless word. I think it imports the meaning expressed by the proviso [the 1929 Act] . . . and that s. 58 of the Offences Against the Person Act 1861, must be read as if the words making it an offence to use an instrument with intent to procure a miscarriage were qualified by a similar proviso.

The judge went on to say that if the act was done for the purpose of saving the life of the woman, or for preserving her health — later clarified to be physical or mental health — then it would not have been done unlawfully. (Cf. the critical examination of *Bourne* by Keown in his book *Abortion, Doctors and the Law,* (1988) Cambridge University Press, pp. 49-59, the thrust of which is that the understanding of 'unlawfully' had been long debated before 1939, and that the interpretation given to it by Macnaughten J was much narrower than authorities preceding the case and than that adopted in two subsequent but little cited cases, of *Bergmann* (1948), unreported and *Newton* (1958), unreported.)

Until the late 1960s, however, the *Bourne* interpretation remained the only source of defence for a person charged with the unlawful procurement of a miscarriage. In 1967 a private member's bill was introduced to provide a limited statutory defence to a charge of unlawful procurement. That Bill became the Abortion Act 1967. It has stood numerous challenges since then (see further Linda Clarke in Robert Lee and Derek Morgan, *Birthrights: Law and Ethics at the Beginnings Of Life,* (1989), Routledge p. 155 and Keown (supra)), and in the 1990 Act, the law has been recast in several important ways. Section 37 of the 1990 Act amends s. 1 of the 1967 Act (the text of the 1967 Act, as now amended, is set out in Appendix 2). That section provides for the first time a statutory time limit for abortion; a limit of 24 weeks being specified in the 1967 Act itself. In England and Wales, the previous 'limit' of 28 weeks was derived only from the presumption provided for in the 1929 Act that a child was 'capable of being born alive' after a woman's continuous pregnancy of 28 weeks. Procurement of a miscarriage after this point would amount to the offence of child destruction, unless within the proviso to s. 1(1) of that Act, outlined above, that the miscarriage was procured with the sole intent of saving the life of the mother. The other fundamental change introduced by the 1990 Act is that in respect of three of the grounds for statutory lawful abortion, no time limit is specified at all, and abortion is lawful if carried out on these grounds up to term.

The debates in the Commons were as passionate and as forceful as consideration of the rest of the Bill had been careful and measured. David Alton, a leading campaigner for abortion law reform and restriction, argued that we should not 'impose quality controls on life' and asserted that 'eugenics is the refuge of a society that has grown uneasy with disability' (House of Commons, Official Report 24 April 1990, col. 225). In reply, Emma Nicholson retorted that 'the pro-life group's calling card rests on its validation of the over-arching importance of life' but doubted whether that was really so (House of Commons, Official Report 24 April 1990, col. 251).

The amendments as passed by the House of Commons mean that there are five separate grounds for a lawful abortion within the terms of the 1967 Act. Section 37 of the 1990 Act substitutes for ss. 1(1)(a) and (b) of the Abortion Act 1967 a new subsection 1. Here we proceed to examine the new abortion law as the 1967 Act now reads.

The New Abortion Law

Before proceeding to examine the reformulated Abortion Act, there are a number of preliminary points to make. First, the Act identifies separate grounds for abortion which were previously run together in the 1967 Act; the grounds are now set out in s. 1(1)(a), (b), (c), (d) and 1(4). Secondly, the way in which two of these grounds have been worded either continues or introduces doubts as to their precise scope and application. Thirdly, and of most importance, in respect of these four initial grounds, the protection given to the pregnant woman and the doctor performing the abortion arises, as before, only where the pregnancy is terminated by a registered medical practitioner and following certification by two registered medical practitioners acting in good faith, that the ground for abortion exists. In an important change, however, s. 37(4) inserts for s. 5(1) of the Abortion Act 1967 a new provision which 'uncouples' the Abortion Act from the Infant Life (Preservation) Act altogether. An abortion performed on any of the specified grounds in s. 1 and having met the procedure requirements is now lawful, whether carried out on a child incapable of being born alive or of one capable of being born alive. It is in this sense that the explicit nature of the underlying eugenic philosophy of the reforms may be most clearly seen. Finally, abortion services are for the first time put under the review of a statutory agency. Previously, the accountability of registered clinics and hospitals was to the Department of Health. Section 8(a) lays upon HUFEA a duty to 'keep under review information about embryos and any subsequent development of embryos . . .'. It was the inclusion of this latter phrase in the long title of the Bill which had enabled the issue of abortion to be included within the purview of the Bill in the first place. Precisely how HUFEA will discharge this duty, and the way in which this form of statutory monitoring will affect the delivery of abortion services remains to be seen (see discussion of this issue at pp. 92–3).

1. Section 1(1)(a) of the 1967 Act

This section now provides that where the continuance of the pregnancy would involve risk, greater than if the pregnancy were terminated, of injury to the physical or mental health of the pregnant woman or any existing children of her family, a lawful abortion may be performed up to the end of the 24th week of pregnancy. In 1988 the equivalent of this ground accounted for 89% of all terminations.

This is the first time that a specific time limit has been written into the Abortion Act. Under the 1967 legislation, the time limit was taken to be 28 weeks (following from the presumption in the 1929 Act) although it had become very rare indeed for any abortions to be performed after 24 weeks (see above) and, according to specialists who gave evidence in *Rance,* unusual for abortions to be performed after 20 weeks.

The voting on the 'pendulum' introduced to secure agreement on the time limit that was for the first time to be written into the 1967 Act is of some interest. The proposals for various time limits were put and voted on until one secured a majority; Patrick Cormack MP was later to refer to it as the 'night of the long votes' (House of Commons, Official Report, 21 June 1990, col. 1196; the voting occupied two and a half hours). The proposals and the votes were as follows:

18 weeks	for 165	against 375	majority 210
28 weeks	for 141	against 382	majority 241
20 weeks	for 189	against 358	majority 169
26 weeks	for 156	against 372	majority 216
22 weeks	for 255	against 301	majority 46
24 weeks	for 335	against 129	majority 206

In the case of the second, third and fourth grounds for lawful abortion, the 1990 Act marks a radical departure from the approach of the 1967 Act. Although the grounds are substantially similar they have been recast and reformulated. But there are two major innovations. The first is that a lawful abortion may be performed on any of these three grounds without any time limit. And secondly, there is a new ground for lawful abortion.

The 'unlimited' grounds are:

(a) that the termination of the pregnancy is necessary to prevent grave permanent injury to the physical or mental health of the pregnant woman s. 1(1)(b);

(b) that the continuance of the pregnancy would involve risk to the life of the pregnant woman, greater than if the pregnancy were terminated s. 1(1)(c);

(c) that there is a substantial risk that if the child were born it would suffer from such physical or mental abnormalities as to be seriously handicapped; s. 1(1)(d).

Each of these grounds, which may be invoked at any stage of the pregnancy until birth, needs separate attention. But two preliminary notes may be entered. Each of these grounds may be used to justify termination of the pregnancy between the end of the 24th week and term. Although they are open textured, in the sense that they will justify all abortions after 24 weeks as long as one of the grounds can be presented each of the grounds is restricted by specific wording. In each case, it will be necessary for the medical practitioners to certify that the proper conditions of the grounds have been satisfied. Otherwise, they will remain open to prosecution under the Offences Against the Person Act s. 58. They may also remain vulnerable to prosecution under the 1929 Act where the foetus aborted was 'capable of being born alive.' Section 37(4) introduces a substitute s. 5(1) in the Infant Life (Preservation) Act. It provides that:

> No offence under the Infant Life (Preservation) Act 1929 shall be committed by a registered medical practitioner who terminates a pregnancy in accordance with the provisions of this Act.

Accordingly, a practitioner who terminates a pregnancy believing, in all good faith, that the foetus if born would suffer from 'such physical or mental abnormalities as to be seriously handicapped' is protected from prosecution even if it later transpires that she has made a mistake and aborted a perfectly healthy foetus. The question of good faith here is, as under any of the grounds, one for the jury to decide on the totality of the evidence: *R* v *Smith* [1974] 1 All ER 376.

Section 1(1)(b); 'grave permanent injury'

This is a new ground for abortion under the 1967 Act. Section 1(4) of the Abortion Act — which is not affected by these present changes — already provides that a pregnancy may be terminated following determination by one medical practitioner alone where it is 'immediately necessary to save the life or to prevent grave permanent injury to the physical or mental health of the pregnant woman.' Examples of such causes would be be conditions such as pre-eclampsia, abruption and placenta praevia. That provision has two important differences from the new sub-section 1(1)(b) introduced here:

(i) the new ground requires two medical practitioners to be of the opinion that the termination is necessary (and not immediately necessary)

(ii) to prevent 'grave permanent injury' to the woman's physical or mental health, falling short of being either an immediate threat to her life (provided for in s. 1(4)), or of the continuation of the pregnancy being a risk to her life greater than if the pregnancy were terminated, provided for in the next sub-section.

Nor is there a need under this ground to balance the risk to the woman against that posed by the continuance of the pregnancy, as in s. 1(1)(a), although here it is necessary to show that the woman would suffer 'grave permanent injury' and not simply 'injury' as in the previous case. This ground was inserted in the Bill in debate in the House of Commons by a vote of 337-146 (House of Commons, Official Report 24 April 1990, col. 291). The effect of it is to put into statutory form the reading given to the Infant Life (Preservation) Act 1929 given by *R* v *Bourne* [1939] 1 KB 687. Recall that Macnaughten J opined that 'the word "unlawfully" is not, [in s. 58 OAPA 1861], a meaningless word'. He held that it imported a meaning similar to that expressed legislatively in 1929, and that the statutory offence of s. 58 should be read as if subject to a defence of acting in good faith solely for the purpose of saving the life of the pregnant woman. And, he continued, it is not necessary to wait until the woman is in peril of immediate or instant death (separately provided for in s. 1(4)). Indeed, he went so far as to suggest that a doctor was not merely entitled, but was enjoined by a common law duty, to intervene to save the life of the pregnant woman. It would include cases where the doctor (and to comply with the provisions now of the 1967 Act, a second registered medical practitioner) is of the opinion, formed in good faith and on the basis of her or his clinical experience, that the woman is in danger of grave permanent injury to her physical or mental health. In such a case, the doctors are justified in proceeding to the termination without having to wait for the events which put the life of the woman at immediate risk. Examples here might include: mild pre-eclampsia; breast or cervical cancer in which the risk to the woman increases during pregnancy because of the hormonal changes which increase with the growth of the foetus; uncontrolled diabetes; conditions which may improve or deteriorate during pregnancy, such as asthma and epilepsy, and conditions such as hypertension, where the woman may run the risk of severe permanent damage to her brain, heart or kidneys. It does appear that although this ground gives access to a lawful abortion after 24 weeks, it does so in such a way that most practitioners would attempt to save the life of a viable foetus if possible.

This goes some way to helping understand what would be necessary to prevent 'grave permanent injury' to the pregnant woman's physical or mental health such as to justify termination at any stage. The wording speaks of a grave, and not a serious risk. It is possible that a jury would be invited to give these expressions a similar, if not an identical meaning. In debate, Frank Doran MP described the test as a 'severe legal test' and dismissed fears that the provision could be used to justify and sanction abortion until birth in a wide variety of cases which would markedly alter the existing law (House of Commons, Official Report 21 June 1990, col. 1185). However, it seems possible to suggest that this provision will enable immediate termination in such cases as discussed, where the continuation of the pregnancy might seriously accentuate or exacerbate the illness to the point at which the woman's health would be permanently affected.

Section 1(1)(c); risk to the life of the pregnant woman

This ground overlaps with that considered under s. 1(1)(b), and is a restatement of the old s. 1(1)(a). However, abortion on this ground is available at any time during the course of the pregnancy where it can be shown that the continuation of the pregnancy would entail a risk to the life of the woman greater than that posed by termination. With the sophistication of abortion technology and the increasing skill of health care practitioners performing abortions, most terminations of up to 12 weeks carry less risk to the life of the mother than continuing with the pregnancy, which always carries with it degrees of risk. As term and birth approach those risks increase, but so do the obstetric risks associated with termination. A similar effect had been provided for in the Infant Life (Preservation) Act 1929 s. 1(1), with a saving for an abortion at any stage of the pregnancy to save the life of the woman.

There is an important similarity, however, which can be adduced between this and the previous ground. It concerns the notion of 'termination.' Recall that s. 1(1)(b) provides for cases in which the termination is necessary to prevent grave permanent injury to the physical or mental health of the woman, where her actual or reasonably foreseeable circumstances may be taken into account. Such a termination may take place, up to term, on a healthy foetus capable of being born alive. Section 1(1)(b) thus provides for the case in which it can be foreseen that termination will be necessary for the benefit of the woman, but which is not at the time the termination is carried out immediately necessary to save her life (since this is separately provided for, see s. 1(4)). Nor is it a pregnancy the continuance of which would put her life more at risk than if it were terminated; that is provided for in s. 1(1)(c). As with s. 1(1)(c), s. 1(1)(b) may be thought of as a 'sacrifice' ground. But the statute does not say in what sense that sacrifice must be effected. It does not say, for example, that the termination must be carried out in such a way as to kill the foetus. What the statute now provides is that there will be a lawful defence to a charge under the OAPA Act when that course is chosen.

Where the termination is carried out very close to term, it may be possible to argue that the pregnancy may be terminated in such a way as to maximise the possibilities of producing a live birth, consistent with achieving the objectives which the termination grounds set out. It is unlikely that this argument would be applied to the serious foetal handicap ground (s. 1(1)(d), below), where the whole purpose of the ground is to relieve the mother or parents of the foetus from the responsibility of caring for it.

This novel argument was indeed proposed by one commentator during the Bill's legislative passage. In her essay 'Abortion Law: Is Consensual Reform Possible?' (in Len Doyal and Lesley Doyal, eds., Legal and Moral Dilemmas in Modern Medicine, (1990) 17 *Journal of Law and Society Special Issue,* 106, at p. 116), Sheila McLean recalled that the time at which viability occurs is a mobile one and foetuses at the upper end of the scale may develop sufficiently to become not potentially but actually salvageable in greater numbers and with greater frequency. It is at this point that the interests of the developing relatively mature foetus and the rights of the woman who is carrying it are seldom so clearly in conflict. Indeed, some philosophers suggest that a proper understanding of sacrifice would entail that it is in circumstances such as this that the woman should be prepared to 'lay down her life' for that of her foetus. McLean's proposal is different however, in that it seeks to challenge two routinely made assumptions:

(i) that this last, post-viability period of pregnancy is sacrosanct and that termination should not be routinely available in the third trimester; and
(ii) that pregnancy termination automatically equates to foetal death.

As we have seen, the first assumption is indeed swept away with the passage of this Act. The second, perhaps equally controversial suggestion is now open for review. McLean observes:

> What is sacrosanct for many about the final stage of pregnancy is, primarily, the fact that the foetus is recognisably 'human' at this stage, that is, it could be born in the shape of a human baby and kept alive. To anti-abortion protagonists, therefore, the well-developed foetus should be saved. At no stage has this lobby argued for any concessions because the anticipated outcome of pregnancy termination at this stage is the destruction of the foetus. . . . On the other hand, the pro-choice lobby, if consistent, would have to argue that pregnancy termination at this stage should be permissible, since the issue is not the development of the foetus but the rights of the woman. However logical it may be, this last position is counter-intuitive for many people. This is because, as the anti-abortion lobby has stressed, it entails the destruction of something which at the moment of destruction could have been saved. . . . this situation is another very clear example of a case where the very evidence used by the anti-abortion lobby can facilitate women's rights, without harming the interests of foetuses. . . . late pregnancy termination is not, and need not be, synonymous with foetal destruction. Indeed, induction, the method commonly used to terminate such pregnancies, is a technique also in wanted pregnancies.

Whether such a proposal, if seriously introduced, would be thought to contribute to the emotional or psychological health or well-being of the woman selecting termination is moot. However, in considering Commons' amendments when the Bill returned to the House of Lords after the summer recess, Baroness Cox sought to amend ss. 1(1)(a)-(c) by introducing a requirement that in aborting a child 'capable of being born alive' under these provisions, the medical practitioner effecting the termination should use 'all reasonable steps to secure that the child is born alive'. (Official Report, House of Lords, 18 October 1990, cols. 1043-87.) The proposed amendment was defeated by 133 votes to 89.

Section 1(1)(d); serious foetal handicap
As originally presented in the Bill, this ground would have been restricted to terminations carried out before the end of the 28th week of pregnancy. That limitation was, however, deleted from the Bill in the course of the controversial 'pendulum' voting provisions introduced to deal with the reforms to the Abortion law, when reference to the Infant Life (Preservation) Act 1929, with its presumption of foetal survivability at 28 weeks, was removed from the Abortion Act 1967 following the introduction of a specific 24 week limit for abortions on all grounds other than foetal handicap (House of Commons, Official Report 24 April 1990, cols. 273-304). This conclusion had indeed been the recommendation of the House of Lords Select Committee in its examination of the Infant Life (Preservation) Act (the Brightman Committee) earlier in the same session (see supra). The Lords' Committee had argued (at p.18) that if an unborn child were diagnosed as:

> grossly abnormal and unable to lead any meaningful life, there is in the opinion of the Committee no logic in requiring the mother to carry her unborn child

to full term merely because the diagnosis was too late to enable an operation for abortion to be carried out before the 28th completed week.

We may abstain for the moment from a detailed examination of the philosophical and ethical assumptions which lie behind this statement. It suffices to remark that the sentiment which it conveys is one which was eventually to commend itself to MPs. An attempt on Report to reinstate the time limit of 28 weeks was defeated by 14 votes (229-215, House of Commons, Official Report, 21 June 1990, cols. 1176-1207).

This is the most difficult of the abortion grounds to interpret, although it is probably that which would have the most widespread public support. Curiously, it is also the one ground under the abortion legislation of 1967 which has not been subject to sustained analysis. (See Morgan, 'Abortion — The Unexamined Ground' [1990] *Criminal Law Review* 687; J K Mason, *Medico-Legal Aspects of Reproduction and Parenthood,* (1990), p. 105 et.seq.) The Brightman Committee reported that DHSS figures supplied to it showed that this ground had been invoked in late terminations of 26-28 weeks with regularity in the 1980s.

26 weeks,	1981 = 15,	1982 = 9,	1983 = 9,	1984 = 7,	1985 = 1,	1986 = 11
27 weeks,	1981 = 2,	1982 = 6,	1983 = 10,	1984 = 9,	1985 = 6,	1986 = 3
28 weeks,	1981 = 1,	1982 = 3,	1983 = 2,	1984 = 3,	1985 = 0,	1986 = 1

Health Minister Virginia Bottomley referred to this ground under s. 1(1)(d) as that about which there was 'widespread agreement that such cases present particular difficulty for several reasons' (House of Commons, Official Report, 24 April 1990, col. 179). Foetal handicap may not be diagnosable until fairly late in the pregnancy, although new medical techniques such as Chorion Villi Sampling, Florescence Activated Cell Sorting and DNA sampling techniques using PCR (Polymerase Chain Reaction) are making the amniocentesis technology less burdensome (for a discussion of these various techniques and some of their implications see Morgan, 'Legal and Ethical Dilemmas of Fetal Sex Identification and Gender Selection' in A A Templeman and D Cusine, *Reproductive Medicine and the Law,* (1990), Churchill Livingstone, pp. 53-77). And secondly, it is the ground about which recent disturbing incidents have been reported, and which excited much critical commentary following the Commons vote in April.

John Finnis and John Keown wrote of that Parliamentary vote that it sanctioned abortion up to term on such flimsy grounds as cleft palate or harelip. In an amendment that was not taken in the House of Commons debates there was a proposal that the foetal handicap ground should be more clearly delineated. A new clause, clause 5 (House of Commons, Official Report 24 February 1990, col. 169; the clause was not moved during debate) provided that abortion could be justified only where 'there is a foetal abnormality with a strong possibility that the child would suffer a condition both incurable and wholly destructive of the quality of life'. A later amendment (No. 28) at Commons Report stage (House of Commons, Official Report, 20 June 1990, col. 1176 et. seq.) would have given an additional regulation making power to the Secretary of State. Under this proposal, the Secretary of State would have been able to make regulations under s. 2 of the 1967 Act requiring a practitioner providing an abortion certificate to include an opinion as to the nature of the physical or mental abnormalities from which there was a substantial risk that the child would suffer if born. A copy of that certificate would then have had to be sent to persons required by regulation to be notified of the termination. The vote on this amendment was tied — the third tie in voting on this Act — at 197-197. The Speaker, as is customary in such cases, exercised the casting vote to leave the Bill in the form in which it came to the Report stage, without the amendment added (House of Commons, Official Report, 21 June 1990, cols. 1176 and 1216-19). The practical effect of the loss of this amendment was diluted by the Secretary of State Clarke's announcement in debate that, if the amendment was defeated, he intended to use existing regulation powers under s. 2 to make it necessary for the nature of the handicap to be specified on the notification for a 'late' abortion after 24 weeks (see House of Commons, Official Report, 21 June 1990, cols. 1199-1200).

In the House of Lords, a final attempt was made by Baroness Cox to reformulate s. 1(1)(d). She moved an amendment which provided that where a termination was authorised on this ground and (i) the 'child is capable of being born alive' and (ii) 'is not suffering from a handicap incompatible with life', then the medical practitioner should take 'all reasonable steps to secure that the child is born alive'. (House of Lords, Official Report, 19 October 1990, cols. 1087-1102). The amendment was defeated by 101 votes to 53.

The 1967 Act specifically preserved the Infant Life (Preservation) Act. This is removed by s. 37(4) of the 1990 Act. In place, a new s. 5(1) is substituted, which provides that, where a registered medical practitioner terminates a pregnancy in accordance with the new provisions, no offence is committed by that practitioner under the 1929 Act. Thus where an abortion is performed within the provisions of s. 1, no prosecution will lie even though the foetus which is destroyed is 'capable of being born alive' within the 1929 Act and the extended meaning given to that phrase in *Rance* (supra). However, where the terms of the 1990 section are not complied with, then the full force of both the Infant Life (Preservation) Act 1929 and the Offences Against the Person Act 1861, s. 58 remain available to police the operation of abortion services. Examples of failure to comply could arise where an abortion is performed and the prosecution can show that if the foetus had been born it would not have suffered from such physical or mental abnormalities as to be seriously handicapped rather than simply handicapped, or disadvantaged, or where the prosecution can show that the injury to a woman's physical or mental health would have been slight or temporary rather than permanent or grave, although a 'good faith' defence will be available, or discussed above (at p. 50).

Selective Reduction of Multiple Pregnancy

One of the late amendments to the Bill in the House of Commons deals with the legality of the procedure which has become known as 'selective reduction' of multiple pregnancy. The Third report of the Interim Licensing Authority described the use of this procedure 'whereby one or more embryos in a multiple pregnancy are selectively killed to allow others to develop.' The technique was originated in discordant twinned pregnancies following diagnosis of severe abnormality or genetic anomaly to stop the development of the abnormal foetus (see, for example, A Aberg et. al., 'Cardiac puncture of foetus with Hurler's disease avoiding abortion of unaffected co-twin' (1978) *The Lancet,* p. 990; Howie suggests that this might properly be regarded as 'selective foeticide': P W Howie, 'Selective Reduction — Medical Aspects' in A A Templeton and D Cusine, *Reproductive Medicine and the Law,* (1990), p. 25). It involves the injection of potassium chloride into the amniotic sac or into the heart of the selected foetus, or foetal exsanguination or aspiration. (For a consideration of the methods of reduction see P W Howie, op.cit. pp. 30-31; for a review of some of the issues see Frances Price, 'Establishing Guidelines: Regulation and the Clinical Management of Infertility' in Robert Lee and Derek Morgan, (eds.), *Birthrights: Law and Ethics at the Beginnings of Life,* (1990), pp. 44-45.) The nature of the Parliamentary concern was captured by the then Health Secretary Kenneth Clarke, (House of Commons, Official Report 21 June 1990, col. 1198):

> The best advice that we can obtain is that selective reduction is subject to the Abortion Act 1967 but that there is considerable doubt about the matter . . . The difficulty of deciding exactly what selective reduction is, when the foetus is killed inside the womb, makes the position different from that of ordinary abortion. Therefore, miscarriage is regarded as the legally correct description.

Commentators have suggested that this procedure is unlawful unless performed in compliance with the provisions of the Abortion Act 1967 (David Price, 'Selective Reduction and Foeticide: The Parameters of Abortion' [1988] *Criminal Law Review* 199, Zelda Pickup, 'Selective reduction, Abortion and the Law' in Templeton and Cuisine, op.cit., pp. 33-39), or further, that the nature of the offence and the limited parameter of the exclusions created by the 1967 Act are such that there are no circumstances in which the reduction may be performed lawfully. On this point John Keown, in 'Selective Reduction of Multiple Pregnancy' (1987) New Law Journal 1165 (see also his opinion at *Voluntary Licensing Authority Third Report* appendix 4, and the reply by Ian Kennedy and Andrew Grubb to this latter point in their *Medical Law: Text and Materials,* (1989), p. 796) has argued that while the offence created in the 1861 Act of 'procuring a miscarriage' has been committed, the requirement for the protection afforded by the Abortion Act 1967, of the 'termination of a pregnancy' has not been satisfied.

There is some confusion in this legal literature which has discussed selective reduction. In what remains the leading article, 'Selective Reduction of Multiple Pregnancy' (1987) New Law Journal 1165, John Keown sets out to rebut the argument that s. 58 of the Offences Against the Person Act 1861 does not apply because there has been no miscarriage. He argues that the understanding of miscarriage on which the contrary analysis is based — that it implies an expulsion from the uterus — incorrectly understands the ingredients of the offence of procuring a miscarriage. His careful argument is that, properly understood, miscarriage does not require the expulsion of foetal remains from the uterus, but speaks rather to the failure of gestation (citing his own close examination 'Miscarriage — a Medico-Legal Analysis' [1984] *Criminal Law Review* 604). Price reaches a broadly similar conclusion; 'it is the causing of foetal death which is the essence of the crime of abortion and not simply the expulsion of the foetus from the mother' (at p. 200). Kennedy and Grubb introduce their discussion of selective reduction by observing that 'the potentially crucial factual distinction between this procedure and other abortions is that when selective reduction is performed the destroyed foetus is absorbed into the mother's body and is not expelled' (p. 793-94). There appears to be no discussion of whether or when the products of conception which have been reduced are expelled from the uterus.

Section 37(5), which amends s.5(2), again refers to the procurement of a miscarriage, or 'in the case of a woman carrying more than one foetus, her miscarriage of any foetus.' In about 1 in 50 reductions, the attempt to reduce the number of viable foetuses causes the spontaneous abortion of all of the foetuses. Almost all reductions will be justifiable on the grounds that there is a substantial risk that each foetus will be born with 'such physical or mental abnormalities as to be seriously handicapped' within s. 1(1)(d), because multiple pregnancy carries with it a significant risk of prematurity with the associated birth risks. If Keown and Price are correct in their interpretation of the notion of miscarriage, then any difficulties of interpretation are lessened. But if the better view is that expulsion of the products of conception from the womb is an essential ingredient of miscarriage then prima facie there remain difficulties.

Selective reduction cannot be performed until after ultrasonic visualisation of a foetal heartbeat. When such a heartbeat is detectable, other foetal organs have begun their process of development. This cannot be earlier than about six weeks following conception. Most reductions are performed between 8 and 14 weeks of pregnancy, although it is common to wait until at least the 11th week to see how many of the foetuses are viable, because one or more of the foetuses may have died spontaneously. In such cases, or those in which reduction is performed, the foetal sac collapses and is squashed to the side of the uterus by the pressure of the growth of the remaining foetal sac(s). The remains of the aborted foetus may be visible as an attachment to the placenta; the selective reduction does not sever the umbilical connection, and the foetal remains will be expelled from the uterus with the placenta at the time of the delivery of the remaining foetuses. Alternatively, if the reduction is performed at an early stage, and the foetal fluid has dispersed, the remaining tissue cells will have been absorbed into the placenta. Similarly, if a foetus dies naturally very early in a pregnancy, the tissue remains gradually degenerate and become absorbed into the placenta. Pathological section of the placenta at delivery can detect these remains, but visual inspection cannot. Where a death or abortion occurs at about 20 weeks, the tissues will not disintegrate but the foetus will lose its fluid and will become a foetus papyracious of up to two centimetres and having a paper like quality, which can be discerned on the placenta to which it has retained its umbilical connection when the woman delivers any remaining normal babies. The form of the foetus will be visible, but it will appear as paper thin. Where a death occurs at 30 weeks, the fluid loss will be such that on delivery of a remaining baby several weeks later, there will be some maceration and skin peeling, but the foetal form will be maintained. Thus, with reduction, it is apparent that the later in the pregnancy that it is performed, the more the likelihood that the foetal remains will be expelled at the time of the delivery of the placenta. It is then that the miscarriage is completed, insofar as the legal understanding of the term requires expulsion (see the authorities reviewed, only to be challenged, by Keown, in his 1987 article). Neither Keown, Price nor Kennedy and Grubb take this point. In a way this is perhaps not surprising, as this facet of selective reduction appears not to have been written up in any of the medical literature which discusses the procedure, although in illustrated presentations the remains of the aborted foetuses are shown clearly. But in early reductions, the concept of miscarriage which relies on expulsion from the womb will remain of dubious legality.

Such was the concern about the health states of women and foetuses in higher order births (triplets or more, of which there were 299 sets in the two and a half years of the study's life; 275 sets of triplets, 24 sets of quads and quins) that the Department of Health commissioned a research study into the effects of such pregnancies. This report, *Three, Four or More* (HMSO, (1990)) was published during the Parliamentary recess after the Bill had failed to gain assent in July. Its disturbing conclusions included the finding that in 6% of triplet cases and 16% of quads and above, the correct number of foetuses in the pregnancy became clear only at birth. In addition, and not surprisingly, the mortality rates of such babies have not fallen as steeply as other preterm births and foetuses are at increased risk of cerebal palsy, especially spastic diplegia (the limited data is review in Howie, op.cit. pp. 26-27).

Against such a background, and with no public knowledge of how many reductions are performed annually, it was perhaps not surprising (although again it illustrated the fluid way in which the Department of Health approached the Bill), that the abortion section was at a very late stage amended to bring such reductions within the ambit of the 1967 Abortion Act. Section 37(5) of the 1990 Act inserts a new wording into s. 5(2) of the Abortion Act. That section now reads as follows (the full text of the amended Abortion Act 1967 is set out in Appendix 2):

> For the purposes of the law relating to abortion, anything done with intent to procure a woman's miscarriage (or in the case of a woman carrying more than one foetus, her miscarriage of any foetus) is unlawfully done unless authorised by section 1 of this Act and, in the case of a woman carrying more than one foetus, anything done with intent to procure her miscarriage of any foetus is authorised by that section if (a) the ground for termination of the pregnancy specified in subsection (1)(d) of that section applies in relation to any foetus and the thing is done for the purposes of procuring the miscarriage of that foetus, or (b) any of the other grounds for termination of the pregnancy specified in that section applies.

This new provision introduces the reformulated grounds of abortion to selective reduction. Such a procedure must now be legally related to one of the grounds for lawful abortion; thus mere numbers alone will apparently not suffice. While the practical effect of such a rewording may be less real than apparent, it is important, nonetheless, to examine this ground in a little more detail.

One ground for 'reduction' is of course s. 1(1)(d) — physical or mental abnormality amounting to serious handicap of any child born. Selective reduction properly so termed — selective foeticide — will fall within this ground. As we have seen, however, usually the doctor will not be able to show that the one or more foetuses terminated would have suffered handicap. This is not the end of the argument, however, for multiple order birth will carry with it attendant risks of abnormality (supra p. 53 et seq.). It may be likely therefore that there is a greater risk that however healthy tests may show the embryos to be, the fact of the multiple order pregnancy may mean that there is a greater risk that, at birth, some of the children will be handicapped. However, the new section 5(2) of the 1967 Act speaks of the application of s. 1(1)(d) of that Act to 'any foetus', while s. 1(1)(d) addresses the handicap to 'the child.' It might be argued that these provisions apply to the specific risk of handicap to a particular child, and that a general risk of handicap to some children of a multiple order pregnancy or birth is insufficient. Alternatively, it might be argued that the attendant risks of such handicap are not 'substantial.'

Such arguments may prove academic. Reduction would seem to be permissible on the other three grounds of s. 1(1)(a)-(c) by virtue of s. 5(2). As reduction is usually carried out early in the pregnancy, and most usually in the first trimester, ground 1(1)(a) — that the pregnancy has not exceeded its 24th week and that its continuation gives rise to the risk of injury to the woman's physical or mental health which outweighs that of the termination — might apply. In general, foetal reduction will reduce the risk of injury to the pregnant woman. In any multiple pregnancy, the threat to the mother's continued welfare will be relieved by each successive miscarriage procured, in the same way that the termination of any pregnancy sufficiently early removes a growing health threat (the foetus) which increases as the pregnancy moves towards term and childbirth. In a higher order pregnancy the risks to the pregnant woman include: hyperemesis (excessive vomiting); high blood pressure, which may produce fits; cerebral haemorrhage or placental bleeding; hydramnios (excessive fluid accumulation in the uterus), which may result in long term bed confinement and bring associated risks of thrombosis in the leg or pelvis veins. The risk of a pulmonary embolism, the passage of a blood clot to the lungs, which endangers the woman's life, is also increased in these circumstances (see Howie, op.cit., pp. 27-28). One problem here, however, is that the risk of the injury to the woman must arise from the continuation of the pregnancy. But if pregnancy means 'the state of being with child,' or 'the status of the uterus in being pregnant,' then following 'reduction', the woman will remain pregnant.

Only a definition of pregnancy which relates to the gestation of a foetus would permit reduction under s. 1(1)(a); the pregnancy (gestation) of certain foetuses is discontinued. Here, we use the word pregnancy to refer to the foetus, yet in more common usage the word describes the state of the woman. This is reflected in the way MP Ann Widdecombe put her understanding of the point in debate:

> I am not sure that the amendment is technically viable, because it refers to a miscarriage. A miscarriage is not an abortion and it is not a selective reduction or a stillbirth. When a woman has a miscarriage she loses her child. In a selective reduction, the child is left in the womb until birth occurs naturally... (House of Commons, Official Report, 21 June 1990, col. 1192)

This point would refer equally to the ground under s. 1(1)(c), which speaks also of the continuance of the pregnancy. This would leave only the ground under s. 1(1)(b) (which uses the word 'termination') as clearly available. It is clear that multiple order pregnancy may pose threats of grave permanent injury to the health of the woman. But it then remains problematic to discuss what is 'necessary' under this ground. Would reduction from three to two foetuses be necessary prevention? Or from eight to three? Triplets are without doubt less risky than a much higher multiple order birth, but would the doctor be able to defend such reduction if it still left the attendant risks to the woman's health that the birth of triplets must pose?

Medicinal Terminations

A second late amendment which was accepted (by 233 votes to 141) introduces a change to s. 1(3) of the 1967 Act. That section provides that an abortion ('any treatment for the termination of pregnancy') is only lawful under the Act if carried out in a hospital vested in the Minister of Health or Secretary of State under the National Health Service Acts or in a place approved by the Minister or Secretary. To this is now added a rider, a new s. 1(3A), which enables the Secretary or Minister to limit approval to a class of places, where the 'treatment for termination' consists of specified medicinal treatment. In addition, it may be required that the termination be carried out only in a specified manner. The new sub-section provides that:

> The power under subsection (3) of this section to approve a place includes the power, in relation to treatment consisting primarily in the use of such medicines as may be specified in the approval and carried out in such manner as may be so specified, to approve a class of places.

The purpose in introducing this section was quite specific. It anticipates the marketing in the United Kingdom of the French manufactured 'abortion pill' RU486, or mifepristone. The administration of the drug involves no surgery or anaesthetic, and yet without the amendment, it would have been necessary for the drug to have been administered in a hospital or approved clinic. The change was introduced to reflect the fact that there was no medical reason for that to be necessary, certainly with RU486, and possibly with other 'medicinal terminations.' The new section does not take the opportunity to clarify the legality of such methods which, essentially, operate so as to prevent the implantation of the fertilised egg. It has been suggested that such destruction amounts to a criminal offence, unless done within the terms of the Abortion Act 1967 (V Tunkel, 'Modern Anti-Pregnancy Techniques and the Criminal Law' [1974] *Criminal*

Law Review 461 and V Tunkel, 'Abortion: How Early, How Late and How Legal' (1979) *British Medical Journal* 253; J Keown, 'Miscarriage: A Medico Legal Analysis' [1984] *Criminal Law Review* 604). In a forceful reply, Kenneth Norrie has observed that the phrase 'termination of a pregnancy' is not synonymous with 'abortion'. 'Abortion in the sense of the law requires something more.' Norrie suggests that that requirement is the intention to destroy potential human life by the termination of pregnancy:

> There are (at least) three elements: destruction, intention to destroy, and the termination of pregnancy. Destruction is a purely factual matter and causes no real problems for the law (except in trying to define what a 'potential human life' is). Intention does cause problems, because it is often very difficult to prove. . . . The real difficulties for the law come about when we try to define termination of pregnancy.' (Norrie, 'Post Coital Anti-Pregnancy Techniques and the Law' in A A Templeton and D Cusine, *Reproductive Medicine and the Law,* (1990), Churchill Livingstone, p. 11 at p. 12.)

Norrie argues that British courts have a long history of deference to the practices and understandings of the medical profession, and that 'medically speaking, pregnancy begins on implantation, that is the completion of the process whereby the fertilised egg attaches itself to the wall of the uterus'. From this he concludes that 'any anti-pregnancy technique that prevents implantation does not terminate pregnancy, because there is no pregnancy, and therefore cannot be abortion' (ibid, p. 13). However, with RU486 there is a further complication. Mifepristone can dislodge the implanted egg at a later stage, as can the IUD. Hence, a medical practitioner who administers RU486 knowing that a woman is pregnant and with intent to end the pregnancy, clearly intends to procure a miscarriage within the terms of the 1861 Act, and will do so lawfully only if within the terms of the Abortion Act 1967.

It is a truism, sometimes shot across the bows of counsel in argument by more belligerent judges, that 'doctors do not write the common law'. And yet Norrie's observation will find general accord amongst medico-legal commentators. Whether in an individual case that would be persuasive, however, is more open to doubt.

Conclusion

We are now presented with a new law of abortion. However, in its incorporation of much of the language of the old law, central definitional problems remain. In particular, these surround what might or might not be construed as a miscarriage; what constitutes a 'grave risk'; what constitutes the termination of a pregnancy, and so on. In each of the parameters which we have examined, these definitional conundrums are of crucial importance. The language of the Act has not been framed in terms of the 'death of the foetus', which is what is really encapsulated in modern medical and lay vocabularies of abortion, but in the more problematic terms of termination, (dis)continuance of the pregnancy and miscarriage. The difficulties to which this area gives rise could, and we believe should, have been resolved with the adoption of a modern statement of what types of medical conduct Parliament wished to bring within the ambit of the Abortion Act and which it wished to leave to the hinterlands of medical and legal uncertainty. The difficulties do not end with those which we have surveyed here. For example, the section protects only (i) a registered medical practitioner (and not any other health care professional, (see s. 37(4), inserting a new s. 5(1) into the Abortion Act 1967) (ii) who (actually) terminates a pregnancy (iii) in accordance with the provisions of the 1967 Act. Does this protection extend to the pregnant woman, the second certifying doctor who does not actually perform the operation, and the nurse who attends or acts upon the instructions of the doctor? (For a comparable problem under the 1967 Act see *Royal College of Nursing of the United Kingdom* v *Department of Health & Social Security* [1980] AC 800.) And what is the scope of s. 38, which reformulates the 'conscientious objection' provision of the Abortion Act to encompass any activity governed by the 1990 Act? (We return to consider this section briefly in Chapter 7.) What we may say with confidence is this. Lord Diplock said of the Abortion act 1967 that:

> it started its Parliamentary life as a private member's Bill, and maybe for that reason, it lacks the style and consistency of draftsmanship both internal to the Act itself and in relation to other statutes which one would expect to find in legislation that had its origin in the office of parliamentary counsel (*Royal College of Nursing of the United Kingdom* v *Department of Health & Social Security* [1980] AC 800, at p. 821).

On this basis, he concluded that the wording of the specific grounds set out in the 1967 Act should not be subjected to too close a textual analysis. That caveat has disappeared with the introduction of a Government re-consideration of the Abortion Act and the introduction of a scheme of statutory review of the provision of abortion services by HUFEA. Accordingly, we think it possible to predict that abortion law reform will remain high on the political and moral agenda, and that the timetable for its consideration will be constrained only by clashes with other equally pressing social concerns. That the courts will be further drawn into the moral controversy which accompanies abortion seems axiomatic from the missed opportunities of 1990. This will, eventually, require that the common law judges declare upon quite fundamental issues of personal moral and philosophical belief. Whether they are well suited to that task remains to be seen.

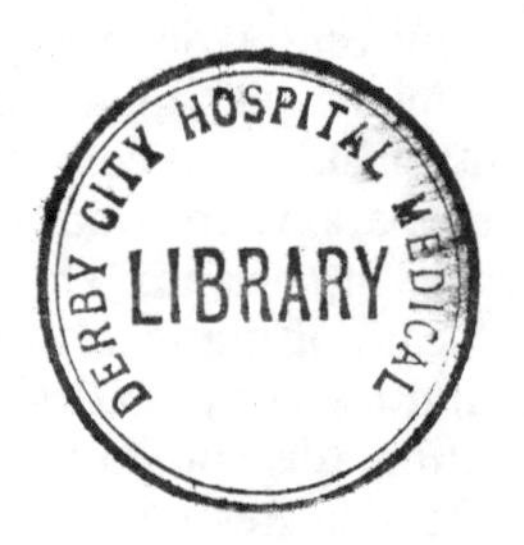

Chapter 3
Embryo Research

The Timing of Early Human Development

Some understanding of the development of the early embryo is useful in understanding both the philosophical and the scientific debates about embryo experimentation. A series of important events in the developments after fertilisation can be expressed in tabular form:

$1\frac{1}{2}$ hours before ovulation LH surge (Luteinizing hormone begins)	
Ovulation	
$\frac{1}{2}$-1 day after ovulation Chemotaxis; sperm moves up a concentration gradient towards the ovum which is attracting it leading to	Fertilisation
36 hours after fertilisation begins	Two cells
48 hours after fertilisation begins	4 cells
4 days	small compact ball of 8-16 cells
4-5 day	blastocyst stage (hollow ball) of 16-32 cells (morula) (formation of inner cell mass)
6-7 days	implantation begins
8-9 days	amniotic cavity forms
7-12 days	trophoblast proliferation and formation of bilaminar disc
11-12 days	conceptus has invaded the uterine wall and become embedded in it
13-15 days	chorionic villi form
15-18 days	primitive streak develops
22-23 days	neural tube begins to close
42 days	first sign of cerebral cortex
56 days	foetal stage begins

(after Anne McLaren, 'Prelude to Embryogenesis' in *The CIBA Foundation, Human Embryo Research: Yes or No?* ((1986), Tavistock Publications p. 15)

The same information may be expressed diagramatically

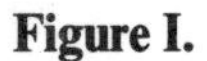

Figure I.

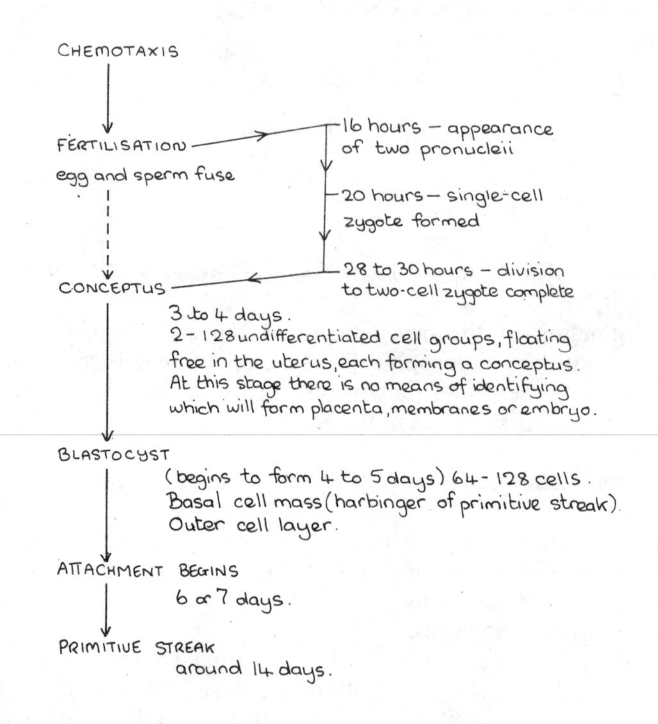

Figure II: The Reproductive Process.

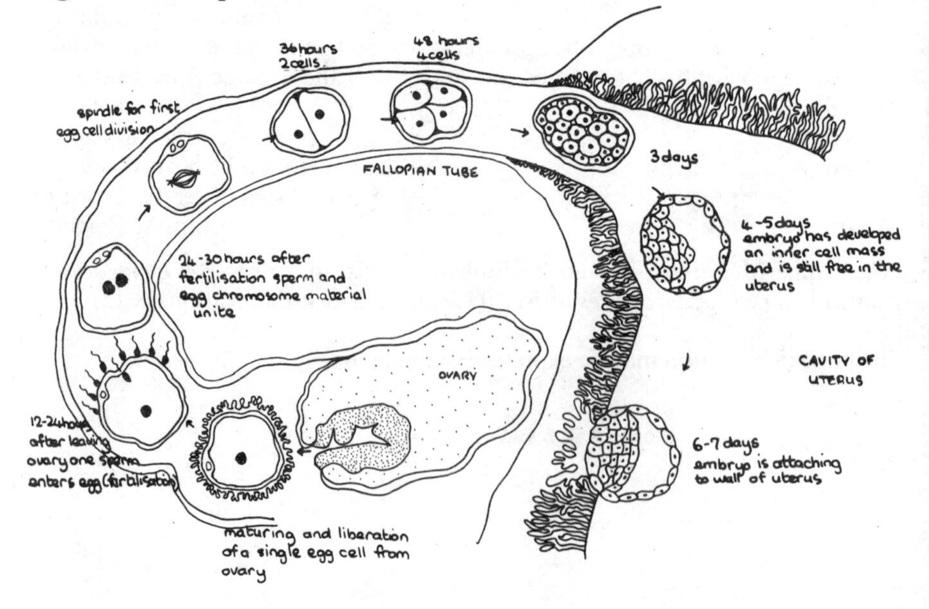

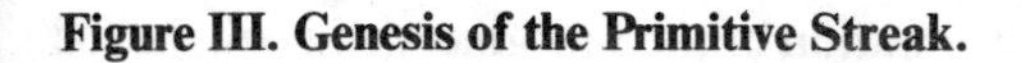

Figure III. Genesis of the Primitive Streak.

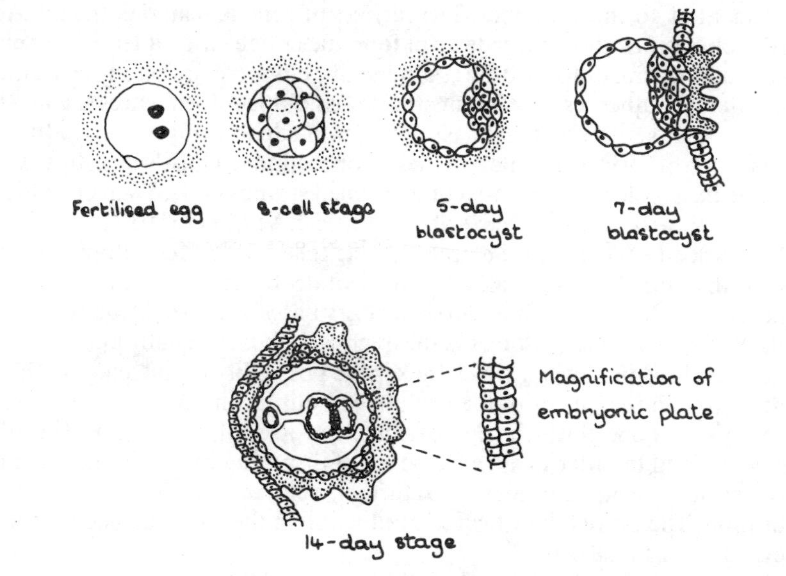

Figure IV: Early Embryonic Development.

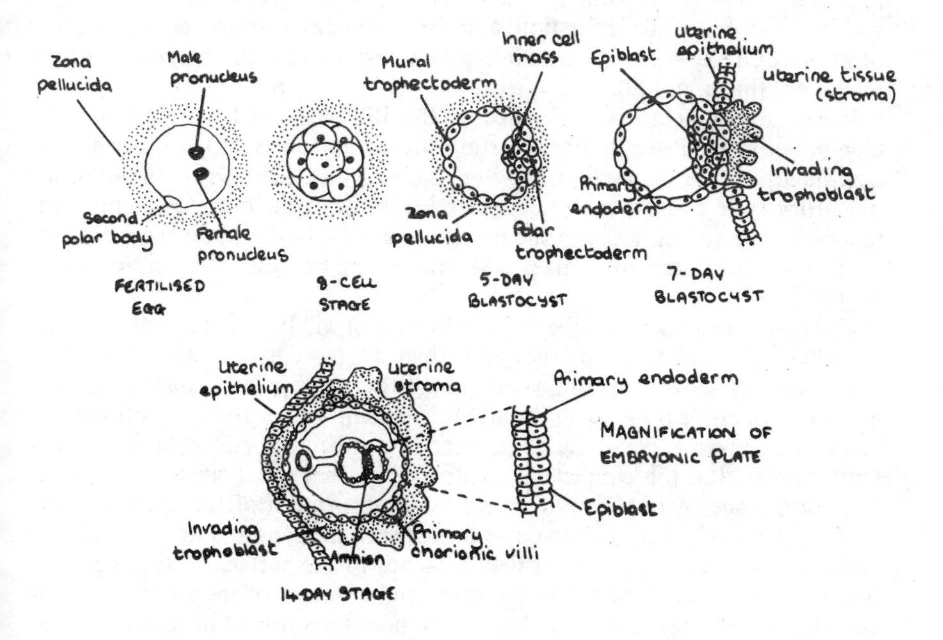

Sperm contain half the genetic information of their producer and ova the full complement of 46 chromosomes. The carriers of genetic material, the DNA — deoxyribonucleic acid — are made up of four nucleotide bases; adenine, guanine, cytosine and thymine, formed on a long chain comprising these four bases in many different sequences. The innumerable possibilities of sequences account for the variety that genetic material has shown itself capable of producing. In their famous work of 1953 Watson and Crick proposed that DNA's structure was a double helix, a molecule composed of two coiled strands (J. D. Watson and F. H. C. Crick, 'A Structure for Deoxyribose Nucleic Acid' (1953) 171 *Nature* pp. 737-38). When DNA replication occurs as the cells divide and multiply, the two sides of the spiral separate and the nucleotide bases are stranded without partners. Then they attract free complementary bases so that eventually two new spirals are formed. Chromosomes in the ovum are divided equally into two polar bodies (it is this complement which makes the possibility of inducing parthenogenesis — the development of the gamete without fertilisation — a theoretical possibility), only one of which takes part in the process of fertilisation. The other is being retained in order to act as a means of disposing of surplus DNA in the newly fertilised egg, and plays no further role in the development after fertilisation. The process by which this reduction in the chromosome number is achieved is termed meiosis.

Fertilisation is the process by which the sperm and the egg interact to produce the zygote. The Act defines the end of this process: 'fertilisation is not complete until the appearance of a two cell zygote' (s. 1(1)). However, it leaves open the question when, as a matter of law, the process begins. This uncertainty has important consequences for the range of treatment services actually brought within the ambit of the legislation, and the crucial, and controversial, question of whether GIFT — gamete intra fallopian transfer — has been regulated or not by the Act (infra, p. 129).

In an important article published as the Bill emerged from its Commons Committee stage, Peter Braude, Martin Johnson and John Aitken described the five stages of the interaction between the egg and the sperm. In a normal ovulatory cycle a single mature egg is released from the ovary and enters the fallopian tube (which leads to the uterus) about 11-16 days into the menstrual cycle. If it encounters and mixes with sperm, the process of fertilisation may begin.

The first contact between the egg and the sperm will be as the sperm meets the cumulus cells which surround the egg. If there are few cumulus cells, they will be readily dispersed by the sperm. Alternatively, the clinician may assist fertilisation in oligozoospermia (low sperm count) by dispersing the cells, either mechanically or using an enzyme. Next, the sperm encounters the zona pellucida, to which it binds rapidly. It is this contact which provides species specificity at fertilisation. The third stage of fertilisation involves the absorption of the spermatozoon through the zona pellucida into the space between the zona and the egg itself (the perivittelline space). The sperm then attaches to the surface of the egg itself, fusion of the two cell membranes occurs, and contents of the sperm enter the cytoplasm of the egg. This stimulus causes the resumption of meiosis in the egg and the second polar body to be nipped off from the egg. The haploid chromosome sets of the egg and sperm (each packaged in a membrane (pronucleii)) come together (syngamy) some 28-30 hours after the introduction of the sperm, and the process of fertilisation is completed and genetic uniqueness begins. Thus the fertilisation process is only completed some 26-32 hours after the first contact of egg and sperm. ('Human Fertilisation and Embryology Bill goes to report stage' (1990) 330 *British Medical Journal* 1410.)

The process of cell division continues. Three to four days after the onset of fertilisation, the number of cells have multiplied from 2 to 128. At this stage the individual cells (blastomeres) are undifferentiated, i.e., they are still pluri- or toti-potential; there is no means of identifying which will subsequently form the membranes and placenta and which will form the embryo, and each appears to have the capacity to form an entire individual. Four or five days after fertilisation, when some 64-128 cell are present, the blastocyst begins to form, in which cells begin to differentiate and a small nodule or basal cell mass, the harbinger of the primitive streak, is identifiable along with an outer layer of cells which begin to be identifiable as the origins of the placenta and membranes. It is possible to remove a single cell from this outer layer and from which the placenta and membranes will develop without damage or detriment to the subsequent development of the remaining cells and determine the sex of the conceptus about 4/5 days after the onset of the process of fertilisation. In normal human reproduction, about 80% of blastocysts are shed spontaneously.

From the morula stage onwards, the toti-potentiality of these individual cells is lost as the foundations of the 'first differentiative event' are laid down.

> The cells of the morula flatten against each other and the junctions between the cells become firm and function like a seal to restrict the passage of material into and out of the centre of the ball of cells. The more central cells of this ball become different from those cells that are left on the outside. These outer cells will contribute cells to the placenta, whilst the product of the inside cells will include the embryo and the remaining parts of the placental membranes (Peter Braude and Martin Johnson, 'The Embryo in Contemporary Medical Science' in Gordon Dunstan, (ed.), *The Embryo From Aristotle to the Modern Day,* (1989), pp. 208, at p. 211; some of what follows immediately draws on Braude's work).

The morula accumulates fluid over the next 24 hours, which causes the formation of a cavity toward the centre of the ball of cells. The inner cells form a discrete mass of cells (the inner cell mass) at one pole of the hollow sphere. The thin layer of cells outside is called the trophectoderm. These developments occur before the pre-embryo has implanted; it is not attached physically to the woman and it floats free on its passage from the fallopian tube to the uterus. Implantation begins when the blastocyst sheds its zona pellucida, about the second week after fertilisation. The trophectodermal cells attach to the lining of the uterus (the endometrium) and, while cell proliferation continues, the trophectoderm invades it and establishes the foundations of the primitive placenta.

From the 6th or 7th day after fertilisation, about 1 in 5 blastocysts begins the process of attachment to the wall of the uterus. The basal cell mass begins to organise itself into a flat, oval two-tiered shape — the embryonic plate. It is still not possible to know whether the fertilisation process has produced anything which will develop beyond a cluster of cells. Each cell, being pluripotential, may go on to develop into an embryo, a hydratiform mole, or indeed, if biopsied at that stage, into many other (cloned) human embryos. Around the 14th day after fertilisation, if the cells have met no other unfavourable conditions in the uterus the inner cell mass which has differentiated initially into a two layered disc composed of endoderm and ectoderm, produces a third layer (the mesoderm). This third layer has become interposed between the ectoderm and the endoderm by a process of invagination from the ectoderm. The site of the invagination can be seen as a line called the primitive streak on the ectodermal surface of the bilaminar disct. It is the development of this groove on which the Warnock Report fixed as the crucial transformation when the rubicon is crossed between molecular matter and potential human being. To this molecular matter scientists later gave the appellation 'pre-embryo'. (For accesible overviews of the scientific literature see Warnock Report, paras. 11.2-7; Penelope Leach, 'Human *In Vitro* Fertilisation' *Annex 3, Voluntary Licensing Authority, First Annual Report,* (1986), p. 39-40; Anne McLaren 'Can we Diagnose Genetic Disease in Pre-Embryos?' (1987), New Scientist 10 December). Braude and Johnson suggest that the importance of the primitive streak is threefold:

(i) it is the time at which the precursor cells for the basic body tissues are laid down in the correct relative position;
(ii) it is the first time at which the embryonic disc has a front and back, left and right and top and bottom;
(iii) it is likely that this is the last stage at which twinning of the conceptus can occur, the number of embryos being determined by the number of primitive streaks that develop.

> For the first time, there are two clearly defined populations of cells in the conceptus. The cells of the trilaminar disc will form the embryo and those around it will form the placental support system. The pre-embryonic phase is over and the embryonic phase begins (op. cit., p. 213).

It is the status of these facts and the values (judgments) which appeal to or dismiss them, which have been balanced against the arguments, for example, of the sanctity of all human life from the beginning of fertilisation. Thus they have provided the kernel of the disputes and arguments which have attended the Act's passage. That many conceptuses are spontaneously lost before implantation in the uterus does not, as some have thought, deal with the question of the sanctity of life, let alone dispose of it. That nature is prodigal is no reason for humans to act in the same way with the products of their creation.

The primitive placenta is one of three sites from which it is possible to do embryo biopsy; another is the second polar body, which is merely a means of disposing of surplus DNA in the newly fertilised egg, playing no further developmental role after fertilisation. Because it represents spare maternal DNA, the second polar body cannot give information on the genetic contribution of the sperm. But it can be of use in some diagnoses. For example, in 80% of all cases of Down's syndrome the extra chromosome is in the egg and not from the sperm; whereas in normal development, one of the maternal chromosomal pair will end up in the egg and the other in the polar body. Another type of biopsy is possible where, in IVF, clinicians usually replace the pre-embryo in the uterus between the 4 and 16-cell stages. A researcher could remove one to two cells at the 8-16 stage to test for genetic defects. The third, later, stage is the blastocyst stage, removing cells from the mural trophectoderm. For a fertile couple this would involve fertilisation after intercourse followed four or five days later by recovery of blastocysts from the uterus by lavage (washing the embryo from the uterus before it has begun the process of implantation into the uterine wall). This carries certain hazards such as damage to the blastocyst and the risk of causing ectopic pregnancy, where the blastocyst implants outside the uterus. But the flushing is said to be no more stressful for the woman than insertion of an IUD. Recovering blastocysts in this way and replacing them gives a good pregnancy rate. In addition, those who favour it argue that lavage is of great importance to research into pre-implatation diagnosis, and they successfully resisted attempts to prohibit the practice (House of Lords, Official Report 6 February 1990, col. 805; Lord Walton).

Some people argue that work of this kind is the thin end of the wedge leading inevitably to the application of genetic engineering to human beings. Anne McLaren, a member of the ILA and a prime scientific mover in the embryo research debate of the last ten years, argues that the opposite is true. At the moment it is impossible to replace a defective gene with a normal one. Any attempt at gene therapy would thus introduce more genetic problems than it solved. It would be pointless, therefore, to attempt gene therapy if we have effective methods of preimplantation diagnosis (see *New Scientist*, 10 December 1987).

When Did I Begin? A Moveable Feast?

The philosophical argument is concentrated on the question 'is this a human being?' Debate is joined about how it is possible to identify a human being; is it a matter of criteria, or of how we feel it is right to treat someone? That is, is it a conclusion reached or a conviction shown? The moral question, which is not dispositively answered by the answer to the philosophical question, is: should we experiment on it? 'Dispositively' here because, as was clear from the Nazi regime, some people thought, at least for some time, that it was morally permissible to experiment on human beings, and even to destroy them, in the supposed name of medical science. Of course, this assumes some intention to produce scientifically useful information and, further, that it might be ethical to use it if it was. But it would seem to suggest that the conclusion that 'as x is a human being, experimentation is unthinkable' is open to much deeper scrutiny, as are the reasons given for experimentation. Notice also that the conclusion 'x is not a human being' does not, of and in itself, make the conclusion that 'x may be experimented on and destroyed' necessarily any more straightforward. The responses to animal research are sufficient to demonstrate that. Indeed, in their understandable zeal to apply a criterial approach to persons, some philosophers are led to argue and conclude that some animals should have more protection than some humans.

This was one of the answers given to the objectors to embryo experimentation, who pointed to the rigourous review procedures in respect of animal welfare safeguarded by the Animals (Scientific Procedures) Act 1986. They argued that whereas with animals one was dealing with mature, sentient beings able to experience pain, with (at least some) embryos or foetuses that was simply not the case. And for some, the question of pain will be dispositive of the moral acceptability of research, whether it is carried out on a human being or not. This will give rise to difficulties in relation to the ethics of researching upon those who are clearly human who but are unable to experience pain, such as the comatose. (Of course one might bring to them an additional series of protections or reasons, which do not apply so compellingly, if at all, to the embryo or to the pre-embryo.)

The weight that is to be attached to the fact that it is not possible to identify which cells will develop in which way(s), and that they appear to be pluripotential until the formation of the primitve streak, was one of the issues which gave rise to the moral disagreements about the significance (or otherwise) of these early stages of development. These scientific facts can only contribute to, and not adjudicate upon, the moral and philosophical disagreements, still less determine them. There is, however, an important way in which the assessment of those facts may determine the moral question of how it is right to treat the human conceptus. It may also be persuasive of the determination of the legal issue; what sort of protection, if any, should the early human embryo be given? (For the distinction between law and morality see Hursthouse's argument, op. cit., pp. 12-25, dealing more specifically with the issue of abortion.)

This important debate is neatly captured in an article by Alan Holland, 'A Fortnight of my Life is Missing: A Discussion of the Status of the Pre-Embryo' ((1990) 7 *Journal of Applied Philosophy* 25) in which he surveys, to dismiss, the arguments of the scientist most closely identified with the development of the work of the ILA, Anne McLaren. His title is reminiscent of a question posed in debate by Lord Rawlinson:

> The question is asked: 'when does life commence?' Surely if it has commenced the killing is not acceptable. To those who reply 'after fourteen days' I say 'fourteen days after what?' (House of Lords, Official Report, 8 February 1990, col. 953).

The assumptions built into this question and the ways in which it is possible to respond to it are important markers in the moral debate which ensued.

Holland's conclusion is an important one, and one which, whether we agree with his arguments, is one to which we broadly adhere:

> [embryo research] should not be defended by relying on the metaphysically dubious notion of the 'pre-embryo'. We should shun at all costs the capture of moral ground by verbal manoeuvres. You and I are human beings. There is only one concept of 'human being' — the biological one. . . . In contemplating

> embryo research we must describe accurately, honestly and without sentimentality what it is that we propose to do. We must not hide from ourselves (what I believe to be) the fact that when we experiment on human embryos we experiment on human beings (ibid., at pp. 35-6).

There are those who believe that all the moral work can be done by the criterial, definitional approach. But as Glover points out, 'any right a pre-embryo may have to life is not diminished by calling it a pre-embryo rather than an embryo' (*Fertility and the Family,* p. 94). He continues with this argument:

> no-one denies that [the pre-embryo] is alive, and that it is surely a member of our species rather than any other. But the problem with this argument is that it applies equally to the unfertilised egg or to the human sperm cell. This argument easily enough proves that the embryo or foetus is a human being, but it is not clear that the status of 'human being' in this minimal sense brings with it any moral rights. It is widely assumed that qualifying as a human being is sufficient to guarantee the possession of a right to life. But this assumption is questionable, and perhaps derives much of its plausibility from our thinking of 'human beings' in terms of our friends and neighbours. An embryo is not the kind of human being you can share a joke with or have as a friend (ibid., p. 96).

Anne McLaren argues that the newly conceived embryo is not yet a human being, not because it lacks the proper form of a human being, but because it has not yet become an individual human being. The point at which the total human being begins is at the formation of the primitive streak.

> If one tries to trace back further than that there is no longer a coherent entity. Instead there is a larger collection of cells, some of which are going to take part in the subsequent development of the embryo and some which aren't (CIBA, *Human Embryo Research: Yes or No?,* p. 22).

This would seem to suggest that the pre-embryo does not have the wherewithal to count as an individual and does not stand in the required relationship to the subsequently developing human being for it to be counted as the same individual.

McLaren's argument depends on asserting that it is only when the primitive streak forms in the embryonic plate that we have 'a spatially defined entity that can develop directly into a foetus and thence into a baby, that we are for the first time justified in using the term embryo' (ibid., p. 22). As the Archbishop of York, John Hapgood, put it in what was to become a highly significant point of reference throughout the legislative debates:

> What is happening embryologically is the creation of persons through a process, which although it begins with genetic union, is not simply about a union of genes but also depends on a certain cellular identity which only becomes apparent at the time of the appearance of the primitive streak (House of Lords, Official Report, 8 February 1990, col. 956).

And, in a passage which could serve as a metaphor not just for embryonic existence and human life but for the whole of the moral debates which these issues engendered, he said:

> By and large a biological approach to life is rooted in gradualism.... The same is true in the development of individual lives. They begin with chemistry and they reach their fulfilment in mystery.... Biologically speaking we are looking at a continuous process. Perhaps I can make the significance of this a little more clear by giving your lordships an analogy. Exactly ten years ago a mathematician called Mandelbrot first discovered what is now called the Mandelbrot set. It is a set of points which can be mapped out as a computer graphic to form the most amazing, beautiful and complex structure that it is possible to imagine. It is a picture of literally infinite depth. If one magnifies the details of any part of the picture, one finds that in them are whole worlds of further detail which are always beautiful, which never repeat themselves and which always reveal more and more detail, on and on, ad infinitum. How is the Mandelbrot set made? It is made by the use of an absurdly simple equation with only three terms. The secret lies in the process. It is a process whereby the answer to one use of the equation becomes the starting point for the next. In other words, it is a cumulative process, just like evolution in which one life form builds on another and just like embryology in which the development of one cell provides the context for the development of its neighbours and its successors (House of Lords, Official Report, 7 December 1989, col. 1020).

This analogy was supported and echoed by Gordon Dunstan, a theological member of the ILA, who was quoted by David Steele in the House of Commons' debate:

> For upwards of 2,000 years the embryo has been said to denote growth of the organism in the womb from the time of the first formation of the body parts until their completion followed by the foetal stage in which the completed baby grows to viability. Now that science has revealed a vital pre-embryonic stage of cellular activity before organogenesis can begin an appropriate name should be given to it. Pre-embryo seems a proper name to describe this stage in development (quoted in House of Commons, Official Report 2 April 1990, col. 936).

One response which has been made to these arguments is of the 'but I'm in there somewhere' type; i.e., that even though it is not possible to identify one, individual, human being in the pluripotential cells, it is sufficient to be able to aver that an identifiable individual will in due course emerge from the cluster. Holland responds to this by arguing that '. . . we live forwards not backwards. The very question, "when did I begin?", encourages one to overlook this simple fact' (ibid., p. 31).

There is a stronger sense of this argument, which is that although no cell in the early stages of development is earmarked for a particular future role, cell commitment is a gradual process. The potency of a cell, the total of the things into which it can develop if put in the appropriate environment, becomes more and more restricted as development proceeds in response to external stimuli. McLaren's implicit allusion, to the lack of a spatially defined entity so far as the pre-embryo is concerned, may well be predicated upon and be a response to the 'I'm in there somewhere' sort of argument. But that argument itself proceeds on the basis of the whole embryo, and not just some special part of it. That many of the cells are destined to be extra-embryonic does not mean that the whole does not contain some very important part.

As we have noted, until the 14th day cells are pluripotential and until the appearance of the primitive streak it is not known whether they will develop into an hydatiform mole; into twins; into one embyro, or degenerate into nothing. It is on this basis that the 14th day is said to be important. But, the response often invoked is that the fact that the cells are pluripotential and that they have a unique genetic encoding from the end of fertilisation tells us only about the limits of our knowledge and nothing about the embryo. Certainly it tells us nothing about how it is right to treat the embryo. Indeed, in terms of selection of biologically revelant dates, the acquisition of further knowledge may affect our approach to research up to the 14th day, or even beyond it. For example, we might push backwards, towards the formation of the basal (or inner) cell mass in the blastocyst, around the fifth day after the onset of fertilisation. Or, we may come to say, (as some already do), that the formation of the primitive streak tells us nothing of moral significance. Here, the argument is that useful knowledge that might be gained can only be acquired from the onset of organogenesis, which will occur from about the 14th day or later. An example of this sort of reasoning is given by Williamson:

> ... organogenesis — whether we are studying limb formation ..., the heart in septum defects, or the nervous system — for the most part occurs at between fourteen and twenty-eight days of embryonic development. It is this area of research, which is central to the understanding of congenital malformation, which in my view would be most inhibited were a strict fourteen-day rule to be implemented ('Research Needs and the Reduction of Severe Congenital Disease' in *Human Embryo Research: Yes or No?* p. 105, at pp. 108-09).

In that sense, we may come to rely on the 14 day moratorium as being only the beginning of the process of organogenesis, whereas what we are (morally) interested in preserving is something beyond that stage.

Thus, we might characterise this sort of claim of pluripotentiality as a weak sense in which the claim to individuation is being made. There is, however, a strong sense in which this claim can be put. If it is the case (if the 'biological facts show') that in a two, four or eight cell stage embryo, any one cell can be extracted and that it will itself divide in order to produce another embryo, and that such cells will sometimes themselves divide naturally, then individuation is not just a sufficient condition, it is a necessary condition for talking of *a* human life, as opposed to the life of a cell.

These opposing arguments can be rephrased by asking 'What weight do we attach to this mass of undifferentiated cells?' In the weak sense (a state of ignorance argument) we can respond by saying that we have no means of knowing which cells are which and that it seems a matter of chance what will develop from which. This sort of argument is most characteristic of that deployed during the Parliamentary debates. It also characterises the scientific arguments on which they are based. However, Evans's suggestion is that there is a strong sense in which the lack of differentiation may be approached. In that, until the 14th day, it is not possible to say whether the cells will form an hydatiform mole; one embryo; two embryos; or even millions of embryos (if cells are progressively biopsied and encouraged to develop to the 16-32 cell stage when more are biopsied and so on). In this sense, there is a strong *logical* difference in talking about a human being before, and speaking about one after, some time of organisation (whether at 14 days or some other time). The point of individuation (14 days or whatever) is when we can describe *a* human life. Before this, as long as the cells are genuinely undifferentiated, we cannot speak of a human life. There is no doubt that there is a fertilised ovum, nor that it may be the pre-embryonic stage of human life. But that is not the same as a pre-embryo, still less an embryo (see Don Evans in *Making and Taking Life,* (1991) Macmillan). The particularly salient aspect of Evans's argument is that it acts as a stopper against the argument that what we are interested in is not the beginning of the formation of the primitive streak, but (at some later point) its completion, in the same way that the beginning of the *process* of fertilisation is now held to tell us nothing. The attraction of this strong sense of individuation is that it delineates the outer ambit of that concept, and not some further moveable feast.

If then, we have spare embryos and no willing woman into whom they could be placed, there arises for some an important philosophical distinction between killing and letting die. If it is possible to do something about the saving of a life, it may be killing if we fail to do that. Where we are incapable of saving the life, then all that can be said is that we have let it die ('allowed it to perish' in statutespeak, see s. 14(1)(c)). If we concentrate only on the consequence (the embryo is dead) then we will find the distinction between the means of death irrelevant. If, however, we think that the distinction between killing and letting die describes the morally relevant difference between the two deaths — for one of which we are indeed responsible (and maybe culpable) but for the other we are not — then we may be morally justified in proceeding to treat the two deaths, and the two ways of dying, very differently.

Arguments Against Embryo Research

Those who oppose all such research, regulated or not, argue that any such 'benefits' are bought at a price which is unacceptable. The fundamental point of objection is that from conception (when the process of fertilisation begins) a unique human being is created with exactly the same rights and interests as any other human being, whether adult or child. A variant is that this full protection attaches from the point of syngamy, when the process of genetic fusion of the sperm and the egg is completed, about thirty hours after the onset of fertilisation. This is the relevant point adopted in, for example, the Australian State of Victoria's Infertility (Medical Procedures) Act 1984 ss. 3(1) and 9A. Research which leads to the eventual destruction of the embryo is, on these views, morally no different from murder. Another variant holds that, even though it is a human person, the embryo is unable to consent to research being undertaken on it. At the least, then, it is only research clearly and demonstrably for the therapeutic benefit of that embryo alone which might be justified. Others object to such research because they claim that animal studies can yield all the same information anyway, or because such 'experiments' with embryos put society on a slippery slope to even more awful possibilities, or because the whole development of embryology amounts to 'playing God' and interfering with human life in ways which recall the abhorrent regime of the Nazi concentration camps. Perhaps the most forceful exposition of this view was put by the Earl of Lauderdale in debate in the House of Lords. Opposing research on embryos he said that:

> My conscience requires that I say that I believe that this legislation is playing God in the most intimate and sacred centre of life itself. If the embryo were not human then experimentation would have little purpose. Thanks to what we have consented to here, life may now be created simply for laboratory experimentation, however noble the purposes of that experimentation may be. The ethics of human vivisection have been condemned ever since classical Alexandria, and I believe that they are implicitly at work here. In exchanging the ethics of the farmyard for those of the family, I believe that human debasement has plumbed new depths (House of Lords, Official Report, 20 March 1990, col. 247).

A forceful argument which was heard occasionally in the Parliamentary debates concerned the extent to which 'destructive' embryo research represented a major derogation from the Helsinki Declaration of 1964 as amended in 1975. That declaration, which is one of the governing instruments of ethical control of medical practice, provides in part that '. . . the interests of science and society should never take precedence over considerations related to the wellbeing of the subject.' Many made it clear that they were opposed only to research which caused the death or destruction of the embryo and not that which was intended for its therapeutic benefit. Even so, it was on the basis of the Helsinki Declaration that the use of the term pre-embryo to describe the conceptus in its first 14 days was regarded as a neologism, a piece of linguistic engineering as dazzling as the reproductive engineering which it was supposed to serve.

Research with human pre-embryos, it was charged, is not and has never been concerned with the treatment of genetic disorder or chromosomal abnormality but with their prevention. It was accepted by supporters of research that embryo experimentation has neither identified or cured any genetic disease. But they responded by suggesting that this was to fail to understand or to have ignored all the arguments which favoured continued research; gene therapy is in its infancy, the ability to 'engineer' faulty genes so that the dysfunction may be overcome is at its dawn. Opponents responded by asserting that the 'fact' that it is only at the 14th day after fertilisation that an identifiable human embryo is present is a failure not of the genetic programming of that embryo but of our own human processes and procedures for assessing identifiable evidence. It is in both senses a failure of our vision.

It is sometimes forgotten that three members of the Warnock Committee expressed their dissent from the majority on some sort of argument which approximated to this.

> The beginning of a person is not a question of fact but of decision made in the light of moral principles. The question ['When does the human person come into existence?'] must therefore be refined further. It thus becomes 'At what stage of development should the status of a person be accorded to an embryo of the human species?' Different people answer this question in different ways. Some say at fertilisation, others at implantation, yet others at a still later stage of development. Scientific observation and philosophical and theological reflection can illuminate the question but they cannot answer it ('Expression of Dissent', Cmnd 9314, p. 90).

Building on this approach, the dissentients held that the special status of the human embryo, to which all members of the Committee were committed, did not depend on the decision as to when it becomes a person. Before that point, its potential for development to the stage where everyone would accord it the status of a human person was sufficient to ensure that nothing should be done to reduce the possibility of a successful implantation of the embryo:

> in the event of there being more embryos than it is judged [by the clinician] right to implant at any one time the remainder should be frozen with a view to implantation at a later date or allowed to die. They should not be used for experimentation. Still less should they be deliberately created for the purpose of experimentation ('Expression of Dissent B', para. 5).

On this latter question of embryos created specifically for the purposes of research, a further four members, while permitting research on 'spare' embryos created during the provision of treatment services, joined in dissenting from the acceptability of embryos created specifically for research purposes (see 'Expression of Dissent C').

In debate, an amendment in the House of Lords limiting research to those 'spare' embryos donated by a woman who no longer had need or desire for them and criminalising any other matter of research, was defeated by 214 votes to 80. Lord Bridge, opposing the amendment, argued that the 'moral scrupulosity' which distinguishes between the propriety of research upon a spare embryo and the iniquity of research upon a specifically created embryo:

> may be an admirable subject for debate in the senior common room but it has no place at all in the dock of the Old Bailey (House of Lords, Official Report, 6 March 1990, col. 1072).

This lacklustre approach was countered more forthrightly by Lord Robertson (ibid., col. 1080), who argued that it would be unthinkable to grow a person through birth to adult life solely for the purpose of carrying out research on her or him. 'The principle is surely the same and the difference is one of degree when one is dealing with an embryo'. Similar arguments were rehearsed in the House of Commons, both in Committee and in the debate on Report, where further unsuccessful attempts were made to limit the practice of research to embryos obtained during the course of treatment services which were 'spare' to that treatment and which otherwise would have perished.

Perhaps the most consistent approach of those opposed to embryo research admitted no concessions in terms of the potential benefits or the lack of specificity with possible alternative to such research. Proponents of this view hold that from the beginning of the fertilisation process the embryo is a new human life — the fusion of the sperm and egg introduces an 'intrinsic organising power' (Lord Harrington, House of Lords, Official Report, 7 December 1990, col, 1070) — which, independent of further outside stimulus, represents a small developing human being. This fact alone should govern its status, dignity and rights under the law. No wrong could justifably be done to this life, even for the right reasons or for a noble cause. To research destructively on it is to discriminate against it on the basis not of its humanity but its size.

In debate this point was most clearly put by Michael Alison:

> . . . the embryonic human individual . . . has been imperceptible, invisible and not in evidence but essentially, logically and potentially there from the moment of fertilisation (House of Commons, Official Report, 23 April 1990, col. 67).

Bernard Braine argued that the human embryo is growing and developing at a tremendous rate. It has an orientation towards growth and is thus different from the previously inert sperm and egg. The simple fact is that the human embryo is a tiny human being, which has all the potential to become a foetus, a baby, a child and an adult, given a favourable environment and appropriate nutrients. He summed up these arguments by arguing that:

> when one bases decision making on the proposed benefits of a type of research, rather than its morality, one will always be under pressure to extend that limit when greater benefits are envisaged. That is no way to make law. The anticipated benefits seem compelling but they are misleading (House of Commons, Official Report, 2 April 1990, col. 934).

And in the House of Lords, Lord Kennet had objected to seeing the beginning of moral worth at 14 days because, he said, it encapsulated a typical reductionist myth: it may be true, but it was not important (House of Lords, Official Report, 7 December 1990, col. 1026).

There were several other types of argument against the use of embryos for research purposes which were deployed. First was that rehearsed by Dale Campbell-Savours. Perhaps surprisingly, he was the only MP to refer explictly to any radical feminist views. When he did so, he quoted from the arguments put forward by FINRRAGE, the Feminist International Network Of Resistance To Reproductive And Genetic Engineering, formed in Vellinge, Sweden in 1985.

Finrrage, while pro-abortion, is opposed to research on embryos and the development and application of technologies derived from embryo research. Its members argue that reproductive and genetic technologies are harmful to all women; they destroy women's physical integrity; exploit their procreativity and attempt to undermine women's struggle for control of their own reproduction (cf. Patricia Spallone *Beyond Conception* (1989) Macmillan p. 1).

A second line of argument and dispute concerned the adequacy of other sources of research, such as the human egg or animals. On the latter, it was argued that it is not possible to extrapolate the results of animal studies to humans because human embryos react differently to other mammalian embryos under various conditions. The differences in their physiological make-up were also stressed.

Thirdly, opponents of embryo research pointed to the experiences of other countries in which research has already been prohibited. For example, in both South Australia and Victoria, in Australia, IVF programmes have claimed increased success rates since restriction, citing 17-18% better success rates than that suggested by the figures for the UK in the *ILA Fourth Report* (1989). Critics of this argument responded by pointing out that South Australia has not banned *therapeutic* research, and also questioned the age (and hence the fertility) of the patients involved in the IVF programmes when compared with UK clinics.

A similar disagreement surrounded claims that embryos were unnecessary for research into genetic disease. Opponents argued that recent US reports suggest that techniques of molecular biology used to diagnose genetic disorder would be better applied to gametes than to the early embryo. The necessity of embryo research was also questioned by pointing to the development and deployment of laboratory based molecular biology and DNA recombinant technology. This, it was said, has been applied recently on blood and tissue samples from consenting human subjects, leading to the identification of the exact chromosomal localisation in the human genome of the abnormal genes responsible for diseases such as cystic fibrosis (the gene for which was discovered in Toronto from research on DNA taken from an ordinary cell); Huntington's chorea; haemophilia; myotonic muscular dystrophy; one form of peroneal muscular atrophy and Duchenne muscular dystrophy, the gene for which was identified in December 1987 at Boston Children's Hospital. In addition, research not involving embryos has produced advances as diverse as that on auto-immune disease (Cambridge, Mass.); sickle cell anaemia (at the National Institute of Medical Research) and on retinitis pigmentosa (Trinity College Dublin). Kay Davies, head of the molecular genetics group at the Institute of Molecular Medicine in Oxford, was quoted in the debates as suggesting that in the next ten years tests will be discovered and developed for the defective genes that cause the most common severe genetic disorders. Indeed, it was argued that the benefits are overstated, in that even if every embryo with cystic fibrosis were discarded, it would take 1,250 years to halve the frequency with which the gene occurs. It was also said that a very high incidence of congenital defects and gene mutations occur in families with no history of disorders and no high risk factors. Hence, screening of all potential parents might be necessary if the effect on disease was to be other than marginal.

Finally, opponents of embryo research pointed to the increasing study of seminal fluids and the functioning of the female immune system, both of which appear to hold out prospects equal to those of the development of IVF, as an alternative approach to the understanding of infertility. Other alternative approaches to infertility treatment, including microsurgery, gene therapy and IVF without superovulation were also highlighted. One clinic, the Jessop in Sheffield, reports that one in four of their patients who are not superovulated and who finally receive an embryo become pregnant, although not all of them run to term.

These alternatives to experimentation were supplemented by appeals to international legislative comparisons; several European countries have already banned research and the European Parliament, following a debate on the Rothey Report, has voted for an eventual ban (although as the Gunning Report makes clear there is presently no uniform position within Europe on this question, see, infra, pp. 86–7). In fact, even if the 'restrictive' provision of the original Bill clause 11(3) had been enacted, and embryo experiments had been prohibited, it would still be permissible under sch. 2 para. 1(d) to screen embryos for genetic defects before implantation.

Arguments In Favour of Embryo Research

Two different types of arguments can be discerned from those who were in favour of embryo research; a response to the criticisms made by those opposed to research, and an advocacy of the value of research. We consider each type of argument separately, although there is some overlap.

1. Responses to critics

Those who argued that embryo research was permissible did so on a number of grounds. Suppose that we could refocus on the question of whether, whatever its status, it was right or permissible to experiment on the human person in embryonic form. Here the question of whether we are speaking of a human pre-embryo or an pre-embryo human becomes important. And here, scientific evidence might enable us to reach a conclusion with which we felt more comfortable; a conclusion with which, quite literally, we thought we could live. That, for example, the embryo is incapable of experiencing pain might be thought to be quite relevant. That it could not envisage its history or its future, for example, or that others to whom it is most closely related, such as its genitors, felt that it was right (not just all right, but morally permissible) to subject it to non-therapeutic research for the benefit of others, might be thought to be highly relevant (if not of itself conclusive). An appeal might here again be made to the 'scientific facts', for reassurance as to what was being experimented on. Fears of the 'slippery slope' kind would be prevented, because the foetus, the neonate, the baby, the child and the adult all differ form the embryo in important and morally significant ways.

The argument was advanced that we accept post-coital contraception, such as the IUD, which acts to prevent implantation of the fertilised ovum. Indeed, the Attorney General has gone so far as to advise that this and other techniques which prevent the implantation are not abortifacients (although this view has not gone unchallenged; see the survey of these arguments in J K Mason, *Medico-Legal Aspects of Reproduction and Parenthood,* (1990), pp. 54 et seq). The arguments proceed that if this practice was condoned, the same entity — the fertilised ovum — could not be given a different status here. Of course, that ignores the different sorts of reasons that one might want to give for favouring, tolerating or opposing abortion and embryo research. Concern to set limits to embryo research is sometimes dismissed on the basis that if abortion is allowed, then concern for the embryo is misplaced. But, if there is no metaphysical frontier, there is 'the possibility that abortion and embryo research should be treated differently, perhaps because the reasons supporting them are of different weight' (Jonathan Glover, *Fertility and the Family,* (1989) p. 101).

Responding to some of the charges made in the attempt to limit research to 'spare' embryos alone, and not to have embryos created specifically for the purposes of research, Lord Walton argued that research into the mechanisms of fertilisation and on chromosomal abnormalities which cause miscarriages or malformations could only be done by investigation of deliberately fertilised normal eggs from normal donors with no intention of providing a treatment service (House of Lords, Official Report, 6 March 1990, col. 1065). A further line of research, known as polar body biopsy, which involves the removal of chromosomal material from the egg before fertilisation and which may eventually be an effective way of avoiding embryo biopsy, could never be justified ethically unless prior validation had been made by deliberately fertilising such biopsied eggs, not in the course of providing treatment services but to see how the biopsy affected their development. The improvement in IVF techniques and the development of freezing techniques will, in any case, mean that the numbers of 'spare' eggs and embryos available will be reduced. Nonetheless, according to Walton, it remained important that embryos donated in the course of treatment services should be available for research. The small number of 'spare' embryos would not be sufficient on their own to allow for the study of the metabolism or the chemical behaviour of the dividing embryo in its early stages, and study of the development of its chromosomes as well as the production of the pre-implantation hormone which promotes implantation in the uterus would be compromised. And, in relation specifically to research into Duchenne muscular dystrophy and cystic fibrosis, he argued that while it is already known that embryo biopsy was possible, the next crucial step is to extract DNA from the single biopsied cell to determine whether or not the dystrophic gene is present. More research is needed to perfect this technique.

In summary, Walton argued for the preventative approach to genetic disease through continued research. It was surely preferable, he said, to identify within that group of cells resulting from fertilisation, the presence of a harmful gene, and to allow that group of cells to degenerate naturally, rather than for a woman to carry a child with a major, fatal, crippling disease. He pleaded that it must surely be preferable to undertake such screening than to allow the pregnancy to proceed to 10 to 12 weeks and then to see whether or not the gene is present and carry out an abortion. And of alternatives to embryo research, such as examining the chromosomal material in the polar body that is discarded by the egg and plays no further part in its development, are said to be unreliable despite advances in DNA technology, as a means of detecting genetic abnormality with any degree of confidence. This work requires the removal of the polar body before it is naturally discarded, and there are fears that such manipulation of the ovum prior to fertilisation might impair fertilisation or produce foetal abnormalities.

2. Advocating Embryo Research

Everyone in Parliament was in favour of regulating embryo research and making it subject to the criminal law. The matter of difference when it arose was at what point it should be banned. Some of the commentators in the debates pointed out that if for some reason the Bill should not pass, embryo research would continue in its statutorily unregulated fashion and ostensibly subject to no law. Indeed, it seemed to be accepted on all sides, and the debates proceeded on this basis, that as the law stood it was entirely up to an individual researcher when research was to be terminated because there was no express legal provision against it.

Given the scheme of protection afforded by the common law and by statute, it would have been surprising if an alternative conclusion had been advanced. Although John Keown has argued that there is nothing in principle to prevent the courts exercising wardship jurisdiction over a fertilised egg or embryo, this is not a popular view. Keown is correct to the extent that he shows that the courts' reluctance to countenance the wardship of an unborn foetus in the uterus — as attempted in *Re F (in utero)* [1988] 2 All ER 193 — proceeded on the basis that the foetus is not a child and that the court had no power to direct the life of the pregnant woman. This latter constraint does not apply to the embryo outside the body. Nonetheless, the courts have refused to expand the ambit of the common law to include a five-month-old foetus (*R* v *Tait* [1989] 3 All ER 682) or even one of eight months (*R* v *Wenham, The Times* 23 March 1990), where a motorist was sentenced to three months' imprisonment for reckless driving, following an accident in which he knocked down a woman who was eight months pregnant causing the death of the foetus, escaped liability for causing death by reckless driving because there was not a life to be lost. Therefore, it is unlikely that it would operate to protect an embryo from research. This conclusion can be reached, of course, without agreement either with the conclusion or the reasoning of the courts in these two recent cases.

Of course, the issues involved here are fundamental to any society and the way in which it orders its moral thinking, argumentation and boundaries. The claimed benefits for continued research are great. It is held to offer potential for improvements in assisted conception (with one contention that it could increase the 'successful' outcomes in IVF from around 10-20% to nearer 70%) and better understanding of causes of unexplained infertility (thought to affect 40,000 couples in the United Kingdom) and repeated miscarriages (with 75,000 miscarriages a year in the UK). Additionally, it is argued that continued research will assist in the development of newer contraceptive techniques — one project has sought to develop a vaccine which would enable the egg to repel sperm from seeking to fertilise it. As we have seen (supra, p. 78) amendments which sought to prevent such research as 'frivolous' were defeated.

However, the greatest potential for continued research is in the development of safe and reliable techniques for pre-implantation diagnosis of genetic abnormalities. Approximately 14,000 infants (2% of all babies) are born each year with a genetic defect and half of those are born with an obvious single gene inherited defect, of which there are over 4,000. Imminent 'breakthroughs' in relation to cystic fibrosis, muscular dystrophy and thalassaemia fuel the present debate (see ILA, *IVF Research in the UK, A Report on Research Licensed by the Interim Licensing Authority for Human In Vitro Fertilisation and Embryology 1985-1989*, (1989)).

General Prohibitions

Section 3 defines activities which are beyond the power of the HUFEA to licence. For example, the Authority may not authorise the use or retention of a live human embryo after the appearance of the 'primitive streak' (s. 3(3)(a)). Unless the embryo is stored by way of freezing (see below), this is taken to be 'not later than the end of the period of fourteen days beginning with the day when the gametes are mixed' (s. 3(4)). This much criticised pragmatic solution was adopted by the Warnock Committee as the point when human life begins to matter morally (Warnock para. 11.2-9).

Similarly, the Authority may not authorise the placing of a human embryo in any animal, the keeping or use of an embryo where regulations prohibit this or nucleus substitution, (sometimes referred to as cloning). This is where the nucleus of the cell of an embryo (which contains the hereditary genetic material) is removed and replaced with the nucleus taken from a cell of another person, embryo or later developed embryo (s. 3(3)(b), (c) and (d)). This latter technique has been claimed to hold important prospects for work with genetically inherited disease and the production of immunologically identical organs for transplantation purposes. But, it raises the spectre of the production of genetically identical humans, clones, or humans with specific characteristics. The Authority will not presently be able to licence such work. Section 3(3)(b) prohibits 'placing an embryo in any animal'. There is, on the face of it, no similar prohibition in respect of placing human sperm and egg together in the uterus of another animal. Section 4(1)(c) prohibits the mixing of human gametes with the live gametes of any animal except in pursuance of a licence, but that is not what is contemplated by placing human sperm and egg in an animal. Such experiments have in fact been reported in Australia, by Carl Wood and Anne Westmore. In their book, *Test-Tube Conception* ((1984), George Allen & Unwin) they recount an experiment in which they introduced human eggs and sperm into the fallopian tube of a sheep. They comment, on the failure of the fertilisation:

> In some ways we were relieved at the failure of this experiment as it may have been difficult to convince the community that the sheep was an appropriate place for human fertilisation and early human development.

Under the Act, it seems that such an experiment would not be totally prohibited. It could, it appears, be done but only under licence. A licence would be required, because the experiment might amount to 'storing' gametes under s. 4(1)(a). Section 2(2) provides that 'keeping, in relation to embryos or gametes, include keeping while preserved, whether preserved by cryopreservation or *in any other way* . . .'(emphasis added) and s. 1(3) provides that 'This Act, so far as it governs the keeping or use of an embryo, applies only to keeping or using an embryo outside the human body'.

But notice the two important limitations to this argument. Section 1(3) applies only in respect of embryos, and although s. 1(1)(b) defines that to include an egg in the process of fertilisation, the point of the experiment is to see whether fertilisation will occur or not. And secondly, the extended meaning given to 'keeping' in s. 2(2), actually applies to keeping while preserved. Unless the gametes in the sheep uterus are regarded as 'preserved' while there, s. 2(2) does not straightforwardly determine whether such an experiment can proceed only with a licence. The problem here is that the outcome or likely outcome of the experiment is determining the need for a licence under the Act. Moreover, s. 2(2) does not purport to give an exhaustive definition of 'keeping', it merely provides some instances which are included. Thus a s. 4(2) licence would be necessary for the storage of gametes in such an experiment. It is possible that regulations will prohibit such an experiment altogether, in which case no licence could be issued to endorse it (s. 2).

Schedule 2 'treatment licences' may authorise a variety of practices designed 'to secure that embryos are in a suitable condition to be placed in a woman or to determine whether embryos are suitable for that purpose' (para. 1(1)(d)), which may in practice look uncommonly like research.

Section 4 provides more contentious reading. Sections 4(1)(a) and (c) provide for offences of storing gametes (ova or sperm) and cross-species fertilisation using live human gametes without a HUFEA licence.

Licensing Human Embryo Research

Any research presently undertaken in the United Kingdom is invited to subscribe to the supervision of the Interim Licensing Authority (ILA), established by the Royal College of Obstetricians and Gynaecologists and the Medical Research Council in 1985. To June 1990 the ILA had approved 38 IVF centres in the UK of which 17 are engaged in licensed *in vitro* fertilisation research. This work involves the use of either 'surplus' fertilised eggs following a woman's superovulation as part of her fertility treatment or unfertilised eggs donated and subsequently fertilised *in vitro*. (See Appendix 8, below.)

To June 1990 the ILA had licensed 66 research projects; 13 new projects in 1989-90 having started with 22 in 1985-86. (It is difficult to make the ILA Annual figures tally with the overall figure; and the data for 1986-87 are not clearly presented; the ILA appears to have approved an additional 10 projects compared with their first report but have only received seven applications.) The aims of these projects were either the improvement of existing IVF provision (on average only 1 in 10 IVF cycles successfully results in a live birth), or the treatment of infertility including the causes of miscarriage. These activities are not themselves uncontroversial, but they are the first practical results of the research work which has been done in the last 25 years. Other applications to which research may be put include the diagnosis of genetic abnormalities in an embryo before implantation (14,000 births annually; see the Royal College of Surgeons' report, *Prenatal Diagnosis and Genetic Screening*, (1989)), and the discovery of improved methods of contraception. The ILA has established voluntary guidelines for such research work, which include provisions for donor consent and prior ethical committee approval of the work. To 1989, only one projected protocol had been refused a licence, and that because the procedure involved the transfer to the uterus of a woman of an embryo on which no check had been taken as to its chromosomal content following research.

HUFEA will take over the responsibility of supervising and licensing research involving human embryos in 1991. Originally, there was nothing in the Bill which would have prevented unlicensed 'research' up to the point of syngamy. Section 1 was amended to deal with this point; it adopts a scientific understanding as its definition of an embryo; in s. 1(1) it provides that references to an embryo are to a live human embryo 'where fertilisation is complete' but that references to an embryo 'include an egg in the process of fertilisation' (ss. 1(1)(a) and (b)). Fertilisation is not complete 'until the appearance of a two cell zygote'(s. 1(1)(b)). The difficulty with this definition, providing as it does a clear indication of when, for legal purposes, fertilisation ends, is that it does not provide when 'an egg in the process of fertilisation' begins. And the difficulties to which this gives rise in the determination of whether an embryo has been brought about partly inside and partly outside the human body for the purposes of s. 1(2) are discussed in Chapter 5.

A licence authorising specific research under the 1990 Act may be granted by the HUFEA for a maximum period of 3 years (sch. 2 para. 3(9)). Any research licence may be made subject to conditions imposed by HUFEA and specified in the licence (sch. 2 para. 3(7)), and any authority to bring about the creation of an embryo, keep or use an embryo or mix human sperm with a hamster or other specified animal's egg, may specify how those activities may be carried out (sch. 2, para. 3(8)). Each research protocol must be shown to relate, broadly, to one of the existing categories of research aim (sch. 2, para. 3(2)), and then again only if the Authority is satisfied that the research is 'necessary for the purposes of the research' (sch. 2, para. 3(6)). These aims are:

(a) promoting advances in the treatment of infertility (para. 3(2)(a));

(b) increasing knowledge about the causes of congenital disease (para. 3(2)(d)); (an amendment seeking to limit this to life-threatening or severely disabling conditions was withdrawn);

(c) increasing knowledge about the causes of miscarriage (para. 3(2)(c));

(d) developing more effective techniques of contraception (para. 3(2)(d)); (an amendment condemning this as 'frivolous' was defeated);

(e) developing methods for detecting the presence of gene or chromosome abnormalities in embryos before implantation (para. 3(2)(e));

(f) more generally for the purpose of increasing knowledge about the creation and development of embryos and enabling such knowledge to be applied (para. 3(3)).

The 'hamster test' referred to in sch. 2 para. 3(5) is used to test the motility and normality of sperm. The hamster is at present the only known animal amenable to such a test. The zona pellucida of the ovum and the tip of the sperm are species specific. Whereas very closely related species such as the horse and the donkey can interbreed, the hamster is the only known exception to possess a removable zona pellucida which would otherwise repel the sperm from another species. The hamster zona can be removed following treatment with an enzyme, and what has become known as the zona free hamster oocyte penetration test performed. The test requires the mixing of 40 hamster eggs with sperm. After 3-4 hours, a judgment is made as to the percentage of the eggs that have been penetrated by the sperm, on the basis of which judgment is made as to the fertility of the sperm. No embryo is formed and the result is immediately destroyed. The provision in sch. 2, para. 3(5) to extend this test to other animals specified in directions sch. 2, para. 1(1)(f), sch. 2, para. 3(5) and s. 24(11) subject to the report of the proposed directions to each House of Parliament by the Secretary of State, anticipates the discovery of any other suitable source of testing. Anything which forms must be destroyed when the research is complete, 'and in any event, not later than the two cell stage' (sch. 2, para. 3(5)). The importance of the test, introduced in the United States in 1976, is its value in studying the chromosomal constitution of human sperm, and hence the male contribution to genetic abnormalities, and to infertility, thought to affect 1 in 16 of the male population. It is said also to be a key part in researching the development of a male contraceptive agent, including in particular a contraceptive vaccine. Lord Houghton enlivened Parliamentary proceedings on debate when he announced that he had 'a small constituency in the animal world' and declared that:

> I must stand up for the hamster. . . . I am simply asking, on behalf of the hamsters of this world, what happens to them when the embryos have been taken away and immediately destroyed (House of Lords, Official Report 13 March 1990, col. 1505).

It has not been possible to trace a satisfactory reply.

Conclusion

HUFEA is placed under a duty to keep under review information about embryos and any subsequent development of embryos as well as of treatment services and other services prohibited or which require a licence under the Act, s. 8(a). This, and its licence granting and supervisory function will attempt to ensure that the limitations (although they are in fact very broadly drafted) of permissible research will be adhered to.

In the international arena, embryo research has already been banned in Eire, Denmark, Portugal, Norway, and the Australian states of Victoria and South

INTERNATIONAL COMPARISONS OF IVF AND EMBRYO RESEARCH — NOVEMBER 1990

Nation	Legislation	Research allowed	Regulatory Body	No. Clinics providing service	No. treatment cycles p.a.	Finance
United Kingdom	1990 Act	Up to appearance of 'primitive streak'	Human Fertilisation and Embryology Authority, constituted 7 November 1990	44	7043 (1987)	Only 2 NHS clinics — charges to patients vary from £250-£2,000
Australia	Victoria: Infertility (Medical Procedures) Act 1984, amended 1987, Regulations 1988 S. Australia Reproductive Technology Act 1989	On fertilisation up to syngamy or on surplus embryos up to 14 days Non-detrimental research to implantation stage	Standing Review and Advisory Committee reviews research Hospitals approved by Ministry S. Australian Council on Reproductive Technology	22	6796 (inc NZ) reported 1987	Approx half costs available on Medicare. Federal funds available for drugs
Belgium	No	Yes — no legal restriction	No	14	Not known	Social Security funds available
Canada	No federal legislation but see the Uniform Child Status Act proposed by the Uniform Law Conference, 1980, adopted in Yukon Territory 1984; Royal Commission sitting	Yes — no legal restriction	No	13	2,000	Provincial funds available only in Ontario
Denmark	Moratorium imposed	Establishing National Ethics Council; see Law on the Establishment of an Ethical Council and the Regulation of Certain forms of Bioethical Research, in Stepan, op.cit., pp. 104-107	No	3	900	IVF available on NHS
France	Draft Bill (1989) not yet officially published	On surplus embryos up to 7 days: Moratorium on embryo biopsy	National Commission (1988) licenses clinics	> 100 (74 approved)	19,000 (FIVNAT)	Social Security reimburses clinical cost — patients may bear laboratory charges
Germany [Federal Republic]	1990 Act, 24 October 1990	No	No	51	14,400 egg collections in 36 clinics	Couples pay or claim on insurance

Italy	No; See Stepan, op.cit., pp. 125–27. Circular letter of the Ministry of Health, 'Limits and Conditions of Lawfulness of Artificial Insemination Services in the National Health Service'	Yes — no legal restriction	No	10 in universities plus other private	Not known	State will reimburse homologous IVF, heterologous in Sicily
Netherlands	No; extracorporeal production of human embryos permitted only where a licence has been issued by the Minister of Welfare, Public Health and Culture; Decree Amending the General Administrative Regulations on Hospital Facilities (11 August 1988 (Stg. 379)); see Stepan, op.cit., pp. 130–31	No legal restriction but no research undertaken	No	30	2,377 (in 21 centres)	Limited Sick Funds subsidy scheme
Norway	Act No. 628 1987 relating to artificial procreation	No	No — clinics reach mutual agreement	7	3-4,000	1 clinic private otherwise state pays 90% of cost
Spain	Law 35/1988 — Health: Law Assisted Reproduction Techniques	Yes on non-viable spare embryos up to 14 days	National Commission for Assisted Reproduction	24	1,500 registered in 1989 (60%)	Available free at public hospitals
Sweden	*In vitro* fertilisation Act 1988	Up to 14 days	No	10	2,000-2,500	18,000 Kr in University 24-27000 Kr in private clinic
USA	No Federal legislation	No Federal funding for research	No — American Fertility Society has issued guidelines	200	14,619 (in 146 clinics)	Patients generally pay or claim on insurance. No Federal Medicaid

Source: Jennifer Gunning, *Op.Cit.*

Australia. In [West] Germany, a Bill before the Bundestag was passed on 24 October 1990 which provides that IVF may be practised only for the purpose of making pregnant the woman from whom the egg(s) was taken; that no embryo may be produced which is not intended for return to its 'mother's' womb; that nothing may be done to harm an embryo outside the womb which is not for its own benefit; that genetic manipulation of human cells is forbidden and that cross-species fertilisation is forbiddden. In the United Kingdom, while a research protocol may seek to alter the genetic structure of a cell while it forms part of an embryo, a licence will only be granted in such circumstances as are to be specified in regulations.

These final UK provisions, even the restrictive ones, are far more liberal than previous attempts to regulate embryo research work. For example, in the Unborn Children (Protection) Bill, presented first by Enoch Powell and then by Ken Hargreaves to successive sessions of Parliament in 1984 and 1985, clause 1 would have prohibited the fertilisation of a human ovum *in vitro* other than for the purposes of subsequent reimplantation, and then only for implantation in a specific woman authorised by the Secretary of State, and then only for a limited period of four months. Interestingly, however, the Bills would have allowed for the Secretary of State to permit the disposal of embryos not inserted, but whether this would have been by perishing was never determined. The person responsible under the licensing provisions of this Act has a responsibility to ensure that proper arrangements are made for the disposal of gametes or embryos that have been allowed to perish (s. 17(1)(c)).

Chapter 4
The Human Fertilisation and Embryology Authority

It is the direct responsibility under the Act of the Secretary of State for Health to appoint the people who are to chair and to act as the deputy and members of the Human Fertilisation and Embryology Authority — HUFEA — established by s. 5 of the Act (sch. 1 para. 4(1)). In addition, the Health Secretary must: approve the Authority's Code of Practice to be published under s. 25 (s. 26); make such regulations as required (s. 45, see below); approve the fee structure to be operated by HUFEA for the purposes of granting a licence (s. 16(1), (6)); and present an annual report of HUFEA's activities and proposed activities to Parliament (s. 7). HUFEA itself will take responsibility for individual licensing decisions and oversee the workings of the statutory licensing scheme. An attempt to make HUFEA merely advisory to the Secretary of State was defeated. This would have brought the procedures more closely in line with those under the Medicines Act 1968. Comparing the status of HUFEA with that of the Committee on the Safety of Medicines, it is clear that the Act cedes away from Parliament less control over the licensing procedure and the grant of licences.

The Composition of HUFEA

The membership of HUFEA is detailed in sch 1. It provides that the Authority shall be informed by the views of men and women, and that at least half of the membership shall be people other than those who:

(a) have been or are a registered medical practitioner;
(b) have been or are concerned with keeping or using gametes outside the human body; or
(c) have been or are directly concerned with commissioning or funding any research which involves keeping or using gametes outside the body.

This limitation in (b) and (c) extends to anyone who has actively participated in any decision to keep, use or research on gametes or embryos. In addition, any person falling within these limitations is excluded from being appointed to chair, or act as the deputy of, HUFEA. This latter formulation disqualifies any member of the Interim Licensing Authority from being invited to chair, or act as a deputy to the person who chairs, HUFEA (sch. 1, para. 4(3)(a)-(c)). In the longer term, restrictions (b) and (c) may be sufficiently widely drafted to exclude 'lay' members with previous experience of serving on ethics committees and professional bodies where these have dealt with embryology issues. Discussions reported to have taken place during the Bill's Parliamentary passage made it clear that few members of the ILA would be invited to serve on the new statutory Authority (see *Times Higher Educational Supplement* 15 June 1990, p. 1), and in the event the 21-member Authority includes only six who had gained experience as members of the ILA or the VLA.

The then Secretary of State for Health, Kenneth Clarke, announced on the 3 July 1990 that Professor Colin M. Campbell, an academic lawyer and Vice Chancellor of the University of Nottingham, had been appointed to chair HUFEA in anticipation of the Bill receiving Royal Assent in July 1990. Lady Diana Brittain, a magistrate in the City of London, a member of the Equal Opportunities Commission and a member of the Board of Management of the British School of Brussels, had been nominated as Deputy to Campbell. Continuing the mixture of bishops and actresses, practitioners, pundits and patients' representatives, the Department of Health announced the remaining complement of the Authority's provisional membership later the same month. In addition to Professor Campbell and Lady Brittain, the full membership of the 11-woman and 10-man Authority is:

Margaret Auld, former Chief Nursing Officer at the Scottish Home and Health Department and Vice President of the Royal College of Midwives, and a member of the ILA

Professor Robert Berry, Professor of Genetics at the University of London

Professor Ian Cooke, Professor of Obstetrics and Gynaecology at the University of Sheffield Jessop Hospital for Women, specialist in reproductive medicine, Chairman of the Fertility Sub-committee of the Royal College of Obstetricians and Gynaecologists and a member of the ILA

Professor Anthony Cox, Professor of Child and Adolescent Psychiatry at the United Medical and Dental Schools of Guy's and St Thomas' Hospitals

Liz Forgan, Director of Programmes at Channel 4 television

Joan Harbison, Senior Lecturer in Education at Stranmills College, Belfast

Dr Stephen Hillier, Director of the Reproductive Endocrinology Laboratory in the Department of Obstetrics and Gynaecology of the University of Edinburgh's Centre for Reproductive Biology, and a member of the ILA

Professor Brenda Hoggett, Law Commissioner and Recorder of the Crown Court, Visiting Professor of Law at King's College, London

The Rt Rev Richard Holloway, Bishop of Edinburgh

Dr Helen Houston, a general practitioner and Senior Lecturer in Continuing Medical Education in the Department of Postgraduate Medical Studies of the University of Wales College of Medicine, Cardiff

Penelope Keith, actress, and neighbour of Health Minister Virginia Bottomley

Angela Mays, a training consultant

Dr Anne Maclaren, Director of the Medical Research Council's Mammalian Development Unit, and a member of the ILA

Rabbi Julia Neuberger, Visiting Fellow of the King's Fund Institute, London, Chairman of the Patient's Association and a member of the ILA

Professor Robert Shaw, Professor of Obstetrics and Gynaecology at the Royal Free Hospital School of Medicine, and a member of the ILA

David Shilson, a senior official of the Bank of England

Professor Robert Snowden, Professor of Family Studies at Exeter University

Christine Walby, Director of Social Services, Solihull

Professor David Whittingham, Professor of Experimental Embryology, University of London and Director of the Medical Research Council Experimental Embryology and Teratology Unit.

The Secretary of State, on whose authority all these appointments are made, was bound to ensure that at least one person from each of the groups (a), (b) and (c) (above) was appointed to serve on HUFEA. The Secretary is charged to ensure that the Authority is chaired and has a deputy chair outside the three excluded categories, and numbers at least one person from each of those categories, as long as these three form at least one third of the other members but not more than half. An attempt to ensure that the membership of HUFEA demonstrated a balance between people in favour of and those opposed to research on human embryos was defeated. Since the purpose of Parliament in creating the Authority was to licence such research, it was evident that this was proposed solely as a wrecking amendment.

Appointments to HUFEA are for renewable periods of three years (sch. 1, paras 5(2), (4)). An appointed member who is absent without HUFEA permission for six consecutive months, or who becomes bankrupt or makes an arrangement with creditors, or who is unable or unfit to discharge the functions of a member of the Authority may be removed (sch. 1, para. 5). A member of the House of Commons is not eligible to become a member of HUFEA, but there is no apparent restriction in respect of a member of the House of Lords.

Arrangements for the remuneration of the person who chairs HUFEA and for the payment of pensions, allowances, fees, expenses or gratuities of any members may be made by the Authority in accordance with the Secretary of State's determination and with the approval of the Treasury (sch. 1, para. 7(1)). The Authority may appoint such staff as it thinks fit, except that where inspectors of premises, or employees whose duties include inspection, are concerned, HUFEA must ensure that they are 'of such a character' and are qualified by training and experience to be a 'suitable' person to carry out the inspections (sch. 1, para. 8(2)). The task of deciding whether prohibited or unlicensed research is being carried on will also be a difficult task, requiring appropriate skills and training, and is not one which can be discharged by the untrained observer. (For an account of the workings of the Genetic Manipulation Advisory Group and the experience and policy issues as perceived in the 1970s and early 1980s, see David Bennett, Peter Glasner and David Travis, *The Politics of Uncertainty: Regulating Recombinant DNA Research in Britain* ((1986), Routledge), esp. pp. 42-125. This work is now undertaken by the Health and Safety Executive with the Advisory Group on Genetic Manipulation.) For example, whether an embryo has been or is being maintained beyond the appearance of the primitive streak might pose more than a few problems for the passenger on the Clapham Omnibus. And deciding whether the bus had even left the garage might puzzle the untutored ticket inspector. So, in determining whether an offence was being committed by a person keeping or using an egg in the process of fertilisation without a licence, observation alone would be insufficient. This is because there are only two points at which the unfertilised egg and the fertilised egg look different. The first is when the sperm is entering the egg, and the second is during a short period about 16 hours later when the two pro-nuclei are present as the final manifestation of the separate chromosome sets from the egg and the sperm before they begin to merge. It follows from this that not only are the personnel of the Authority crucial, but so are their powers (see below, 'HUFEA licences').

The Developing Role of HUFEA

The explanatory financial memorandum estimates the expected costs of establishing and running HUFEA, and this is thought to have been a major factor in the decision to leave GIFT outside the immediate licensing and monitoring powers of the Authority (see further 'Access to Treatment Services' below at chapter 5). In addition to the licensing and supervision of treatment, research and storage, s. 8 requires HUFEA to keep under review information about:

(i) embryos,
(ii) the provision of treatment services,
(iii) the prohibited activities of ss. 3 and 4, (prohibitions in respect of embryos (s. 3(3)) or gametes (s. 4)), and
(iv) the subsequent development of embryos.

In respect of each of these s. 8 functions, HUFEA may be called upon to advise the Secretary of State if asked to do so. Of particular significance is s. 8(a) which requires HUFEA to 'keep under review information about embryos and any subsequent development of embryos'. This would seem to include a responsibility to accumulate and collate information about the provision of abortion services so as to introduce for the first time statutory review of abortion services provided under the Abortion Act 1967. The manner in which the Authority should discharge this duty was not discussed in Parliament. Presumably the regulations or directions to be made under the Act, or the matters to be covered in the Code of Guidance under s. 25, will provide for this responsibility. However welcome the proper monitoring and dissemination of information about abortion services may be, it is odd that it attracted so little interest or comment during the debates. A regulatory provision of this kind has been thought lacking by many, at least since the introduction of the Abortion Act 1967. It would seem that the consequences of the s. 8(a) duty were not fully appreciated during the Parliamentary passage of the Act.

There are four ways of monitoring the work of HUFEA, allowing simultaneous review of medical and scientific practice. The first is through the licensing committees and their functioning (s. 9, see below) and through the system of annual inspections of licenced premises (s. 9(8)). Secondly, the Authority's Annual Report must include information about its activities in the preceding 12 months and those it proposes to undertake in the succeeding 12 months (s. 7(1), (2)). The Report is intended to cover all the licences issued; any advice given by HUFEA to the Secretary of State under s. 8(a); the number of staff employed by the Authority; and changes in HUFEA membership and developments in the work covered, whether in treatment or storage. The Minister when pressed was not able to confirm that a much wider range of information would necessarily be provided. Members of the Standing Committee debating the Bill wanted to ensure that the Authority's Annual Report would provide:

(1) full details of the licences granted;
(2) details of licensed centres including:
(a) the numbers of patients treated and retreated,
(b) the rates of superovulations, embryo transfers, pregnancies and multiple pregnancies;
(c) details of eugenic and therapeutic abortions and selective reductions following IVF, embryo transfer or treatment with donated gametes;
(d) any known complications, whether for women or their children following licensed treatment services;
(3) details of individual licensed centres, including statements of their fees and costs, something which the Interim Licensing Authority has refused to publish as not being in the public interest;
(4) details of the number of inspections of licensed premises and those applying for a licence, of which under the ILA scheme there are about 10 per year, how and when the inspections are carried out, what they uncover and whether the inspections reveal breaches of the rules governing research, storage or the provision of treatment services in the laboratories.

In addition, amendments sought to have the proceedings of HUFEA's licence committees heard in public, or their proceedings made public. These detailed amendments were resisted, partly because the records maintained by Centres and the services they provide will contain personal and confidential information which, it was argued, it would be improper to make available to full public scrutiny.

Thirdly, through the powers in the Act to make changes by way of regulations under s. 45 (see below), there are some provisions in the Act which are regarded as providing protections so fundamental to the integrity of the scheme agreed on that they may not be changed without Parliamentary scrutiny. Such scrutiny takes two forms; what are called in constitutional parlance the 'negative' and the 'affirmative' resolutions of the Houses of Parliament. Under the former, the statutory instrument will be laid before Parliament and will take effect unless there is a 'prayer for annulment' which then receives a favourable vote. This seldoms happens. Under an affirmative procedure, the draft stautory instrument will not take effect until approved by affirmative resolution and Parliamentary time must be found for this. Three activities (considered in the following paragraph) are subject to change only under the 'affirmative' resolution procedure, requiring that the draft instrument be laid before, and approved by each House before it comes into force.

Section 45(4) provides that the Secretary of State may not make regulations which would permit the hitherto prohibited keeping or use of an embryo (under s. 3(3)(c)) without the opportunity for full Parliamentary consideration secured by the 'affirmative' resolution procedure. A similar reservation is made in respect of any proposal to relax regulations prohibiting the storage or use of gametes (s. 4(2)) or any changes proposed under sch. 2 para. 1(1)(g) or 3(3). These latter provisions concern, respectively, the practices which may be authorised in a treatment licence, and a condition in a research licence which authorises the alteration of the genetic structure of an embryo cell. If any amendment is proposed to either of these provisions, it must be the subject of affirmative Parliamentary scrutiny.

There is a further range of matters which, while important, it was thought suitable to leave to the less stringent safeguard of the 'negative' resolution procedure (s. 45(5)). This provides that where regulations are made which have not been subject to prior scrutiny and approval, a copy should be lodged in the office of the Clerk to each House and come into force 40 days after lodging if they have not been subject to a resolution for annulment passed in either the House of Commons or the House of Lords. There are five sorts of amendments which might at some time be thought desirable which are subject to this form of review. They concern any additional functions to be undertaken by HUFEA (s. 8(d)); the composition of HUFEA licence committees, (s. 9(5)); changes in the licensing procedure (s. 10(1)(2)); any proposed increase or decrease in the permitted period for the storage of eggs or embryos (s. 14(5)); and any changes in the information which HUFEA is obliged to disclose to an applicant under s. 31 of the Act (s. 31(4)(a), 45(4)).

The fourth and final information source regarding HUFEA concerns finance. Although the accounts of HUFEA will not be open to public inspection as such, the full accounts will be audited by the Comptroller and Auditor General and a copy of that official's report will be laid before Parliament (s. 6). Financial provisions also control the functioning of the Authority in two ways. First HUFEA must bring many of its plans back to the Secretary of State for approval and Treasury ratification; and secondly, the public funding of the whole project may be so insufficient that it functions more like a door keeper at an exclusive club than a park-keeper on a vast and extensive moorland.

In conclusion, the legislation which Parliament has enacted has endorsed the architectural plans, and laid the foundations, of the laboratory which will accommodate scientific contributors to the reproduction revolution. It has also decreed that certain structural and design specifications may not be altered without the express or implied approval of Parliament. However, it has left HUFEA with a fairly open plan in which to construct the detailed interior design. This will be found in the exercise of the power given to HUFEA to make directions about particular matters under s. 23 and a similar power for general directions under s. 9(4). In addition, s. 25 provides that HUFEA shall maintain a Code of Practice which is to give guidance about the proper conduct of activities carried on under licences granted under the Act.

HUFEA Directions

Section 23(1) gives the power to make directions; ss. 23(2) and (3) specify what effect these directions are to have; and ss. 23(4) and (5) deal with the means of communicating these directions to parties who will be affected by them. Failure to comply with directions issued by HUFEA in respect of any licence is a ground for the licence's revocation (s. 18(1)(c)) and in one instance constitutes an offence. Section 9(4) provides that any person, committees or sub-committee discharging functions of HUFEA are to do so in accordance with general directions of the Authority. The particular matters in respect of which HUFEA may issue directions and the purposes to be achieved by them are best indicated by the following table:

sections	providing for
12(d)	maintenance of proper records by licensed persons in a form specified by HUFEA
12(e)	authorisation of payment or other benefit for gametes or embryos unlawful under s. 41(8) unless in accordance with such directions (the intention is that only expenses should be authorised and that a commercial market in gametes or embryos prohibited)
12(f)	information to be supplied to the licensed recipients of gametes or embryos
13(a)-(f)	information to be recorded in pursuance of a treatment licence (see below s. 24(2))
13(4)	length of time for which information must be kept (subject to s. 24(1)), information to be kept for at least 50 years if the provider of treatment services does not know whether a child was born)
14(1)(d)	records dealing with the storage of gametes or embryos to include the consents required for their storage under sch. 3, the terms of those consents and the circumstances of the storage, and (sch. 3 para. 2(3)) any other matters which HUFEA specifies

14(2) length of time which information about the storage of gametes or embryos must be preserved

15(2) information to be maintained in research licence records

15(3) the length of time for such information to be held

24(2) and 13(2)(a)-(e) in respect of every treatment licence under sch. 2, para. 1 which involves either:

(a) bringing about the creation of an embryo *in vitro,*
(b) keeping embryos,
(c) using gametes,
(d) any therapeutic practice with an embryo to ensure it is in a suitable condition for transfer to a woman,
(e) placing any embryo in a woman,
(f) using the hamster or other specified test to determine the fertility or normality of sperm, or
(g) any other specified practice, information be recorded and given to HUFEA in respect of:

(i) the persons for whom any of those services have been provided,
(ii) the services provided,
(iii) the persons whose gametes are kept or used for those purposes or the bringing about the creation of an embryo,
(iv) any child appearing to the person responsible to have been born as a result of the licensed treatment service, and
(v) any mixing of egg and sperm or taking of an embryo from any woman or other acquisiton of an embryo from another licensed person, whether inside or outside the United Kingdom.

24(4) the receipt or despatch of embryos or gametes from or to outside the United Kingdom to be subject to specified conditions and that the provisions of ss. 12-14 be modified accordingly

24(5)-(7) licence committees to direct what is to happen when a licence is to be varied or cease to have effect because it has expired, been revoked, suspended, or otherwise (including surrender). It is an offence under s. 41(2)(d) to fail to comply with a direction under s. 24(7)(a), requiring the continued discharge of duties under a licence which has expired, been suspended, revoked or surrendered. A person guilty of such an offence is liable to a maximum penalty of two years' imprisonment or unlimited fine or both, if tried on indictment or, if tried summarily (i.e. before magistrates) to a maximum of six months' imprisonment or to a fine not exceeding the statutory maximum (presently £2,000), or both

26(5) the draft code approved by the Secretary of State shall come into force as laid out in the directions

24(11), sch. 2, para. 1(1)(f), sch. 3, para. 2(4) the egg of an animal other than the hamster not to be used under a treatment or a research licence to test the fertility or normality of sperm until proposed directions have been reported by the secretary of State to each House of Parliament.

In addition to the requirement to issue directions a primary responsibility of HUFEA is the granting, supervision, and where appropriate, revocation, suspension or variation of a licence granted under the Act. This deserves separate consideration.

HUFEA Licences

Section 11 provides that HUFEA may grant any one of three types of licence authorising either:

(1) activities in the course of providing treatment services (s. 11(1)(a)) and sch. 2, para. 1);
(2) the storage of gametes and embryos (s. 11(1)(b) and sch. 2);
(3) activities for the purpose of a project of research (s. 11(1)(c) and sch. 2, para. 3).

A licence granted by HUFEA can authorise the specified activities only under supervision of an individual named in the licence and to be carried on only on premises which the licence specifies (s. 11(2) and sch. 2, para. 4(1)). No licence can authorise more than one research project — each proposed project requires a separate licence (s. 11(2) and sch. 2, para. 4(2)(b)). No licence can authorise more than one individual who is to be responsible for the licensed activities (s. 11(2) and sch. 2, para. 4(2)(c)), nor apply to premises in different places (s. 11(2) and sch. 2, para. 4(2)(d)). A licence authorising treatment services or a licence authorising research can also permit the storage of embryos or gametes, but a treatment licence cannot authorise research, nor a research licence, treatment; each activity must be considered in a separate licence application (s. 11(2) and sch. 2, para. 4(2)(a)).

The legislation precludes the granting of licences for certain types of activity. Under s. 3(3) a licence cannot authorise:

(a) keeping or using an embryo after the appearance of the 'primitive streak' — taken to be not later than 14 days after gametes have been mixed, but excluding any time when the resulting embryo has been preserved by freezing (s. 3(4));
(b) placing a human embryo in any animal;
(c) keeping or using an embryo in contravention of regulations;
(d) nucleus substitution, sometimes called cloning.

These provisions are more fully discussed in Chapter 3.

There is also a specific and important restriction in respect of the grant of research licences. A single research licence cannot authorise both the bringing about the creation of embryos *in vitro* together with the keeping or use of them and the alteration of the genetic structure of a cell while it forms part of an embryo (s. 11(2) and sch. 2, para. 4(2)(a)). A research project which proposes to alter genetic cell structures of an embryo may only be granted — if at all — in accordance with regulations approved under the 'affirmative resolution' procedure, s. 45(4); (see 'The Developing Role of HUFEA', (supra)). Even if such regulations are made, a research licence which is to permit work under these regulations must be the subject of a seperate licence consideration, and fulfil the requirements laid down in regulations for the grant and supervision of such licences. Schedule 2, para. 3(5) makes it clear that the Authority must not grant any research licence unless it is satisfied that the purpose of that research could not be achieved in any other way. Additionally, s. 13(7)(b) provides, in relation to treatment licences that consideration shall be given to the use of practices not requiring the authority of a licence as well as those which do. It will be incumbent, therefore, for HUFEA to keep abreast of all developments.

The 1987 White Paper announced that the Government did not intend to specify in legislation the 'detailed criteria' which were to be applied in granting licences (Cm 259 para. 22). However, certain key features were to be spelt out, and s. 12 of the Act provides for a number of general conditions which are to be incorporated into every licence granted by HUFEA, whether for treatment services, research or storage.

1. All licences will provide that the licensed activities may be carried out only on licensed premises and under the supervision of the 'person responsible' (s. 12(a)). This is the individual under whose supervision the activities authorised by a licence are carried out (s. 17(1)(a)).

2. Proper records must be maintained in the form specified by HUFEA (s. 12(d)). Copies of extracts from those records or any other specified particulars are to be supplied to the Authority when and how it specifies (s. 12(g)). These powers are to be exercised in directions relating to required information made by HUFEA under s. 23.

3. The written consent requirements of sch. 3 must be complied with (s. 12(c)). The requirements in respect of storage licences are dealt with below (see pp. 115–16). The other consents requirements are dealt with in 'Treatment Services' (at pp. 118–124).

4. No money or other benefit may be made or received in the supply of gametes or embryos other than in accordance with authorisation given by HUFEA in directions (s. 12(e)). This important provision originally provided only that 'no person providing gametes for the purposes of a treatment service should be given any money or money's worth for doing so'. This had three immediate limitations: it did not extend to embryos; applied only to providing gametes in the course of a treatment service; and prohibited only payment in money or money's worth. This gave rise to fears of the development of an unregulated 'market in gametes

or embryos.' These fears appeared to have been comfirmed during the summer Parliamentary recess. *The Mail on Sunday* carried reports of a trade in human embryos, intended for use in an international surrogacy arrangement (see, *The Mail on Sunday*, 9 September 1990, p. 19). The ILA were reported to be very disturbed about these developments, although efforts to identify the clinic involved, which presumably held an ILA licence, were unsuccessful. The present wording was settled upon in order to prohibit inducements in respect of gametes and embryos, unless specifically authorised by HUFEA.

Particular concern had arisen because the original provision would not have prevented the sorts of 'inducements' which prompted the Interim Licensing Authority to action in 1989-90. Following newspaper coverage of some clinics' practices, in its Fifth Report (1990), the ILA drew attention to the ethical problems of possible inducement offered to a woman who is being sterilised to encourage her to donate her eggs. The ILA stated clearly that 'Financial inducement is not acceptable' (Dame Mary Donaldson, 'Foreword', p. 2). However, they were also concerned at payment in kind such as jumping an NHS waiting list or alternatively being offered treatment in a private hospital. While they recognised that there was both a shortage of eggs and also women who were willing to become donors when undergoing sterilisation, the ILA were concerned to ensure that 'no undue pressure is exerted on any woman to persuade her to alleviate this shortage by becoming a donor' (ibid). Accordingly, they added two new guidelines, which we review in Chapter 5. In debates on the Bill Lord Donaldson (a relation) suggested that the waiving of charges for private treatment in consideration for donation of eggs would be the waiving a payment for advantage and not a 'payment in money or money's worth.' Hence it would not have been subject to the precursor to s. 12(e).

That section now provides that HUFEA may authorise payments where it is desirable to allow particular expenses incurred by donors to be repaid. It is generally understood that this will enable HUFEA to ensure that donors do not incur any financial costs as a result of their donations, but the Act does not specify, nor was any indication given, of how far this will extend. Although the directions or Code of Practice may deal with this point, and it is unlikely that the Authority will countenance significant payments, the scope that the directions should take is unclear. For example, although we might expect (say) travel costs to be reimbursed, might the payment cover the loss of wages or other payments in connection with time and inconvenience? Will it extend, in cases such as ovum donation, to compensation for discomfort? There is a good case for allowing financial benefit to be greater where more invasive procedures are used. However, the medical profession has generally distained payments calibrated according to risk, (where human volunteers are used in drug studies, for example). This would seem to militate against large sums of money being offered for the supply of healthy eggs or ova. A person to whom a licence applies and who gives or receives any money or other benefit, other than in accordance with HUFEA directions, commits an offence under s. 41(8). This is punishable with up to six months' imprisonment or a fine not exceeding level 5 on the standard scale (presently £2,000). A nominal licensee (s. 17(3)), (that is, a licence-holder who is not the person responsible for supervising the licensed activities under s. 17(1)) may also be caught by this provision.

5. Where gametes or embryos are supplied by one licence holder to another, the supplier shall give to the recipient such information as HUFEA specifies in directions (s. 12(f)). This is to ensure that where gametes or embryos are moved around, the information held by one centre about the genetic identity of the donor, the nature and extent of the consents given, and the purposes for which the gametes or embryos are to be used, will be passed from the first to subsequent custodians of the gametes or embryos. It will presumably also be necessary for the supplying licence-holder to be required to offer sufficient information concerning the transfer to enable the donor or gestators quickly to be able to contact the new holders. This would be necessary to enable them to revoke or vary their sch. 3 consents.

6. Any member of HUFEA may, at any reasonable time and on producing identification if necessary, be allowed entry to licensed premises to inspect the premises, any equipment or records, or to observe any activity taking place at the centre (s. 12(b)). In addition to this licencing provision, members or employees of HUFEA are given further powers to police licensed premises or services, treatments or research. Section 39 provides that any member or employee of HUFEA entering and inspecting licensed premises may take possession of or take away anything (including information) which they believe, on reasonable grounds, to be relevant to the grant, variation, suspension or revocation of a licence, or which they believe may be required for the purpose of evidence of an offence under the Act. Section 39(3) specifically protects a member or employee of HUFEA who, in the discharge of their functions, keeps an embryo or gametes without a licence. This will also protect such a person who keeps an embryo beyond the 14 day limit specified in s. 3(3)(a). An additional provision (s. 43) provides that a person such as a police officer who keeps gametes or embryos as evidence for a prosecution is exempt from these general prohibitions. Section 40 provides that a member or an employee of HUFEA may obtain from a justice of the peace (or, in Scotland, a sheriff), a warrant to enter and search premises and to take possession of anything which the member or employee has reasonable grounds to believe may be required in evidence in proceedings for an offence under the Act.

Licensing Functions and Licensing Committees

The Authority is charged by s. 9(1) to establish one or more committees to discharge its licensing function under the Act. According to Health Minister Bottomley, 'the licence committees will be the cutting edge of the Authority. . . . [they] are the central force behind the Authority' (House of Commons, Official Report Standing Committee B, 15 May 1990, cols. 113–14). HUFEA may discharge any of its other functions by committee, or through its members and employees, and it may appoint sub-committees to carry out the work. With the exception of a licence committee, any committee or sub-committee may co-opt a minority of people who are not members of HUFEA (sch. 1).

The size and composition of the licence committees are to be determined by the Secretary of State in regulations. Unlike other committees, the licence committees will not be able to delegate their work to sub-committees and must be composed wholly of members of the Authority (ss. 9(3) and 9(5)). Section 9(5) provides that the licence committee must not be dominated by clinical interests, and must include at least one person who is not presently authorised to carry on or participate in any licensed activities. A similar exclusion applies in respect of any member of HUFEA who has a licence application outstanding for their own work.

When an application for a licence is received by HUFEA, a licence committee must arrange for an inspection of and report in respect of the premises in respect of which the licence is sought (s. 9(7)). This applies where an application is made to carry on activities not already licensed or to carry on previously licensed activities in as yet unauthorised premises. Where the application comes from a licensed person and the premises have been inspected within the previous twelve months, then the licence committee may dispense with a second inspection. This could occur if a further licensed activity is proposed at existing licensed premises, since different licences must be applied for and granted in respect of research, treatment or storage. Equally, it may be necessary if premises change ownership and a previously unlicenced person makes an application. HUFEA is required to ensure that licensed premises are inspected once in each calendar year (s. 9(8)), unless a licence committee considers that an inspection is unnecessary. This might be the case where, for example, research or storage or treatment services have for some reason been suspended and work is not actively in progress for that year or a large part of it.

The Secretary of State is empowered to regulate the proceedings of licence committees and of HUFEA acting as an appellate body in respect of a determination by a licence committee. In addition, regulations may provide for the admissibility of evidence (s. 10(2)(b)) and the attendance of witnesses and production of documents before a licence committee (s. 10(2)(a)). In debate, Ann Widdecombe unsuccessfully sought assurances on the workings of the licensing committees. Specifically, she wanted the Code of Practice to ensure that: HUFEA had suitable procedures to make its work open and public; that the public would indeed be invited to submit evidence on licence applications; that the hearings would be in public or the proceedings published; that details of all licences granted would be made public, and that there should be a procedure for the public appeal against the awarding of any licence (House of Commons, Official Report Standing Committee B, 15 May 1990, cols. 123-24). The Minister made it clear that HUFEA is given authority to regulate its own proceedings (sch. 1, para. 9(1)) and discharge its functions in accordance with such arrangements as it thinks appropriate.

Thus, it will fall to HUFEA to decide whether the proceedings of any of its committees, including licensing committees, should be heard in public or in private. The Franks Committee (Cmnd 218 (1957)) recommended that hearings should be in public except where there are matters of public security, intimate personal or financial detail, or professional reputation to be discussed. Thus, under their regulations Family Health Service Authority Committees and Social

Security Appeal Tribunals sit in private. As for other tribunals, most tribunal rules provide for either private or public hearings as needs dictate and at the discretion of the chair. The starting point of Franks seemed to be that since tribunals are an essential part of the machinery of justice, prima facie they ought to hold public hearings. Similarly, HUFEA will need to decide whether notice of applications which it has received should be publicised, and whether and from whom evidence may be taken regarding, for example, the requirements of sch. 2 in respect of research licences.

Paragraph 2 of sch. 3(6) provides that a research project which is shown to relate to one of the permissible categories of research (sch. 2, para. 3(2)(a)-(e)), shall not be granted a licence unless HUFEA is satisfied that 'any proposed use of embryos is necessary' for the purposes of the research. Schedule 2, para. 3(3) provides that in each case the purpose must increase knowledge about the creation and development of embryos, or disease or enable such knowledge to be applied. This does not mean, however, that HUFEA will grant licences only if it is satisfied that the objectives of the research could not be achieved in any other way. A statement to that effect by the Minister was later withdrawn (House of Commons, Official Report Standing Committee B, 8 May 1990, col. 59). It is unclear what standards are to be applied by HUFEA under provisions such as para. 6 of sch. 2. In deciding that they are 'satisfied' of the necessity of using embryos, thresholds are significant. A 'balance of probabilities' approach might allow more room for some type of risk/utility analysis leading to a possible decision that notwithstanding other options, embryo usage was necessary. A 'beyond reasonable doubt' approach may be more problematic in the context of rapid medical advance. The withdrawal of the ministerial statement would seem to indicate acceptance of the 'balance of probabilities' criterion.

In respect of any licence application, any member of HUFEA who is directly or indirectly interested in a licence must disclose that interest to the Authority (sch. 1, para. 10(1)). This would apply to the colleague of an applicant, or someone who sits on the local ethical review committee of a hospital putting forward an application for a treatment licence. A person who has made such a disclosure is prohibited from taking further part in deliberations or decisions affecting the licence otherwise than in accordance with procedures to be established by HUFEA under sch. 1, para. 9(1). Any decision or deliberation in which a person takes part after having made disclosure shall be of no effect unless protected by HUFEA procedures (para. 10(3)), although no provision is made for a case in which an application is heard and granted where a member of the Authority does not declare a relevant interest. Doubtless, if an application is refused in such circumstances, this would be a ground for seeking to have the determination set aside as in breach of natural justice (see p. 108 for a consideration of this question.)

Procedure of Licensing Committees

Sections 16–22 inclusive detail in further depth the procedures to be adopted, the requirements to be satisfied and the safeguards available in the granting, revocation and suspension of licences. Controversy has stalked these particular provisions because of the fee requirements attached to the licence applications. This raises a wider question of access to treatment services, and is dealt with in that section in the chapter on Treatment Services (below at p. 141 et seq.).

Section 16 provides that an applicant for any licence must file in an approved form an application accompanied by an 'initial fee.' This is the fee set by HUFEA and approved by the Secretary of State and the Treasury for entertaining a licence request (s. 16(1) and (6)). A variable fee scale may be set according to circumstances, such as: whether the applicant intends to offer storage facilities as well as treatment services; the number of treatment cycles it proposes to perform annually; and the ability to reclaim all or part of its cost from patients. This final consideration is significant because some NHS facilities or university departments may not be permitted to 'charge' patients. On the other hand, a private hospital can pass on the full economic cost of complying with HUFEA costs to all of its patients. Moreover, some research projects may be carried on without offering treatment services through which costs can be recovered (of the 45 Centres licensed by the ILA, three are licensed to conduct research without offering a clinical treatment service, of either IVF or GIFT).

Before a licence committee can grant a licence it must be satisfied as to a number of conditions. These are spelt out in s. 16(2). The application must name an individual who is to be responsible for supervising the activities, whether they are treatment services, research or storage, under the licence (s. 16(2)(a)). Section 17(1) labels this person the 'person responsible' and imposes on him or her a number of specific duties set out in that section.

The proper functioning and enforcement of the licence conditions is one of the tasks entrusted to the 'person responsible' under s. 17 (s. 17(1)(e)). That person is the individual (i.e., it must be a named natural person under s. 17(1) and not a body corporate or other legal person) under whose supervision the licensed activities are carried on. Such a person has the duty to secure (not ensure, i.e. it is a duty which can be delegated) that any other persons to whom the licence applies are suitable to participate in the licensed activities. These are the persons responsible themselves, any person acting under their direction, and any person either designated in the licence, named in a notice given to HUFEA or anyone acting under the direction of such a designated person (s. 17(2)). In each case, the person responsible must take into account the character and qualifications of any such person (s. 17(1)(a)). This will include staff involved with counselling under s. 13(6), nursing staff, and laboratory staff. This is a matter which has been of continuing concern to the ILA. In its 4th Report (1989) it observed that 'as a result of the increasing number of clinical centres undertaking IVF there is a shortage of laboratory staff with the relevant expertise in embryology' (p. 13). In particular they noted that for newly appointed members of staff an appropriate biological background was not of itself sufficient. In addition, the ILA advised that new laboratory staff should receive 'appropriate training', preferably in an approved centre, before they are employed on a clinical programme. This concern was repeated in the Fifth Report in 1990 (p.13).

The person responsible will be required to ensure that all staff are so qualified, and also that proper equipment is used (s. 17(1)(b)) and that suitable practices are used in the course of licensed activities (s. 17(1)(d)). A particular duty is to ensure that proper arrangements are made for keeping gametes and embryos, and that attention is given to the arrangements for the disposal of gametes or embryos that have been allowed to perish (s. 17(1)(c)).

The application must show that the applicant is the person responsible (s. 16(2)(b)), or at least that it is made with the consent of the applicant (s. 16(2)(b)(i)) and, in either case, the licence committee must be satisfied that the applicant is a 'suitable person' to hold a licence (s. 16(2)(b)(ii)). In addition, the committee must be satisfied as to three other matters: the fitness of the person responsible under s. 17; the suitability of the premises to be licensed (s. 16(2)(d)); and that all other requirements of the Act have been complied with. Section 16(2)(c) requires the licence committee to be satisfied that the person responsible has the necessary 'character, qualifications and experience' such that they can discharge their duties imposed by s. 17. This curious formulation is a common one in licence application conditions laid down in statute; it occurs, for example, in the Animals (Scientific Procedures) Act 1986 s. 4, which demands that a person in authority at premises used for animal experimentation should have a knowledge of the biological and other relevant qualifications, and of the training, experience and character, of any applicant whose licence is endorsed. An example in a non-medical or scientific context is in the Insurance (Registration) Act 1977 s. 3, which dwells also upon qualifications and experience as well as 'character and suitability'. Such provisions are designed, broadly, as a form of quality control over the sorts of person to whom licences can be awarded. The further provisions of s. 17 are dealt with below. In the same way that s. 17(1)(a) places a duty upon the 'person responsible' to be satisfied as to the character, experience and training of any staff who do work covered by the licence, so the committee will want to ensure that only suitably qualified, experienced and, where necessary, trained people are permitted a licence. The Committee may call for further information if it thinks it necesssary to consider an application (s. 16(4)), and if it intends to impose any conditions on a licence, those conditions must be acknowledged in writing by the applicant, and, if a different person, the person responsible.

In respect of each type of licence, a licence committee is given power to impose such conditions as it may specify in the licence. Such conditions in a treatment licence, for example, would include the statutory conditions in ss. 12 and 13, and under the authority of sch. 2, para. 1(2), any special conditions attaching to that application or applications of that kind. A treatment licence could be made subject to a maximum number of patients at any one time. A ceiling on the number of treatment cycles which could be attempted in any one year could be imposed because of factors disclosed in the report submitted to the licensing committee following inspection of the proposed premises under s. 9(7). Similar powers are given in respect of storage licences, which must include the statutory conditions (ss. 12 and 14) and may include any special conditions including storage in a specified manner (sch. 2, para. 2(2)). In respect of research licences, ss. 12 and 15 and sch. 2, para. 3(7) make similar provision for incorporation of the statutory conditions and any special conditions. However, in respect of research licences alone, HUFEA (i.e., not just a licence committee) must additionally be satisfied that the research is 'necessary' (sch. 2, para. 3(6)).

Appeals and Judicial Review

There are two ways in which a person may seek to challenge the exercise of the statutory powers laid upon licence committees by the Act. The first, and most straightforward, is where a committee has imposed on an applicant a condition which he or she or it does not like or accept. Here, an application may be made under ss. 18(4) and 18(6)(a) for a variation of that condition. The procedure for such variations is provided for in s. 19, which we discuss below. However, the wording of ss. 19(1) and (2) and ss. 20(1) and 20(2) is such that if a licence committee determines not to allow the application for variation in respect of a licence condition, the applicant is given no right of appeal to HUFEA. The full Authority has the power to hear appeals from a refusal of a licence or a refusal to vary a licence, but only where the variation sought under s. 18(5) is to designate another person in place of the person responsible (ss. 19(2) and 20(2)). A licence-holder who dislikes any other condition imposed by a committee which the committee refuses to vary must rely on the second and doubtless more expensive and time consuming method of seeking judicial review of the committee's decision.

Where a statutory body such as HUFEA is given this sort of power to grant licences, without which an activity may not lawfully be performed, it is subject to a general public law scrutiny in order to ensure that it does not abuse its licensing powers. However, the courts have struck a balance to ensure that review does not usurp the power which Parliament has appointed a public authority to discharge. As with any other such body, HUFEA is subject to a duty to impose only such conditions as could be considered 'reasonable' under a test established in *Associated Picture Houses* v *Wednesbury Corporation* [1948] 1 KB 223. This is not, as Wade explains (W. H. Wade, *Administrative Law* 6th ed., (1989), Oxford University Press, p. 363) the negligence standard of the reasonable passenger on the Clapham omnibus, but it is the standard indicated by the true construction of the Act in question. It distinguishes between the proper and improper use of power. The formulation of the *Wednesbury* principle was given by Lord Greene (at p. 229):

> It is true that discretion must be exercised reasonably. . . . Lawyers familiar with the phraseology used in relation to exercise of statutory discretions often use the word 'unreasonable' in a rather comprehensive sense. It has frequently been used and is frequently used as a general description of the things that must not be done. For instance, a person entrusted with a discretion must, so to speak, direct himself properly in law. He must call his own attention to the matters which he is bound to consider. He must exclude from his consideration matters which are irrelevant to what he has to consider. If he does not obey those rules, he may truly be said, and often is said, to be acting 'unreasonably.' Similarly, there may be something so absurd that no sensible person could ever dream that it lay within the powers of the authority. Warrington LJ in *Short* v *Poole Corporation* [1926] Ch 66 gave the example of a red-haired teacher, dismissed because she had red hair. This is unreasonable in one sense. In another it is taking into consideration extraneous matters. It is so unreason-

able that it might almost be described as being done in bad faith; and, in fact, all these things run into one another.

So, the sorts of conditions that a licensing committee may lawfully impose on an applicant or person responsible are wide-ranging, but not without limit. In considering whether a condition is unreasonable, regard has to be had to the statutory background and purpose, but that considered, the ability of a licence committee to impose rigorous limiting conditions is wide, and the ability of an applicant to object to them is available only through judicial review, and not by way of appeal to HUFEA under s. 20, as we shall see. A sense of the legal standard of reasonableness may be understood from a review of the judgments and speeches in the case of *Secretary of State for Education and Science* v *Tameside Metropolitan Borough Council* [1977] AC 1014. There, judges in the Court of Appeal and the House of Lords discussed the error of confusing differences of opinion with unreasonableness on the part of one side or the other. To exceed a statutory power, a party must be 'so wrong that no reasonable person could sensibly take that view' (Lord Denning, at p. 1023). Lord Diplock said that:

> The very concept of administrative discretion involves a right to choose between more than one possible course of action upon which there is room for reasonable people to hold differing opinions as to which is to be preferred (at p. 1064).

Particularly pertinent in this discussion is the judgment in *Commissioners of Customs and Excise* v *Cure and Deeley Ltd* [1962] 1 QB, in which the court struck down purchase tax regulations which were excessively drastic and oppressive. So a licence committee may lawfully write into a licence conditions which relate to such matters as:

(a) the procedures to be adopted in determining the quality of sperm received from a donor;
(b) even the frequency with which donated sperm may be used;
(c) the types of emergency resuscitation measures and equipment which must be available in a centre;
(d) the number of eggs or embryos which may be transferred in the course of any given treatment cycle, or indeed the number of treatment cycles to which a woman may expose herself overall;
(e) the frequency with which treatment services may be offered;

and so on, but perhaps not the size of a bed which a patient receiving treatment services must occupy, or the number of television sets which should be available for patients if admitted to the licensed centre during the course of a service. Other examples can be given which would illustrate the general point, that as long as a condition is properly related to the aims and scheme of the regulatory statute, then it will be very difficult to persuade a court by way of judicial review that a licence committee has exceeded its powers. In relation to such conditions, it will presumably be open to a committee to take into account the character, attitudes and behaviour of an applicant towards the voluntary licensing scheme of the ILA over the previous years in deciding whether and on what terms to grant a licence. That this has acute implications for some treatment centres, which have not always been assiduous in their ready adherence to ILA advice or guidelines is obvious.

Thus far, what has been said is that, in the context of the parent Act, irrelevant considerations, errors of law, and unreasonable conditions may be such as to render administrative actions by HUFEA ultra vires. In such instances, the substantive provisions of the regulations would fail to fulfil the general purpose(s) of the statute. There are a number of other types of substantive ultra vires which may be relevant. A clear example would be bad faith, although instances of successful cases of bad faith are rare, and the burden of proof upon those making such allegations is stringent: see *Cannock Chase DC* v *Kelly* [1978] 1 WLR 1. Another obvious example of substantive ultra vires arises out of the improper exercise of discretion. A good example of this in the present context arises from the provision, in s. 9(3) and (5), that the licensed committees cannot delegate their work to sub-committees. Such statutory requirements will be rigorously upheld by the courts, and even without the express prohibition of statute, the general line in administrative law would be that a body given a discretion under statute must exercise that discretion (see *Vine* v *National Dock Labour Board* [1957] AC 488).

Another method by which the licensing authority might neglect the true exercise of their discretion would be to continually fetter their discretion. This might be so, for example, if a licence committee took an early decision that a certain category of research laid down in sch. 2, para. 3(2)(a)-(e) could never be appropriately pursued using embryos. In such cases the courts generally take the view that the person exercising the power should always be willing to hear representations before making a decision (*R* v *Secretary of State for the Environment ex parte Brent LBC* [1982] QB 593). The courts may uphold general policies which are pursued for administrative convenience, but only if the body in question can show that they are always willing to hear from particular applicants on why the policies should not apply in the instant case (see *British Oxygen Co Ltd* v *Board of Trade* [1971] AC 610).

In a piece of legislation which is so detailed in the procedures which it lays down, it is important to consider not merely substantive but also procedural issues which may lead to ultra vires action. In this context, procedural ultra vires is likely to take two forms: failure to follow the directions of the Act, and failure to meet principles of natural justice. As regards directions under the statute, there are both mandatory and directory provisions governing the action of the Authority. The distinction between the two is crucial. Where the statute lays down that a licence committee must follow a particular procedure, then this is a mandatory requirement, failure to comply with which will render the decision invalid. Examples of this might include: a determination by a licence committee which is improperly constituted in breach of the regulations determining the composition of such committees (see s. 9(5); or where a licence committee fails to give notice of a determination of a licence application contrary to s. 19(5).

Where, however, procedures are merely directory, (for example where a licence committee may by notice suspend a licence under s. 22(1), the courts will not generally find committees bound by such directory provisions and failure to meet the procedural requirements will not generally be fatal to the validity of the action. It should be noted that action on the part of the committee may be enforceable, even where dealing with directory provisions. For example, under s. 9(8) HUFEA is required to ensure that licensed premises are inspected once each calendar year. This inspection may be foregone if the licence committee considers it unnecessary. It is likely, however, that someone with sufficient locus standi could at least require the remedy of mandamus to cause the Authority to consider whether they ought to inspect where it appears that they have not directed their minds to the problem.

There are certain classes of procedural requirements which the courts are vigilant to uphold. Thus, for example, where licensed premises change ownership, and a previously unlicensed person makes an application for the transfer of the licence, then there is little doubt that a decision by the licensing authority without consultation or hearing to refuse to transfer the licence would be reviewable. This is because, in practice, provisions to consult, inform or offer hearings are treated as though they were mandatory requirements (see *Agricultural Training Board* v *Aylesbury Mushrooms* [1972] 1 WLR 190). Here the procedural requirements of the statute slowly merge with the background principles of natural justice, and a broad duty to act fairly. Many of the principles of natural justice, such as the right to be heard, are encompassed within the procedures of the Act itself or will be contained in future regulations (see s. 10(2) on licence committee procedures). There are similar protections within the statute against bias. For example, sch. 1, para. 10(1) states that a member of HUFEA who is directly or indirectly interested in a licence must disclose that interest to the Authority.

In the GCHQ case, *Council of the Civil Service Unions* v *Minister for the Civil Service* [1985] AC 374 at 414, Lord Roskill proposed that the phrase 'natural justice' be 'replaced by speaking of a duty to act fairly.' It is true to say that it is now more common to talk of broad duties to act fairly rather than strict principles of natural justice. In particular, the courts will be prepared to uphold broad principles of fairness in situations in which persons have legitimate expectations (such as that a licence may be renewed in the absence of changed circumstances), and where what is vested in a person is a particular right or privilege which the holder might expect would be safeguarded by clear principles. This is all the more true where statute gives a clear inference (as is the case with the Act) that it wishes strict and fair procedures to apply. In the context of other sorts of licence-holders, there are clear examples of the strict applications of such principles; see *R* v *Barnsley MBC ex parte Hook* [1976] 1 WLR 1052; *Wheeler* v *Leicester City Council* [1985] 3 WLR 335; and *Congreve* v *Home Office* [1976] QB 629.

One important remaining question in relation to judicial review is precisely who may have standing to bring a case. This is because 'the law does not see it as the function of the courts to be there for every individual who is interested in having the legality of an administrative action litigated' (*R* v *Secretary of State ex parte Rose Theatre Co* [1990] 1 All ER 754, 768). In the leading case of *IRC* v *National Federation of Self-Employed and Small Businesses Ltd* [1982] AC 617, the House of Lords decided that rather than have a rigid test of locus standi which would be unconnected with the precise facts of each case, the courts should use their general discretion to determine the applicant's status in accordance with the strength of the case in all respects. In the view of Lord Diplock in that case, rights were given in public law actions not merely to 'people aggrieved', so that the notion of 'interest' should be a wide one and a matter for the court's discretion. However, the majority of the Law Lords did not go that far. Lord Scarman thought that the person would only have status if they were owed some form of duty which was recognised by law, and Lord Fraser too focused on the applicant having a right to complain, although this might in his view be express or implied. Both Lord Wilberforce and Lord Roskill focused on the nature of the statutory duties, and seem to regard as significant whether or not the applicant was within the scope of the duties owed. Interpreting these principles in the *Rose Theatre* case, it was said that not every member of the public can complain of a breach of statutory duty by a person making a decision under statute; to rule otherwise would be to deprive the phrase 'sufficient interest' of all meaning. In the view of Schiemann J in this case, while a direct financial or legal interest was not required, it was helpful if the applicant had a right given under statute such that she or he might have that duty performed. Merely to assert an interest was not sufficient, and the fact that a pressure group asserted its particular concern with a matter did not of itself create a sufficient interest. To allow otherwise would be to open jurisdiction widely to those people who simply campaigned on any particular issue.

These observations have obvious significance in the context of the background debate on embryo experimentation. Clearly, there are many interest groups which might seek to challenge decisions of licensing committees. The *Rose Theatre* case suggests that, of itself, that is not enough, even though those interests groups may have been campaigning on, for example, right to life issues for many years. On the other hand, on the test of Lord Diplock in the *Self-Employed* case

> it would be a grave lacuna in our system of public law if a pressure group . . . were prevented by outdated technical rules of locus standi from bringing the matter to the attention of the courts to vindicate the rule of law and get the unlawful conduct stopped.

This view would seem however to be an exceptional one, and the remainder of the judges in the House of Lords in the *Self-Employed* case based their approaches, one way or another, upon either some implicit right to complain or upon some recognisable duty arising out of the statute. Again, in this context it is not clear precisely which duty an interest group might claim would give them a sufficient interest to intervene by way of judicial review. Of course, the situation might be different if the complainant were a party in some way connected to the provision of infertility treatment.

Revocation, Variation and Suspension of Licences

A licence committee may revoke a licence or vary any terms of a licence which it would otherwise have the power to revoke (s. 18(1), (3)). The circumstances in which a licence may be revoked or varied are set out in s. 18, and the procedures to which a committee must adhere in either refusing, revoking or varying a licence are set out in s. 19. The Act also gives limited grounds upon which a licence holder may apply for changes to the licence. Sections 19 and 20 provide mechanisms whereby parties interested in revocation or variation of a licence may be entitled to be heard before a committee determines the application. It would seem clear on the principles of *Ridge* v *Baldwin* [1964] AC 40 that the licence-holders at least would have this right, but so too might interested third parties in appropriate cases (see *R* v *Hendon RDC ex parte Chorley Taxi Fleet Operators' Association* [1972] 2 QB 299). Sections 19 and 20 provide limited grounds upon which an appeal from such a determination can be taken, in the first instance to the full body of HUFEA, and thence, on a point of law, to the High Court.

The grounds for revocation or variation are that:

(a) any information given in a licence application was false or misleading in a material respect (s. 18(1)(a));

(b) the licensed premises are no longer suitable for the licensed activities (s. 18(1)(b));

(c) the person responsible has failed to discharge, or is unable because of incapacity to discharge the s. 17 duty, or has failed to comply with any directions given in connection with any licence (s. 18(1)(c));

(d) there has been a material change of circumstances since the grant of the licence (s. 18(1)(d));

(e) there has been an application by the person responsible or the nominal licensee (s. 18(4)).

A licence can only be varied to the extent that it affects activities authorised by licence, by changing the manner in which the licensed activities are conducted or by changing or removing conditions which a licence committee have attached to a licence (s. 18(6)(a)). To the extent that the licence authorises the conduct of activities on licensed premises, the licence can be varied only so as to extend or restrict the premises to which the licence relates (s. 18(6)(b)). In other words, an application to vary a licence cannot seek to add new, previously unlicensed premises to the licence, nor to add new services to an existing licence, nor to authorise the conduct of an activity which needs a separate application for a new licence. There is one exception to this provision, which is where a nominal licensee applies to vary a licence to designate another individual in place of the present person responsible for overseeing the licensed activities and securing the discharge of the s. 17 duties. Here, as long as the application is made with the consent of the proposed person responsible and a committee is satisfied as to that person's character, qualifications and experience to supervise the licensed activities and discharge the duty, then the committee may vary the licence as requested (s. 18(5)).

Section 18(2) provides three additional grounds of revocation only, and not variation. These are where a committee ceases to be satisfied that the character of the person responsible or the nominal licensee (see s. 17(3)) is such as is required for the supervision of licensed activities. It could be, for example, that such a person is convicted of an offence unrelated to the Act but which casts general doubt as to that person's continuing suitability (s. 18(2)(a)). The second and third grounds may occur either where the person responsible dies or is convicted of an offence under the Human Fertilisation and Embryology Act 1990 (s. 18(2)(b)).

In any case where a licence committee has reasonable grounds to suspect that a s. 18 revocation of a licence would be warranted and believes that matters are sufficiently serious to warrant an immediate suspension, it is given power in s. 22(1) to suspend the licence immediately for a period not exceeding three months. Section 22(2) provides that such a suspension is to be effected by giving notice either to the person responsible or, if she or he has died or appears to the committee to be incapable of discharging the s. 17 duties, to the nominal licensee or to any person to whom the licence applies (as defined in s. 17(2)(a)-(c)). A suspended licence, which may be further suspended for periods not exceeding three months (s. 22(2)), is of no effect (s. 22(3)), but while it is suspended an application may be made by the nominal licensee under s. 18(5) for a new person to be designated as the 'person responsible' (s. 22(3)).

Section 19 details the procedures to be followed where a licence committee proposes either:

(i) to refuse a licence or to refuse to grant an application for variation to designate a new 'person responsible' (s. 19(1)); or
(ii) where a licence committee proposes to vary or revoke a licence.

In the first case the committee must give notice of the proposal to the applicant and include the reasons for its proposed refusal (s. 19(1)). In the second case the committee must give notice of its proposal and the reasons for it to the person responsible under s. 17 and the nominal licensee (but not to anyone, such as a member of the public, who has applied for the variation or revocation) (s. 19(2)). In both cases, the notice must indicate that the recipient may within 28 days give notice to the committee of their intention to make representations (s. 19(3)). If such a wish is expressed, the committee is obliged to give the person or someone acting on their behalf an opportunity to make oral representations at a meeting of the committee or written representations or both before it reaches its determination (ss. 19(3), 4(a), (b)). The licence committee must give notice of its determinations and reasons for it to the relevant parties (s. 19(5)(a)-(c), (6)). This provision may be significant, for it has been said that there is no general legal principle stating that reasons must be given (*Payne* v *Lord Harris of Greenwich* [1981] 1 WLR 754, 765). Having said that, the more judicial the setting the more likely the requirement for reasons — simply as the basis of appeal and as part of the duty to act fairly (supra).

In any case where a committee proposes to suspend, revoke or vary a licence, or where a licence has been varied, has expired, been suspended, revoked or otherwise ceased to have effect, the licence committee may make directions ensuring the continued discharge of the duties of the person responsible under the 'old' licence (s. 24(6), (7)). In particular, such directions may require anything kept under the old licence to be transferred to HUFEA or to any other person. This could include instruments, gametes, stored embryos or information generated under the terms of the old licence (s. 24(7)(a)). In addition HUFEA may secure through directions the continued discharge of the duties under the Act by a person taking over from the person responsible. HUFEA must be satisfied that that other person fulfils the requirements that would be demanded if they were an applicant to be a person responsible under a licence. They must consent in writing to taking over (s. 24(7)).

Refusal of Licences

In any case where a committee's determination is to refuse a licence or to refuse to grant a variation designating another person as the person responsible, the applicant may appeal to HUFEA on giving notice to the committee and the Authority of that intention within 28 days of the service of the committee's determination on them (s. 20(1)). Notice, as discussed above, there is only one ground on which appeal lies against a committee's refusal to accede to a request to vary a licence. However, where a committee determines to allow a variation of a licence, an appeal lies at the suit of any person on whom notice of the determination was served. The appeal may be against the extension or the limitation of a current licence. There is however a restriction upon appeal by persons who have no other interest except that they applied for the variation. This means that although a concerned member of the public may bring to HUFEA's attention the existence of grounds for investigating a licence holder, they may not appeal against the committee's determination. Where an appeal does lie, again 28 days notice of the intention to appeal must be given to the committee and HUFEA.

Any appeal under s. 20 must be heard by the full Authority; the appellate function cannot be delegated to a committee, member or employee of HUFEA, the quorum for an appeal is five members of the Authority (s. 20(6)) and any member of HUFEA who took part in the work of the licence committee which resulted in the determination under appeal is disqualified from sitting on the appeal (s. 20(3)). This accords with ordinary principles of natural justice (see *R* v *Barnslay MBC ex parte Hook* [1976] 1 WLR 1052). An appeal takes the form of a rehearing (s. 20(3)) and the appellant is entitled to representation (s. 20(4)(a)), as are the members of the licence committee (s. 20(4)(b)). HUFEA is charged to consider any written representations made by the appellant or any licence committee member and to take into account any matter which the licence committee could have taken into account. Thus HUFEA is precluded from taking into account anything adduced by a member of the public, other than the grounds for their original complaint. The Authority must give notice of its determination to the appellant, and where the appeal has concerned an unsuccessful application for a licence under s. 16 or an unsuccessful application to vary a licence under s. 18(5), HUFEA must give reasons for its decision (s. 20(5)). In any case where the Authority decides under s. 20 to refuse a licence, to refuse to vary under a s. 18(5) application, or to vary or revoke a licence, an appeal on a point of law lies to the High Court, or in Scotland to the Court of Session (s. 21).

The provision that an appeal takes the form of a rehearing dictates the function of HUFEA as an appellate body. Without this provision, it might be assumed on general principles that HUFEA should review only the legality of the decision. Appeal by way of rehearing allows a consideration of all relevant and available evidence with a right of the appellate body to reach its own conclusions (see *Sagnata Investments* v *Norwich Corporation* [1971] 2 QB 614).

The Code of Practice

An important part of HUFEA supervisory functions will be to draw up and maintain in force a Code of Good Practice for licensed centres and individuals. The Code will give guidance about the proper conduct of licensed activities and of the discharge of the functions of the individual under whose supervision those activities are carried on and of any other persons to whom a licence applies (defined in s. 17(2)). In particular, s. 25(2) states that the Code will give guidance to those licensed to provide treatment services about the account which is to be taken (under s. 13(5)) of the welfare of children born following treatment services. The Code will specify also the account which is to be taken of the welfare of any other children affected by the birth of children of assisted conception.

The Parliamentary debates indicate that the Code will deal with such matters as the counselling arrangements which have to be made available to those about to undergo treatment services under s. 13(6) and those about to donate gametes or embryos under sch. 3, para. 3(1)(a). Included here will be matters such as the qualifications which would be necessary for those undertaking the counselling to possess. The Department of Health has commissioned research from the Institute of Population studies at the University of Exeter to prepare a report on the current provision of counselling in IVF centres in the UK, and that report will clearly form part of the background to the drafting of the Code. In addition, the Department has commissioned a booklet for women and men undergoing treatment services which will contain information about the prospects of triplets and other higher order multiple births. This is being produced in the Child Care Development Group in Cambridge.

The Code will also include provisions which deal with: the confidentiality of records maintained in pursuance of the Act; the arrangements which will be made for securing the necessary consents under sch. 3; screening procedures for sperm and egg donors and guidance on limits to be placed on the number of uses of donated sperm and eggs; the appropriate laboratory standards to be maintained, and the qualifications and experience of staff to be employed in licensed centres. The means of involvement of local ethical research committees will also be included in the Code. The degree of autonomy allowed to individual centres to develop services as they see fit is reflected in this outline of the provisions which the Code will contain. After consultation and discussion within the Authority, it is likely that its ambit will be markedly extended, but it forms an important aspect of the regulatory system which the Act establishes. Two different levels of 'enforcement' of compliance with the Code are envisaged.

Failure of any affected person to observe a provision of the Code is not, of itself, sufficient to render a person liable to civil or criminal proceedings. But a licence committee may take into account the provisions of the Code and their observance or breach when it is considering whether or not to vary or revoke a licence under s. 18 (s. 25(6)(b)). And a committee must when considering whether there has been a failure to comply with licence conditions (a breach of the duty which is imposed on the person responsible by s. 17(1)(e) for which a committee may revoke or vary a licence (s. 18(1)(c), (3)) take account of any relevant provision of the Code, especially where those licence conditions require anything to be 'proper' or 'suitable' (s. 25(6)(a)).

The legislation is littered with such adjectives. These include 'proper records' (s. 12(d)), 'proper counselling' and 'relevant information as is proper' under s. 13(6) and sch. 3, paras. 3(1)(a) and (b); 'suitable opportunities for counselling' under s. 13(6) and sch. 3, para. 3(1)(a), 'suitable procedures' under s. 13(7)(a) and (b) for determining the matters there referred to. They do not include 'suitable person' (s. 16(2)(b)(ii)) or 'suitable premises' (s. 16(2)(d)) because they relate to a condition for the grant of a licence and not a licence condition, nor similar words used in s. 18 which deal with the conditions for revocation or variation of a licence. But they may include the duty imposed under s. 17. If the discharge of the duty imposed on the person responsible under s. 17(1) is regarded as a condition of a licence, then these must be taken into account under s. 25(2)(a). Such duties may include those to ensure: the employment of 'suitable persons' (s. 17(1)(a) and the use of 'suitable practices' in the course of licensed activities (s. 17(1)(d)); that 'proper equipment' is used (s. 17(1)(b)); and that 'proper arrangements' are made for keeping gametes and embryos and disposing of those which have been allowed to perish (s. 16(1)(c)). In addition to the reliance on the Code by the committees, it may be utilised by both the civil and criminal courts as an appropriate evidential yardstick. This may be in the context of the judicial review of, for example, the reasonableness of a decision to refuse or revoke a licence. In relation to the criminal law provisions of the Act, the Code may be taken as a measure of the appropriate standards of conduct. The growth of codes published under statutory authority by statutory bodies has grown considerably in recent years. It is clear from such contexts as employment law that Codes of Practice from both ACAS and the Secretary of State have an effect such that for practical purposes they can be regarded as a statement of the requirements imposed both by the tribunals and the courts.

The Code is to be published following the approval of a draft by the Secretry of State (s. 26(1)) and come into force in accordance with directions under s. 23 (s. 26(5)). The initial draft must be drawn up after consultations, both with parties nominated by the Secretary of State and with any other persons which HUFEA thinks appropriate (s. 26(3)), and delivered to the Secretary of State within twelve months of the establishment of HUFEA under s. 5 (s. 26(1); HUEFA came into being on 7 November 1990 (see 'Commencement' below,

p. 184. An approved draft must be laid before Parliament, and the Secretary must give reasons if it is proposed to reject the draft (s. 26(1), (4)). It is not clear if this refers to a rejection of the whole or any part of the code, a distinction which appears in s. 25(4) empowering the Authority to revise the Code, but not in s. 26(4). It appears that the Secretary of State must give reasons to HUFEA for not approving any individual provision, for in not doing the draft is disapproved of, no matter how minor the disapproval. A revised or further draft Code likewise needs the Secretary of State's approval (s. 26(2)).

Storage Licences

Treatment licences and licences authorising a specific project of research are dealt with, respectively, in the chapters which cover Treatment Services and Embryo Research. Here, however, it will be convenient to deal with the conditions under which a storage licence may be issued, and the effects of such licences.

A storage licence may be issued in its own right or in conjunction with a research or a treatment licence. A storage licence, which may authorise the storage of both embryos and gametes (sch. 2, para. 2(1)) may be granted for any period up to a maximum of five years (sch. 2, para. 2(3)). It will permit the freezing and storage of gametes for 10 years (s. 14(3)) and embryos for 5 years (s. 14(4)), after which they must be allowed to perish (s. 14(1)(c)). An embryo which is created from stored gametes may itself be stored for the full length of the applicable storage period. Thus, an embryo created from gametes which have been stored for say, eight or nine years, or right up to the ten year limit, may then be frozen and stored for the maximum period allowed for the storage of embryos. Hence, an embryo could be used in the provision of treatment services or for the purposes of research for a maximum period of up to 15 years after the egg or sperm from which it derives was donated. No gametes, nor any embryo which was created *in vitro,* nor an embryo obtained by lavage may be stored unless there is an effective consent by, respectively:

(i) the person whose gametes they are,
(ii) the people whose gametes were used to create the embryo or the woman from whom the embryo was obtained, and unless
(iii) the gametes or embryos are stored in accordance with those consents (s. 12(c), sch. 3, para. 8(1)-(3)).

Section 14(5)(a) contains a power to provide in regulations for a shorter maximum period of storage, and s. 14(5)(b) envisages the occurrence of a particular case or type of case in which a longer period may be thought appropriate. This may arise where a young person, usually a man, presents for certain type of treatments which may render him sterile, and where he (and his partner) may wish to store his sperm enabling its later use in a treatment service. Such an example might occur in treatments for Hodgkin's disease or testicular cancer.

Section 14(1) envisages four types of provider for embryos or gametes which may then be stored:

(i) sperm donation;
(ii) egg donation;
(iii) an embryo created *in utereo* and obtained following lavage;
(iv) an embryo created *in vitro*.

In respect of (i), (ii) and (iii), the gametes or the embryo may only be placed in storage if received from a consenting donor or from another licensed centre (s. 14(1)(a)).

Embryos created *in vitro* by someone other than the licence holder (a storage licence may also authorise bringing about the creation of an embryo under sch. 2, para. 1(1)(a)) may be stored only if it is acquired from another licensed person. Section 14(1)(a) is ambiguous on the point of whether that licence must be one which authorises the creation of embryos *in vitro*, or, as the section provides ex facie, whether they are licensed only for the purposes of storage, or for providing treatment services or research, either of which may authorise the bringing about the creation of an embryo *in vitro* (sch. 2, paras. 1(1)(a) and 3(1)(a)). The wording of s. 14(1)(a) seems to contemplate that an embryo may be placed in storage by a duly authorised person even if it is created by someone who is not licensed to bring about the creation of an embryo, as long as they are 'a person to whom a licence applies.' The section contains no limitation such as 'a relevant licence' nor does it say that an embryo created *in vitro* may only be placed in storage if received from a person who is licensed to bring about the creation of embryos *in vitro*. It is true that it would be more consistent with the general scheme of the Act for the section to be read in the more restrictive way, and for an embryo to be stored only if it is received from a person who is licensed to bring about the creation of embryos. The other interpretation contemplates the storage of embryos even if they are received from a person who is not licensed to create them, and who may indeed commit an offence if that creation is done deliberately.

However, s. 41, which makes further provision with respect to offences, ensures that a person accused of the offence of unlicensed creation of an embryo (under s. 3(1)) has a defence in showing that they took all such steps as were reasonable and exercised all due diligence to avoid committing the offence (s. 41(11)(b)). So the wider interpretation of s. 14(1)(a) may be to make provision for a person who is licensed to provide treatment services, but who does not have the necessary facilities or personnel to carry out proper *in vitro* fertilisation, and who mistakenly produces an embryo which may then lawfully be passed on to a licensed storage facility. The storer may later pass on the embryo to another treatment facility and the embryo may be lawfully used for the purpose of assisting a woman to become pregnant.

Embryos may not be placed in storage at all if they have been created *in vitro* by an unlicensed person (s. 14(1)(a)) and an embryo which has been 'appropriated' for the purposes of any project of research may not be kept or used other than for such a project (s. 15(4)), whether it has in fact been used in such research or not.

Chapter 5
Regulating Clinical Practice: Treatment Services

In this chapter we turn to consider the areas of clinical practice with assisted conception the Act seeks to regulate and those which it is suggested are excluded from review. We also consider the statutory limitations on access to licensed assisted conception centres introduced by s. 13(5), and the the requirement of s. 13(6) that before certain treatment services are offered to a woman or a couple they should be provided with the opportunity to receive counselling. And we examine the question of consent to which all assisted conception services give rise. Here, we consider the requirements of the Consent schedule, sch. 3, and the background common law aspects of consent which are relevant to a proper understanding of Assisted Conception Law. We also argue that the focus of attention upon embryo research and abortion has detracted from a proper examination of the scope of clinical regulation which the Act envisages.

The layout of this chapter is as follows:

1. What are 'treatment services'?
2. Why regulate treatment services?
3. IVF, IVC and GIFT
4. Consent to Treatment
5. Issues of Clinical Freedom
6. Consent requirements of sch. 3
7. Posthumous treatments
8. Treatment licences, s. 13
9. Access to treatment services: s. 13(5) and the concept of welfarism
10. Counselling: s. 13(6)

Treatment Services and Treatment Licences

What Are Treatment Services?

Treatment services are medical, surgical or obstetric services provided to the public or a section of the public for the purpose of assisting women to carry children (s. 2(1)). A treatment service may only be provided to a woman when 'account has been taken' of:

(i) 'the welfare of any child who may be born as a result of the treatment (including the need of that child for a father)'; and
(ii) 'any other child' who may be 'affected by the birth.' (s. 13(5)).

The Government's clear intent in its introduction to the legislation was to place a restraint on the provision of certain modes of assisted conception to certain groups or types of women or couples. In spite of the clarity of intent, the actual wording of the section gives rise to considerable levels of ambiguity which we address in our discussion of 'Access to Treatment Services' (infra).

The Act covers five main types of 'infertility treatment' or as we term it, assisted conception:

(a) AID — artificial insemination by donor;
(b) Egg donation;
(c) Embryo donation;
(d) IVF — *in vitro* fertilisation, where an embryo is created outside the human body;
(e) GIFT — gamete intrafallopian transfer — where either the sperm or the egg being used has been donated.

Two main types of assisted conception are excluded from the ambit of the Act:

(i) AIH — the artificial insemination of a woman with the sperm of her husband, and AIP — the artificial insemination of a unmarried woman with her partner's sperm, neither of which involves the use of donated gametes from outside the treated couple; and
(ii) GIFT where the gametes (egg and sperm) come from the woman being treated and her husband or partner.

This new lexicon of life has given rise to the need to provide a quick guide to the treatments considered and related matters. We have attempted to do this in the Glossary. It is fashionable to refer to artificial insemination, whether by donor or husband or partner, simply as AI, to avoid confusion of association with AIDS. We have retained the more precise formulations in this chapter.

The inclusion and exclusion of certain types of treatment is ensured by the wording of ss. 1(2) and 4(1)(b). These provide respectively that:

> This Act, so far as it governs the bringing about the creation of an embryo applies only to bringing about the creation of an embryo outside the human body, and in this Act —

(a) references to embryos the creation of which was brought about *in vitro* (in the application to those where fertilisation is complete) are to those where fertilisation began outside the human body whether or not it was completed there . . .

and

No person shall in the course of providing treatment services for any woman, use the sperm of any man unless the services are being provided for the woman and the man together or use the eggs of any other woman except in pursuance of a licence.

Hence, the intention is to regulate IVF (s. 1(2)) and IVC (s. 1(2)(a)) and not GIFT unless it involves the use of donated sperm or eggs (ss. 1(2), 4(1)(b)). We consider whether this intention has been effected by this wording, infra. Hence, it is apparent that this Act is not meant to be a comprehensive code covering all the legal and ethical issues to which the 'reproduction revolution' has or may give rise. This was recognised by Lord Mackay when he said that this was a limited measure when set in the context of infertility treatment as a whole (House of Lords, Official Report, 7 December 1989, col. 1004). For a comprehensive account of the legal regulation even of assisted conception, one would need also to consider other statutory provisions such as the Surrogacy Arrangements Act 1985 and regulations to be made under the authority of this Act, and, more broadly speaking, the general civil law, which would include such matters as negligence, strict product liability, probate and property rights, contract law, liability of donors for the provision of goods or of services in respect of egg or sperm donation, family law provisions and so on.

Why Regulate Treatment Services?

In their Foreword to the *Fifth Annual Report of the Interim Licensing Authority* (ILA), established by the Royal College of Obstetricians and Gynaecologists and the Medical Research Council, Mary Donaldson wrote:

We have been disturbed at the increase in the number of small IVF centres seeking to establish themselves without the necessary facilities, adequately trained staff or the requisite specialist supervision. We are also aware of the poor success rates in a number of established and licensed centres. In the interests of women seeking treatment the Authority has decided that those centres whose pregnancy and 'take home' baby rates show little or no success over the next 12 months will be warned that their licences might be withdrawn (p. 2).

Mary Donaldson here identifies two separate problems. The first is the standards — physical and professional — of those engaged in the provision of treatment services, and of the plant and associated services which they can offer. The second is the whole enterprise of assisted conception itself. It has, indeed, a low 'success rate'; the provision of service is little known or discussed outside a very limited circle, and the fundamental issues which lie behind treatment services, such as embryo research, have not until late been the subject of exhaustive and thoroughgoing examination and debate. Much of that has changed in the course of one Parliamentary session.

In the ten years which ensued after the birth of Louise Brown in 1978, various national governments began to get to grips with the legal, social and moral issues at stake in the 'reproduction revolution.' It did not go entirely without question that the provision of assisted conception treatments was an unqualified human good; and in particular the debate about the use of human embryos for the purposes of non-therapeutic research was strongly contested (see Chapter 3). But for a long time, the major questions about the provision of 'treatments' for or to circumvent 'infertility' were conducted, at an official level at least, with an air of critical indifference. Feminist analysis was both most sympathetic and most questioning of the nature, methods and rationale of assisted conception (for a selection of this voluminous literature see Renata Duelli Klein, *Infertility,* (1989), Pandora Press; Patricia Spallone, *Beyond Conception,* (1989), Macmillan; Gena Corea, *The Mother Machine,* (1988 ed.), The Women's Press, cp, Michelle Stanworth, *Reproductive Technology,* ch. 1). Established religious responses, while not uniform, were not overtly sympathetic to the project (cp. the contrasting approaches of the Roman Catholic Church, best expressed in *Instruction on Respect for Human Life in its Origin and on the Dignity of Procreation,* (1987), and of the Church of England in *Personal Origins, The Report of a Working Party of the Board for Social Responsibility on Human Fertilisation and Embryology,* (1985)).

The types of risk to which IVF may give rise were reviewed by Chris Anne Raymond in '*In Vitro* Fertilisation Enters Stormy Debate as Experts Debate the Odds' (*Journal of the American Medical Association,* 22-29 January 1988 pp.464-65). In this, Raymond noted that the miscarriage rate for IVF pregnancy is 20-35%, which is approximately equal to the miscarriage rate for normal pregnancy. Of the risks associated with treatment, she pointed out that ovarian hyperstimulation can give rise to the development of ovarian cysts, with accompanying abdominal discomfort or severe pain. Ovarian cysts may rupture, resulting in bleeding into the abdominal cavity which may require surgery and the removal of all or part of the affected ovary. Ovarian hyperstimulation can also lead to temporary or permanent ovarian dysfunction. (For further catalogues of the physical and emotional costs of IVF see Linda S Williams, 'No Relief Until the End' in Christine Overall, (ed.), *The Future of Human Reproduction* (1989), The Women's Press) pp. 120-38 and importantly, Lesley Brown and John Brown, with Sue Freeman, *Our Miracle Called Louise* ((1979), Paddington Press; it is often forgotten that the Browns had a child of his first marriage. We discuss other health risks to which a woman undergoing assisted conception may expose herself in, infra, p. 128.)

These concerns were echoed in an important exchange in *The Lancet* in late 1989. It is illustrative of the nature and moment of this debate. In a paper entitled 'Are *In Vitro* Fertilisation and Embryo Transfer of Benefit to All?' Marsden Wagner of the World Health Organisation European Office and Patricia St Clair from the Department of Health Services at the University of Washington raised fundamental questions about the provision of assisted conception treatments (*The Lancet,* October 28, 1989, p. 1025). The response which their essay provoked was spirited, and taken together with the original article help to understand why the need to regulate infertility treatments had come to be seen as pressing.

In their article, Wagner and St Clair argued that the efficacy, costs and benefits of IVF and embryo transfer (ET) were not sufficient to suggest that programmes should be continued. They argued — in common with other previous critics — that resources should be concentrated on the prevention of infertility. IVF and ET programmes and associated assisted conception procedures had not been screened and monitored in a way which was appropriate to their experimental status. They raised major questions about the efficacy of treatment programmes. For example, they suggested that when outcomes are related to all stimulation cycles, reported studies revealed between 11.6 clinical pregnancies and 8.3 livebirth pregnancies per 100 stimulation cycles, to 10.3 livebirth pregnancies per 100 stimulation cycles for IVF/ET and GIFT combined. They concluded that: 'There are no reliable data on the number of healthy babies per stimulation cycle, although it is estimated to be 4-5%' (ibid, p. 1028).

In questioning the safety of assisted conception programmes, they reviewed the risks to the foetuses associated with multiple pregnancies, and then commented on the risks to the pregnant woman:

> Complications linked with the induction of superovulation by fertility drugs include ovarian hyperstimulation syndrome, cysts, coagulation abnormalities leading to thromboembolism, stroke, myocardial infarction, molar pregnancy, and ovarian cancer. Ectopic pregnancy rates are high, but it is not clear whether this is due to IVF/ET or to pre-existing tubal disease (ibid).

They reviewed data for the costing of assisted conception, in which they factored not only the successful treatment outcomes, but also the failures. With a success rate of about 1:10, they estimated that the true cost of each live born child following assisted conception to be at least $40-50,000, with associated public and private health care costs, many of which are hidden in private caring, stress and grief. In discussion, they raised the question of whether the costs and the benefits were not completely disproportionate:

> To the few infertile women who give birth to healthy babies as a result [of treatment], and to the clinicians who assist them, the benefit is enormous. But policy makers must balance such benefits against the disadvantages to society. No country can afford to transplant every failing heart, dialyse every failing kidney, or offer IVF/ET to every infertile woman. If money is spent on IVF/ET, then some other service cannot be funded. . . . Until full appraisal of the short-term and long-term risks and estimation of efficacy, IVF/ET must be considered experimental, and public and private insurance funds for health services should not be used for IVF/ET' (ibid. p. 1029).

Issue was quickly joined with many of the assessments and the data on which Wagner and St Clair based their conclusions (see the collected letters in *The Lancet,* December 2, 1989). In these, more recent data for outcome were reported, the costs figure suggested earlier was questioned, and Wagner and St Clair's (under)estimation of the strength of people's desire to have children was attacked. The results of a small sample survey which assessed the trade-off functions of people in their desire to have a child was used as the basis of an argument that 'the resources allocated to chemotherapy of solid tumours, which at best may delay death by a few months or years, could be better directed to the treatment of infertility' (Dalton and Lilford, at p. 1327); while Page and Brazier argued that the cost per QALY (Quality Adjusted Life Year) calculation for infertility 'compares favourably with other medical procedures'. (Ibid, p. 1328). All of the responses, however, agreed with the need for accurate information about efficacy, risks and costs, and for the objective assessments of those data. In a particularly forceful response, Braude, Johnson and Aitken took issue with Wagner and St Clair's data and conclusions, but then entered a strong case for full and effective regulation:

> When Wagner and St Clair discuss social and medical issues they make a curious distinction. Cancer, leprosy, and syphillis were all 'social issues' until they became treatable. Application of this distinction implies that we never make progress. Progress means research, control and audit. These are the pleas of Wagner and St Clair and sentiments of the Warnock Report. Medical scientists have for many years been asking for responsible legislation so that these goals can be achieved under a supervisory body. Restrictive legislation, which bans research on fertilised eggs and the early pre-embryo, will slow improvements in the efficacy of IVF and GIFT and in the methods of preventing higher order multiple pregnancies as a consequence of IVF and GIFT, and will stop the development of techniques for preimplantation diagnosis of genetic disease and safer contraception (ibid., p. 1329).

In a rejoinder (*The Lancet,* December 16, 1989), the original authors countered the arguments presented by the clinicians. Particularly, they took issue with the high valuation placed on infertility treatments when compared with, say, cancer or neonatal intensive care (citing a survey by Louis Harris reported in 'What to do in Covering Conception', *Business Health,* August 1989, 45-54). And they counter attacked the medicalisation of infertility and the application of a medical model in discussing it. Current provision does 'infertile people' a disservice, they argued:

> The inability to conceive a child may be emotionally traumatic but it is not a threat to health. Moreover, cancer, leprosy, and syphillis did not stop being social issues when they became treatable, and neither will infertility. Social and preventive solutions, therefore, must have first priority.

This exchange, coming relatively late in the debate about reproductive technologies and assisted conception, is important. It helps to illustrate some of the most salient arguments in the opposing considerations of the acceptability and advisability of assisted conception. But it also demonstrates that the debate is an organic, dynamic one, which needs some occasional reference points and benchmarks. The development of technological capability and therapeutic sophistication since the watershed publication of the Warnock Report in 1984, which foreshadowed eventual legislation, made the present case for formal regulation pressing. But, as we have argued in Chapter 1, it is a temporary marshalling of arguments and evidence. The enactment of a statutory licensing scheme with a supervisory body — HUFEA — now gives a focus and a channel through which that evidence and those arguments can be filtered. Whether HUFEA becomes subject to the classic public law weaknesses of capture or underfunding remains to be seen.

One simple example will suffice to illustrate the way in which the need for legislation became more apparent. Until the Act comes into force there are no legislative limits on the number of times which a given donor's semen may be used in order to attempt to produce a fertilised egg or an embryo. In debate, the Government defeated an amendment which sought to oblige the Secretary of State to lay down in regulations a limit to the number of times that donated gametes could be used in order to try to lessen the chances of 'unwitting incest', between children of a particular individual or even between a donor and one of his genetic offspring. The Warnock Report (1984) had recommended that there should be a maximum limit of ten donations (para. 4.26), but the White Paper delivered the view that the Government thought that this would be 'virtually impossible' to enforce, given the difficulties of identifying births following donations and the gap between donation and any resulting birth (para.87).

This was one of the consequences following on the White Paper's discussion and rejection of the suggestion that there should be a statutory duty placed on the recipients of treatment services to report any subsequent birth either to the treating clinic or directly to HUFEA. This was dismissed as 'an unacceptable intrusion on the privacy of couples,' (para. 86) and no further debate on this point seems to have been seriously mooted. Hence, it will be left to HUFEA to devise ways of recording information about 'any identifiable individual [who] was, or may have been, born in consequence of treatment services' (s. 31(2)). The Government has indicated that a restriction on donation uses is something which HUFEA will incorporate into its Code of Practice by way of guidance to clinics. The fear which many people have in respect of unlimited donations was the type of 'freak occurrence' brought to the notice of the House of Lords by Lord Jackobovits discussing a press report from the *Los Angeles Times,* (see House of Lords, Official Report, 7 December 1989, col. 1074). The report stated that the father of a woman who was about to be married told the groom that his daughter had been born following artificial insemination. The middle-aged groom made further enquiries as to when and where the insemination had taken place and discovered that his intended bride was his own genetic daughter, born following his sperm donation twenty years earlier. Whether this story is apocryphal, represents the rather clever manipulation by a man who disapproves of his daughter's choice of intended husband, or carries a contemporary moral warning about cross-generational marriage is unclear. It was sufficient to illustrate dramatically the point at issue (or the issue in point).

We turn now to consider how the statutory scheme introduces the regulation of treatment services.

IVF, IVC and GIFT

In debate on the Bill it was stated explicitly by the Government that only assisted conception involving the manipulation of the human embryo outside the body, or which in any way involves the use of donated gametes, was to fall within the scope of the Act. As we have already argued, this applies to IVF, where the embryo is created *in vitro*. It applies also to the other major form of treatment provision, GIFT, but only where that involves the use of donated gametes. Where GIFT is provided for a woman, or for a woman and a man together, using their own egg and sperm, it appears that the Government's intention was to bow to clinical pressure and exclude the service from the remit of HUFEA.

The Act also applies to IVC, intravaginal culture. This relatively new refinement of IVF was described in 1988 by Ramoux and colleagues at the Port Royal Hospital, Paris. They reported in *Fertility and Sterility* a new simplified method of IVF, which involved collecting eggs from a woman and placing them, with her partner's sperm, in a small tube containing culture fluid. The tube was sealed and placed into the patient's vagina and held in place with a contraceptive cap. After 48 hours the contents were removed and assessed; if fertilisation had taken place, the pre-embryos were replaced in the uterus as with standard IVF. Ramoux reported 100 treatment cycles, with 20 clinical pregnancies, and 15 deliveries involving 15 children. A randomised trial of 160 patients with standard IVF showed no difference in fertilisation rates, pregnancy rates or delivery rates etween the two procedures. IVC, while producing pregnancy rates no higher than with IVF may enable IVF treatment to become more widely available, and also to permit small GIFT Centres to transport their spare eggs to larger units with cryopreservation units. (When ss. 14(1)(a) and (b) of the Act come into force, this possibility will only be able to continue if the providing and the receiving hospital are licensed under the Act; a centre carrying out unlicensed GIFT will not be able to avail itself of this service to improve the clinical service which they offer, because they will not hold a licence as required under s. 14(1)(a)). IVC is covered by the Act because, although the gametes are placed together in a test tube in the woman's body, the creation of the embryo is in fact outside her body. (On IVC more generally, see Jonathan Hewitt, 'Intravaginal Culture (IVC)' in ILA '*Report of the Meeting for Centres and Ethics Committees — February 1990*' p. 4.)

In one clinic in Liverpool, Hewitt has provided GIFT since 1988 with a clinical pregnancy rate of 31%. IVC was introduced in 1989 and in that year the Unit performed 47 IVC cycles with 42 transfers and 8 clinical pregnancies. From January 1990 onwards, a further 8 cycles have produced 4 pregnancies. To date, 2 babies have been born, with one spontaneous abortion and the rest on-going pregnancies. IVC has two major advantages over GIFT; in the latter the fertilisation cannot be checked or assessed as it can with IVC and IVF, and the quality of the implanted embryo cannot be judged. Secondly, even if GIFT is performed, there may be a large number of spare oocytes which have to be disposed of, unless the clinic has cryopreservation facilities, which many do not. With IVC, it is possible to insert the intravaginal capsule the day following a GIFT procedure, and a woman so treated can then travel to another centre which has facilities and opportunities to assess the outcome of the IVC and, if fertilisation has taken place, to freeze the remaining pre-embryos. Such a collaborative programme has been undertaken by a hospital in Manchester and one in Liverpool.

There were several attempts during the Parliamentary debates to amend the Bill and bring GIFT within the purview of the Authority. An amendment at Committee stage in the House of Lords seeking to bring GIFT within the Authority's remit was withdrawn on assurance that the question would be reconsidered. Following that, in a division on a Commons amendment in Standing Committee to include GIFT, the amendment was defeated only on the casting vote of Michael Shersby, in the Chair, after the Committee divided 8/8 (House of Commons, Standing Committee B First Sitting, 1 May 1990, cols. 3-25). The Government announced its intention to resist these pressures to amend the Bill. When the Bill went to the Commons, Health Minister Virginia Bottomley reiterated the Government's aim to exclude GIFT. In the House of Lords Lord Mackay claimed that to regulate GIFT using the couples' own gametes would be the first step which could logically lead to a much greater degree of statutory regulation of medical treatment than envisaged in the White Paper (House of Lords, Official Report, 6 March 1990, col. 1089). He added that to licence GIFT would be the first step to licensing the use of the superovulatory drugs themselves. These arguments were not only a flawed appeal to the 'slippery slope' (is it a conceptual or logical slope which he has in mind, or is he fearful of an empirical slope?), it ignores crucial aspects of GIFT itself. For example, GIFT differs fundamentally from the use of such drugs alone because large numbers of eggs are removed from a woman and a decision is taken as to how many to return in a treatment cycle. The use of superovulatory drugs alone involves neither the manipulation of gametes nor clinical decisions as to their use.

The 1990 Act stands in interesting contrast with, for example, the comprehensive Spanish Law 35, Health: Assisted Reproduction Techniques of 22 November 1988, which regulates IVF, AI and GIFT. Despite the regulation-making powers which were introduced late in the parliamentary process (see now ss. 4(3), (4) and 25(3); the effects of which were elaborated by Lord Mackay, see House of Lords, Official Report, 18 October 1990, cols. 1110–11), this results in a less comprehensive regulatory code than in jurisdictions with more experience of attempts at self-regulation. The case of the Australian State of Victoria is instructive. Here, GIFT was brought within the statutory scheme of regulation after several years of trying to supervise it only through clinical good practice; see Infertility (Medical Procedures) Act 1984, s. 13A (introduced by the Infertility (Medical Procedures) (Amendment) Act 1987 (q.v. Stepan, *op.cit.*, pp. 157 et.seq., and 67–69). This present position adopted in the 1990 Act has important consequences for clinical practice (see *New Scientist* 31 March, 19 May 1990), which we discuss below.

In respect of GIFT alone the Government developed an extraordinary auditory defect. The careful formulation of policy advice based on scientific or biological criteria from interested parties such as the ILA, the MRC, embryologists, and those working in infertility, threatened to deafen those who came with an open mind and to drown out the issues of philosophy and ethics to which the legislators were more properly tuned. But in respect of GIFT that advice went unheeded. It is true that the chorus of that advice was not harmonious. For example, the Royal College of Obstetricians and Gynaecologists expressed their fear of excessive statutory regulation of clinical practice, and argued that to have included GIFT would have jeopardised the vote on embryo research. Some of the disagreement obscured central lessons which GIFT illustrates, that all assisted conception procedures, with the possible exception of AID and surrogacy, carry with them hazard, cost, invasiveness and low success.

A woman will usually have been on a regime of superovulatory drugs in order to stimulate the production of eggs, occasionally producing up to 20 in one menstrual cycle. GIFT involves obtaining ova (the female gamete or egg) or oocytes (female cells which have not yet developed into ovum) from a woman using ultrasound imaging. The gametes are then injected, with her husband's or donor sperm, directly into her fallopian tube, where fertilisation takes place. The most common use of GIFT is in the treatment of women who are infertile because sperm is prevented from fertilising naturally-produced ova by a blockage of mucus in the cervix of the uterus or womb.

GIFT appears one of the most clinically straightforward and financially accessible assisted conception services. However, there is concern that these potential benefits are being bought at a price which is medically unacceptable for the women involved, and emotionally extortionate in terms of the often unexplained or unexplored hazardous consequences of GIFT. There are doubts about its legality and the wisdom of leaving the resolution of such a difficult question to the courts.

Where GIFT is practised using donated gametes, it is within the ambit of the Act. But it is argued that GIFT using the couple's own gametes is not.

Why Should GIFT Be Regulated?

There are two distinct types of reason for arguing that GIFT should be subject to the same sort of statutory regulation as IVF. First, there are a number of problems which surround GIFT procedures which are virtually indistinguishable from those attendant upon IVF. We here identify three. Secondly, there are dangers associated with the use of GIFT itself which, we argue, give rise to sufficient concern for statutory rather than professional self-regulation to have been introduced.

First, then, the similarities with other, regulated, assisted conception treatments:

1. The critical issue at stake here is not only a concern with the embryo or foetus which is produced, but with the welfare and interests of the woman or the couple using this form of treatment service. The 'infertility work up' which a woman has to undergo is similar in GIFT to that in IVF. Both involve the use of superovulatory drugs to stimulate the production of multiple eggs. This carries

with it a small risk of ovarian hyperstimulation syndrome, which might well be missed in a small clinic providing few treatment services on an annual basis, compared with the many hundreds provided in a duly licensed centre which offers both IVF and GIFT.

2. The only real difference between GIFT and IVF is that the sperm and the egg mix to form a fertilised egg inside rather than outside the body. While it is true that this does not give rise to exactly the same problems with respect to the embryo, it does involve the same sort of clinical manipulation of gametes. The similarity is such, with attendant risks for the health of a resulting embryo and for the continuing health of the woman, that the monitoring, supervision and licensing, the keeping of records and making returns, the assessment of the fitness of the clinicians in charge to run such programmes, involve so closely related issues that GIFT should be within the licensing scheme.

3. One report, which combined data from clinics in nine countries, ranked the chief diagnosis among GIFT patients as unexplained infertility. Allied with this were endometriosis and male infertility. Overall, 29% of the stimulation cycles resulted in clinical pregnancies, making GIFT biologically competitive with, if not superior to IVF. It is unlikely, however, that GIFT will replace IVF because in most cases of damage to the oviducts GIFT is not an available option. With GIFT the gametes need to be placed in the oviduct, whereas in IVF the fertilised ova are placed in the uterus, it is only in certain types of infertility that GIFT is possible. On the other hand, it might be thought that GIFT is more likely to gain ground as it poses fewer technical barriers. Unlike IVF, no requirement exists for expertise in or a facility for handling embryo culture. But its major clinical drawbacks are that it provides no diagnostic information where pregnancy does not result; defects in the fertilising ability of the sperm or oocytes that might have been identified during IVF can go unnoticed; and unlike IVF, GIFT usually requires the woman to undergo general anaesthesia.

Now we turn to consider intrinsic reasons why GIFT should be the subject of statutory regulation rather than left to the vagaries of the common law. We identify four such arguments, three of which relate to the problems of higher order pregnancies — where three, four or more eggs are transferred as part of the treatment. First, however, there is the broad question of the proper maintenance of clinical standards. In the Fourth Report of the ILA, published in 1989, the Authority expressed its view that GIFT treatments should be included in any regulatory scheme and that presently it is not always practised 'in a satisfactory setting with the necessary back-up facilities' (p. 2, Foreword; and see p. 13 para. 5.2 and pp. 17-18, Table II). Furthermore, while the current ILA Guideline 12 provides that no more than three eggs (or pre-embryos in IVF) should be transferred in any one treatment cycle, unless there are 'exceptional' reasons justifying the transfer of four, there is evidence that in the absence of effective regulation practitioners are transferring four or more eggs without good clinical reason.

The second reason for monitoring GIFT follows from this. Multiple transfer of eggs, (some reports suggest up to 15 in the last few years) increases the risk of triplet or higher order pregnancy. This may occur either because: all the eggs fertilise and implant; or because one or more of the fertilised eggs may divide, increasing further the number of embryos; or because not all of the eggs were successfully extracted after superovulation, thus creating the risk that some of those may be fertilised as well as those replaced during the GIFT treatment. It is suggested that these higher order transfers are being undertaken in order to increase the 'success rates' of clinics' treatment service programmes. Multiple pregnancy is then either maintained, with increased risks to the pregnant woman, or some of the foetuses are aborted in a procedure which has become misleadingly known as selective reduction and which is more accurately called 'random reduction'. This carries risks for the pregnant woman, and for the remaining foetuses which are not aborted.

The third major cause for disquiet is that these higher order pregnancies are attended with major risks of morbidity and mortality. For example, the risk of stillbirth is 6 times higher than for a singleton pregnancy and the risk of death in the infant's first year is about 10 times higher. The rate of death below the age of one is 8.5 per 1,000 for singletons. With twins this rises to 44.7 per 1000, and for triplets and other higher order births the rate is 92.5 per 1,000. A similar discontinuity is evident in the risk of stillbirths, where the figures per 1,000 are respectively 5.0, 18.3 and 32.9.(See OPCS, Mortality Statistics [for 1986], Series DG3.) This data can now be supplemented with the figures obtained from the Report of the MRC Working Party on Children Conceived by *In Vitro* Fertilisation, a summary of which appears in (1990) *British Medical Journal* 1229-33 and in the ILA Fifth Report, pp. 31-34. These data lend support to the conclusions suggested by the OPCS:

> Overall, perinatal and infant mortality rates were about twice the national average at 27.2 per 1,000 births and 23.7 per 1,000 live births respectively. However, once allowance is made for multiplicity and maternal age, the observed numbers of deaths were similar to those expected on the basis of national rates. The perinatal mortality rates were 11.7 per 1,000 in singleton, 39.7 per 1,000 in twins and 79.3 per 1,000 in triplets and higher order births. The corresponding numbers for infant mortality were 10.7, 34.1 and 69.2 per 1,000 live births, respectively. . . . In summary, the evidence from this study suggests that the most important determinant of the health of these children in the perinatal period is the high frequency of multiple births (ILA, p. 34).

Compared with singletons, twin, triplet or higher order pregnancies have much higher rates of congenital malformations visible from birth. And in addition to the demands made by such births on chronically stretched neonatal intensive care facilities, the ongoing financial costs to the health services are considerable; one private IVF clinic has entered into an agreement with the local district general hospital to fund extra provision in its paediatric facilities. But most poignant are the costs, usually hidden, to the erstwhile hopeful and expectant parents. Only recently, when some of the aggressively marketed successes have been eclipsed by the failures and the frustrations of multiple births of children with massive debilitating disablement, has this factor entered into the equation. The widely reported experiences of Helen Pusey must give any clinic pause in its treatment zeal to consider its legal liability. Helen Pusey suffered temporary blindness, kidney failure and pleurisy at the end of her quadrupule GIFT pregnancy waiting for an emergency caesarean. Two of the Pusey quads died, one twenty minutes after birth the other at five months; the two 'surviving' have multiple handicaps (see, for example, *New Statesman and Society,* May 1990).

Fourthly, triplet and other higher order births carry considerable financial and social consequences. Unless GIFT is included in a statutory scheme, couples opting for, or being directed towards GIFT will enjoy no statutory access to counselling. Arguably, these are the very people who are most likely to benefit from it; the Victorian legislation provides that counselling should be available prior to *and* after the GIFT procedure has been carried out (Infertility (Medical Procedures) Act 1984, s. 13A(3)(e)(ii)). Not only does counselling enable them to have a structured opportunity to consider the risk that the procedure may result in multiple birth and the implications which that has for them, but it provides a brake on the clinical zeal with which GIFT may be offered. In addition to its use where there is an identifiable reason for infertility, it is thought that GIFT is frequently offered for couples where the infertility remains unexplained. In other words, it may be that GIFT is coming to be seen as the treatment service of last resort, and that it is being offered where there is no good clinical indication for its use.

Has GIFT been excluded?

The Act prohibits several activities in the absence of a licence from HUFEA. It is an offence to provide 'treatment services' without a licence, unless the gametes are those of the couple being treated. And it is an offence to 'bring about the creation of an embryo' without an HUFEA licence. The Act as originally drafted provided no 'protection' to the developing conceptus until the end of the process of fertilisation, some 30 hours after its commencement. This caused concern and consternation, particularly amongst those implacably opposed to research of any kind. The Bill was consequently amended, and now defines an embryo as including 'an egg in the process of fertilisation.' In comparable Australian legislation fertilisation is defined as complete on the coming together on the first mitotic spindle of two sets of chromosome (see the Infertility (Medical Procedures) Act 1984 as amended by the Infertility (Medical Procedures) (Amendment) Act 1987). This 1987 amendment was introduced to bring GIFT within the ambit of the Standing Review Committee and to allow research on the process of fertilisation before syngamy on eggs not destined to be replaced. (Syngamy being defined to mean 'the alignment on the mitotic spindle of the chromosomes derived from from the pronuclei.')

Suppose that the UK Government has successfully negotiated their preferred view through the legislative process. Does it follow that GIFT is totally unregulated? We think not. In addition to the professional guidance which the Royal College of Obstetricians and Gynaecologists has now issued to its members, GIFT, as with other assisted conception techniques is subject to the law of consent. Here we now review questions which arise in respect of consent to treatment, before we consider the specific consent requirements introduced by s. 12(3) and sch. 3 of the Act.

Consent to Treatment

That there are certain acts which cannot be consented to is accepted law. (These are reviewed most recently in the Court of Appeal judgments of Lord Donaldson MR, Neill and Butler Sloss L JJ in *Re F; F* v *West Berkshire Health Authority* [1989] 2 WLR 1025, upheld on different grounds on appeal, [1989] 2 All ER 545, HL.) While the doctrine is sometimes thought of as highly paternalistic, (and for the most part so it is), it also serves moral purposes, wishing actively to discourage certain types of conduct or behaviour. One class of such is the deliberate exposure to risk of harm. It is held that it is not in the public interest that people should cause, or try to cause, actual bodily harm to others, without good reason. The determination of the public interest is a matter for the courts, applying (and this is of crucial importance here) any relevant statutory provisions, whether directly or by analogy, to the common law. With GIFT there is extant the ILA's own Guideline 12 which would almost certainly provide the precursor for the statutory regime under the eventual legislation in respect of GIFT using donated gametes. In addition, the RCOG '*Guidelines on Assisted Reproduction Involving Superovulation*', issued in August 1990, carries five important recommendations (see Appendix 5 for the Guidelines). Importantly, these include that prospective parents must be aware of the problems of multiple pregnancy and the potential risks which this carries during the antenatal, intrapartum and and neonatal periods, as well as the social and medical problems which can arise thereafter. In respect of GIFT and IVF, the advice follows that of the ILA and probably anticipates that of HUFEA, that not more than three oocytes in GIFT or three embryos in IVF should be replaced, except under exceptional circumstances, when a maximum of four may be transferred. The advice also reminds clinicians that:

> In 1988, more multiple pregnancies in the UK resulted from GIFT than IVF. Results in older women (over the age of 39), or when a male contribution to infertility occurs, are poor, so there is a natural temptation to replace more oocytes or embryos which should be resisted.

The analogous guidelines will determine how many eggs or embryos may lawfully (and this is the crucial point) be transferred. It seems inconceivable that these would not form the analogy to which any court would appeal in considering the legality of GIFT involving multiple egg transfer. The known increased risks to mother and to each established foetus in a higher order pregnancy have already been considered. In view of this and considering the existing ILA and RCOG Guidelines it is by no means impossible that, in certain circumstances, GIFT is, and will continue to be, unlawful at common law. It is difficult to outline these circumstances in depth, but it might be anticipated that the responsible clinical practitioner should seek to transfer fewer rather than more eggs, and if necessary, to perform fewer rather than more random reductions of multiple implanted pregnancies. At some point, the tolerance of the law to countenance certain acts might be stretched to the point that consent to multiple transfer would not be regarded as legally effective to defend against a later charge of trespass, whether raised by the woman herself, or by some third party. Recent reports of the routine transfer of four, five and even six eggs raise grave legal doubts; the transfer by one clinic in 1990 of seven eggs gives rise to clear cause for concern. And while legal uncertainty remains as to whether selective reductions constitute an abortion, the provisions of the 1967 Abortion Act should be complied with.

There is a second sense in which the law of consent impinges on the conduct of GIFT, again illustrated by Helen Pusey's case (*New Statesman and Society*, 11 May 1990, p. 12). According to her, the possibility of multiple birth following GIFT was mentioned only once, early in the morning minutes before the operation. Even the meagre legal requirements for disclosure of information and advice about a surgical procedure do not appear to have been complied with. Failure to discharge this duty may render a practitioner liable in negligence.

It is interesting to note that English law has developed notions of negligence rather than those of trespass, which we have just been considering, to address questions of consent. In *Chatterton* v *Gerson* [1980] 3 WLR 1003, the court refused to accept any notion of informed consent beyond the necessity of informing the patient in broad terms of the nature of any intended operative procedure. This judgment was endorsed, most notably in *Sidaway* v *Board of Governors of Bethlam Hospital* [1985] 1 All ER 643, where the wider point of precisely which risks ought to be disclosed by a doctor was canvassed. In this case, the House of Lords subsumed the duty to offer a patient sufficient warning under the general head of the doctor's duty of care in negligence. This means that a duty is owed, in practice, to each patient treated, but in determining whether that duty has been met the test is based much more upon what the doctor chooses to disclose rather than what the patient might want to know.

This results from the application, in determining the appropriate standards of care, of the principles in *Bolam* v *Friern Hospital Management Committee* [1957] 2 All ER 118:

> A doctor is not guilty of negligence if he has acted in accordance with a practice accepted as proper by a responsible body of medical men skilled in that particular art.

In the context of warnings and consent, the standard, once we govern these matters by negligence, therefore becomes such warnings as a responsible body of practitioners consider accepted practice, in this case in relation to infertility treatment services.

There are a number of obvious objections here, quite apart from the helplessness (not to say impotence) of the patients in controlling their therapeutic destiny. Implicitly the doctrine allows the doctor to dictate the standard to the court. The House of Lords show some consciousness of this in *Sidaway*, where they were at pains to stress that where it came to warnings, as opposed to diagnosis or treatment, the courts would remain the final arbiters of the test to be applied. Nonetheless, Lord Scarman was in dissent in his view that the standard should be based upon risks which the prudent patient would wish to be disclosed as significant.

This majority view prevailed in *Gold* v *Haringey Health Authority* [1987] 2 All ER 888, which involved the absence of warning of the risk of failure of a sterilisation operation. The question arose in this case as to what might be expected of a doctor in advising contraceptive services:

> The [*Bolam*] principle does not depend on the context in which any act is performed, or any advice given. It depends on a man professing skill or competence in a field beyond that possessed by the man on the Clapham omnibus. If the giving of contraceptive advice required no special skill, then I could see an argument that the *Bolam* test should not apply. But that was not, and could not have been suggested. The fact that (if it be the fact) giving contraceptive advice involves a different sort of skill and competence from carrying out a surgical operation does not mean that the *Bolam* test ceases to be applicable. It is clear from Lord Diplock's speech in *Sidaway* that a doctor's duty of care in relation to diagnosis, treatment and advice, whether the doctor be a specialist or a general practitioner, is not to be dissected into its component parts. To dissect a doctor's advice into that given in a therapeutic context and that given in a contraceptive context would be to go against the whole thrust of the majority of the House of Lords in that case. So I would reject the argument of counsel for the plaintiff under this head, and hold that the judge was not free, as he thought, to form his own view of what warning and information ought to have been given, irrespective of any body of responsible medical opinion to the contrary (per Lloyd L J at p. 894).

In the context of infertility treatment, with attendant risks of multiple order birth, this might imply a duty to warn of the possibility of more than one child (the experience of Helen Pusey, discussed supra), though not, for example, the social consequences of twins, triplets or quads. The possibility of superovulation or infertility treatment giving rise to a multiple pregnancy and birth would not be something, in the words of Lloyd LJ, within the common understanding of the passenger on the Clapham Omnibus. The social, physical and financial, and possibly the psychological costs of caring for multiple children would be thought to be.

All of this, however, assumes that a responsible body of medical opinion would warn of multiple order birth, or that this risk was 'substantial.' Both Lords Bridge and Templeman in *Sidaway* were of a view that certain risks were of such a magnitude that there could be no doubt that they must be disclosed to the patient. In the words of Lord Bridge, the court:

> . . . might in certain circumstances come to the conclusion that disclosure of a particular risk was so obviously necessary to an informed choice on the part of the patient that no reasonably prudent medical man would fail to make it (at p. 663).

The kind of risk which he had in mind was one such as a brain operation an operation involving a substantial risk of grave adverse consequences, such as a stroke. (Ibid)

Lord Bridge's own example here is interesting. He said that a 10% risk of serious adverse consequences would be 'substantial' such that the risk ought to be disclosed, irrespective of whether disclosure was the commonly accepted practice within the profession or not.

If we apply these arguments to the multiple pregnancy rate associated with GIFT and the consequent risks of disability or mortality in the resulting foetus or child, it is clear that these are obvious candidates for compulsory disclosure. To protect against liability in negligence for non-disclosure will mean time for discussion, reflection and judgment. That is precisely what the counselling opportunity demanded by the Act seeks to provide. Again, it will form the analogy against which a non-licensed centre's standards are judged.

Issues of Clinical Freedom

There are important issues of medical politics being played out in these debates and discussions. If unlicensed GIFT procedures can be performed at the burgeoning number of clinics not presently amenable to ILA review, this will represent a major threat to the financial viability of those programmes which will be subject to statutory control. The superficial attractiveness of centres which can offer what appear to be reduced cost treatment services will push many, and perhaps completely unsuitable women and couples, into unregulated GIFT programmes. The suggestion from the RCOG that procedures for monitoring GIFT should be established in a voluntary Code of Guidance prepared by HUFEA is undoubtedly an improvement on its unsupervised provision, and it is possible that an 'indirect' form of regulation is made possible by the late addition of GIFT to the matters on which HUFEA may give guidance in its Code of Practice (s. 25(3)), non-observance of which may be 'take[n] into account' by a licensing committee (s. 25(6)(b)). But whether that will afford anything more than a veneer of protection to women presenting for treatment services or indeed for participating clinics is doubtful.

For some couples or women, appearing to question the value of, or merits of, any treatment service, to highlight the risks and the costs, may come periously close to looking the proverbial gift horse in the mouth. There is real and increasing concern that the GIFT horse may be a Trojan horse. In truth, each of these procedures is so experimental as to justify proper regulation within the statutory scheme. It is widely thought that GIFT ought not to be left to develop in a haphazard and piecemeal way, to be offered to women in an indiscriminate and untutored fashion, and to be subject to loose professional or legal monitoring. The question raised is whose freedom is more important here; that of the woman undergoing the treatment service or of the clinicians to be able to develop services without a full understanding and disclosure of the complex risks, side effects and potential psychological damage which may follow. Unfortunately, early reports of the experiences with GIFT are not encouraging.

For example, in a paper entitled 'Early experience with gamete intrafallopian transfer (GIFT) and direct intraperitoneal insemination (DIPI)' published by M Doolet et al in (1988) 81 *J of the Royal Society of Medicine* 637-39, a favourable 29% pregnancy rate per treatment cycle and a 33% pregnancy rate per patient is reported. However, the the major caveat entered towards the beginning of the assessment is that: 'The individual cause of infertility was similar in both groups with the majority of patients having unexplained infertility' (p. 637; this accounted for over 60% of such patients).

The ILA's concern was clearly demonstrated in the responses which it had made, to the Government White Paper in its Third Report issued in 1988, where the ILA commented (at p. 42) that they found it 'inconsistent' that GIFT should be included within the remit of HUFEA only where donor gametes are used:

> For GIFT to be successful gamete preparation and quality control are essential. There also needs to be a restriction on the number of oocytes replaced and strict control of what happens to spare oocytes. It would be proper to licence all centres performing GIFT.

However, the ILA has consistently reported that it does not have the finance or the personnel to enable it to carry out this task. And in its Fifth Report issued in June 1990, it reports that:

> The number of centres offering GIFT is increasing; there are currently 36 licensed IVF centres offering this treatment and a further 45 centres unlicensed but registered with the ILA as offering GIFT. . . . It is a source of concern that many of the new 'IVF clinics' applying to the Authority for licensing in fact undertake a minimal amount of IVF but a substantial amount of GIFT (at p. 12).

When the ILA comes on to analyse the data provided by returns from licensed centres it reports that:

> the overall treatment and outcome data [show] the perinatal mortality rate [deaths] is 26.4 [per 1,000] and this is more than three times the national average. Prematurity associated with the high incidence of multiple births would be a major contributory factor to this wastage (p. 18).

The apparent freedom from review, vaunted by the RCOG, is more illusory than real. Faced with the Scylla of statutory control and the Charybdis of the common law, it is remarkable that the medical profession should want to sail through the channel on the raft of clinical freedom rather than in the more securely built, more easily navigable HUFEA. While s. 4(3) and (4) enables GIFT to be brought within the ambit of HUFEA, it is likely that that will take a number of years to achieve and there can be no guarantee that a Secretary of State for Health would accept a HUFEA recommendation to that effect anyway. Following any delay in implementing the Act, the monitoring procedures which the RCOG has said it will establish in respect of self-regulation of GIFT, and then reporting the results, will take time. Subsequent debate and further decisions about whether GIFT should then be licensed, together with Parliamentary inertia, debate and lobbying, ensure that bringing GIFT within the statutory scheme will take a matter of years rather than months.

Whatever the legislation has achieved, (many clinicians appear to believe it to be in their interests or that of their patients that GIFT be excluded from review), it is clear that there is a major policy issue at stake. GIFT is a straightforward obstetrical service which can be offered at District Hospital level. It has advantages for women concerned; it is quick, easy, and can ensure mobility soon after the procedure. It is claimed to offer the major flexibility that a woman can decide how many eggs she wishes to have transferred, (up to 15 have been publicly acknowledged), with subsequent reduction of established foetuses to the number she desires. But there are serious doubts as to the legality of this procedure, (as we discuss in Chapter 2 dealing with Abortion). As one commentator has argued, even compliance with the Abortion Act 1967 may be insufficient:

> . . . [that] act only affords protection when, in the words of section 1(1) 'a pregnancy is terminated.' As selective reduction results in the destruction of one or more but not all the foetuses, a court might rule that it does not terminate a pregnancy, and that compliance with the Abortion Act is ineffective (ILA, Third Annual Report, Appendix 4, p. 41).

We are doubtful whether the provision adopted in an attempt to resolve this confusion has been successful in this respect. It is important to note in this respect that the opinion of a majority of the Court of Appeal in *R* v *Salford Area Health Authority ex parte Janaway* [1988] 2 WLR 442, (a case involving the scope of the 'conscience clause' in the 1967 Act), that s. 1(1) created a defence whenever an offence would have been committed under s. 58 of the 1861 Act but for the existence of the 1967 Act, was rejected by the House of Lords when *Janaway* went on appeal ([1988] 3 All ER 1079).

As we have seen, one stated reason for seeking to exclude non-donated-gametes-GIFT is that it would both complicate the provision of superovulatory drugs and that it would have implications for the provision of AID or AIH services. The Government stated that this would involve unwarranted intrusion into family privacy. Neither of these are convincing reasons; either to exclude GIFT or to leave unregulated by HUFEA any other aspect of assisted reproduction. It has been suggested that one forceful reason why the procedure remains out with the statutory framework is in an effort to secure the compliance of the obstetricians and gynaecologists with the other regulatory aspects of the legislation. If this is true, it is another example of the clinical profession dominating input into the legislative process. It also illustrates the extent to which Parliament was prepared to defer to professional interest groups in order to find some way of taking on board some of the equally pressing issues raised by the original Warnock report, and of responding to the technological challenge posed by developments of the more recent past.

The Consent Requirements of the Act: Schedule 3

The consent requirements which are elaborated in sch. 3 play an important part in the determination of some substantive points of principle and practice which arise. Paragraph 4(1) provides that the terms of any consent in the third schedule may be varied or withdrawn at any time, unless the embryo has already been used in providing treatment services or for research purposes.

Section 12(c) requires that the provisions of the consent schedule 'shall be complied with as a licence condition'. Failure to observe the provisions of sch. 3 will breach the duty laid by s. 17(1)(e) upon the 'person responsible' for the licensed activities to ensure that the conditions of the licence are complied with. A breach of such duty, by proceeding (for example) without an effective consent, is presumably meant to be one ground for revocation of the licence under s. 18(1)(c). That section originally spoke of revocation where the person responsible 'is not discharging . . . the duty under section 17 . . .' It seems unlikely that this was meant to achieve the effect of revocation being possible only where there is a continuing course of conduct. Yet interpretation of an analogous provision, s. 210 of the Companies Act 1948, confirmed that the requirement that the affairs of the company 'were being conducted' in an unfair manner could not give rise to a complaint about a one-off infringement or a course of conduct which had now ceased. It seemed desirable to clarify this point otherwise the only remedy left against a 'responsible person' who had ignored the requirement for continuing consent would be an action for breach of statutory duty, with all the limitations and pitfalls of that procedure. The Act was subsequently amended in the light of representation to provide that a ground for revocation is that 'the person responsible has failed to discharge . . .' their duty (s. 18(1)(c)).

The consents provisions of sch. 3 are not just limited to the formal process of protecting the providers of treatment services. All consents must be in writing, and before consents to use or storage of gametes or embryos are given, a person must be given a 'suitable' opportunity to receive 'proper' counselling about the implications of such a step and 'such relevant information as is proper.' The consent includes the right to vary or withdraw consent by notification, unless the gametes or embryos have been used in treatment or research (sch. 3, paras., 3(1)(a)(b), (2) and (4)(2)(a), (b)). The vagaries of the adopted wording lead to the hope that there will be clarification by HUFEA in directions made under para. 2(3). Good practice, however, might dictate, at the least, that licence holders reaffirm the consents before proceeding with any irrevocable treatments or research, and that 'relevant', 'proper' information include such matters as the procedures' success rates, degrees of risk, alternatives, and the Centre's adopted policies (cp. the counselling requirements set out in the State of Victoria's Infertility (Medical Procedures) Regulations 1988, sch. 3). More challenging is the proposal that, given a Centre's financial interests in these procedures, the counselling be provided by trained, professional counsellors, independent of the Centre concerned (see, infra, p. 151). Given the fiscal burdens that the proposed legislation places on licensees, (see s. 16(1)), this requirement seems fundamental. In addition, the procedures of the Centre must ensure that 'inducements', such as a reduction or waiver of fees for the donation of 'surplus' eggs or embryos cannot be countenanced unauthorised unless within the scope of directions under s. 12(e).

Consents for the use of any embryo must specify to what use(s) it may be put and specify any conditions to that consent (sch. 3, para. 2(1)). An example might be whether gametes or embryo may be used only for the consent giver, or for any other people requiring treatment services or for the purposes of research.

In respect of gamete or embryo storage the maximum period of agreed storage must be specified in the consent. In addition, and importantly, the consent must address the question of what is to happen to stored gametes or embryos if the consent giver dies or becomes incapacitated and unable to revoke or vary their consent. The Act does not provide what should happen, it requires only that the consent giver(s) address the issue. This provision is inserted to obviate difficulties such as exemplified by the 'Rios embryos' and also requests for use of the embryos or gametes after the death of one consent giver. In the *Rios* case, the Rioses were Californian citizens and genitors of frozen embryos held in store in Melbourne when they were killed in a plane crash. They died intestate and the Californian intestate succession laws appeared to apply, giving a share of the estate to Mr Rios's son by a previous marriage and to Mrs Rios's mother. In December 1987, the California Superior Court declared Mrs Rios's mother to be the sole heir. The Medical Centre in Melbourne then declared that the embryos would be thawed and allowed to perish. This led to an outcry, culminating in the intervention of the State Minister of Health, who had to make special provision for them. In the event, the embryos were to be held in storage until a suitable recipient could be found, although the chances of survival were put at less than 5%.

It seems desirable that the powers granted to the Authority under para. 2(of sch. 3 to provide for other matters which must be dealt with in the consen include specific questions that should be addressed. For example, in the event death, does the surviving partner have the right of access to the gametes embryos? While s. 28(6)(b) provides that a man whose sperm, or an embryo derived in part from his sperm, is used after his death is not to be treated as the father of any resulting child, this is not directly relevant to the point here. Similarly, should the gametes or embryos be allowed to perish, or may they be used by the Authority? (see infra, pp. 138–39, Posthumous Treatments).

An important point of difference arises in respect of consent when dealing with embryos created *in vitro* and those obtained from a woman following lavage (recovering the embryo by flushing the uterus) or laparoscopy (a micro surgical technique which permits the recovery of the embryo instrumentally). The continued storage of embryos will depend on how the embryos were 'brought into being.' With an embryo created *in vitro* following gamete donation, the embryo may not be kept in storage without the effective consent (written consent which has not been withdrawn) of both gamete donors (sch. 3, para. 8(2)). Withdrawal of the consent of either donor to the embryo's creation appears to mean that it must be allowed to perish, although this does not appear explicitly stated. (This is the effect of reading together s. 12(c) and s. 14(1)(c), with sch. 3, para. 4(1) and 8(1), (2). Again, clarification would be welcome.)

Where the embryo has come into being in the woman's uterus and is subsequently extracted, not only may it not be used for any purpose unless the woman alone gives consent for that use (para. 7(1)), it may not be stored unless there is an effective consent by her, and her alone (para. 8(3)). This and the preceeding paragraphs appear to be the Government's chosen way of avoiding the litigation spawned over cryopreserved embryos in the divorce proceedings of *Davis* v *Davis* (15 Family Law Reporter 1551 (1989); on appeal West Law 130807 (Tenn App) (1990)) in the Tennessee Circuit Court and Court of Appeals. In the first instance, the Court had awarded 'custody' of seven cryopreserved fertilised ova to the now divorced wife in a divorce suit and declared that she should be 'permitted the opportunity to bring these children to term through implantation.' On appeal, the Court remanded the case to the Circuit Court to enter judgment vesting joint control in the former husband and wife (both now remarried) and giving them equal voice over their disposition. The Appeals Court held that awarding sole custody to Mary Sue Davis, such that she could attempt implantation without her former husband's consent, was impermissible state action. Judge Franks, writing the leading opinion, held that such an award infringed Junior Davis's constitutionally protected rights concerning procreation; in particular, that it might force him to become a parent against his will. The Appeals Court could find no compelling state interest to justify ordering implantation against the will of either party. To this extent, the lower court's action usurped the exercise by Junior of 'the decision whether to bear or beget a child [which is] a constitutionally protected choice' (Judge Franks, citing *Carey* v *Population Services International* 431 US 678 (1977) at 685 and *Griswold* v *Connecticut* 381 US 479, 485 (1965)). However nascent, this seems to recognise an emergent sphere of men's rights to control their fertility and conception, which will lead to a direct clash with women's rights (as in this case) and any emergent notion of foetal rights.

A consideration of the fertility treatment centre's handling of the case discloses some lessons from which the Government have clearly learnt. For example, there was no discussion between the Davises and the centre about the consequences of separation or divorce occurring while the ova remained frozen, nor were the Davises required to sign any agreement as to the terms of storage or disposition at the time the fertilised ova were cryopreserved. The 1990 Act attempts to address these questions. In the first case, where the embryo is brought about outside the body, under the Human Fertilisation and Embryology Act the woman's partner can effectively require the perishing of the embryo by withdrawing his consent; in the second case of an embryo recovered by lavage, he cannot (sch. 3, paras 4(1), 6(3), 8(3)). In both cases the woman can achieve this result (sch. 3, paras 4(1), 6(3), 7(1), 8(2), 8(3)).

Posthumous Treatments

The effect of reading together ss. 14(1)(b) and 4(1)(b) is that where a clinic decides, or the treatment services contract or agreement provides, that the death of one of the partners is to terminate the provision of treatment services, the other partner will have no *right* to insist on the clinic making available to them any stored gametes or embryos. If the clinic decides that it will, for example, honour the wishes which the now deceased partner was required to express as to use of stored gametes or embryos following their death (sch. 3, para. 2(2)(b), written consent '. . . must . . . state what is to be done with the gametes or embryo if the person who gave the consent dies . . .') that appears to be a matter for the exercise of clinical judgment and discretion. Otherwise, an embryo created *in vitro* may only lawfully be kept 'in storage' (cryopreserved in liquid nitrogen) with effective consent of both partners, whereas as an embryo which was formed within the woman's body and subsequently recovered surgically, (by lavage or laprascopy), may only be stored with the consent of the woman from whom it was obtained (sch. 3, para. 8(2) and 8(3) respectively).

Treatment Licences

A treatment licence will provide for monitoring of the provision of 'treatment services.' Every treatment licence must have the general conditions of s. 12 and the specific conditions of s. 13 incorporated into them. (We deal with the provsions of s. 12 in Chapter 4, at pp. 98–100.) Section 17(1)(e) imposes a statutory duty on the person under whose supervision the authorised licencesd activities are carried on ('the responsible person') to secure that the conditions of the licence are complied with. Section 18(1)(c) and (3) provide that if the person responsible under the licence has failed to discharge or is unable because of incapacity to discharge any s. 17 duty, then a licence committee may revoke a licence or vary any of its terms.

A treatment licence is one granted under the provisions of s. 13 and sch. 2, para. 1 of the Act. There are a defined number of activities which such a licence may permit. They are as follows:

1. the 'bringing about the creation of' an embryo *in vitro;*
2. keeping embryos; a phrase which is wider than simply storing embryos by freezing;
3. using gametes;
4. the therapeutic screening of embryos for subsequent implantation purposes, in order to ensure that they are in a suitable condition for implantation: although the Act does not define what is meant by 'suitable condition' an amendment seeking to prohibit selection on any other grounds than likelihood of survival was withdrawn. It was made clear that it is not the intention of this provision to mean that the embryo must conform to parental specification, but only to ensure that 'defective' embryos are not placed in a woman. 'Suitable' here should be read to mean 'medically suitable' and not merely 'acceptable';
5. the placing of an embryo in a woman;
6. the testing of sperm fertility by assessing its ability to penetrate the eggs of other species, but on the condition that anything which forms is destroyed by the two cell stage.

In each case the Authority must be satisfied that the proposed activity is necessary or desirable in providing the treatment service (sch. 2, para. 1(3)).

Treatment licences may be granted for a period of up to five years (sch. 2, para. 1(5)), and in addition to the general prohibitions of ss. 3 and 4, a licence under this paragraph cannot authorise altering the genetic structure of any cell while it forms part of the embryo (sch. 2, para. 1(4)).

Section 13 imposes a further three types of condition of which licence holders are obliged to take cognizance. First, s. 13(7) requires the licence holder to institute suitable procedures for determining the gamete or embryo donors, so that the licence holder has some form of 'quality control' and reference back capabilities (s. 13(7)(a)); and s. 13(7)(b) requires the licence holder to give consideration to use of practices which do not require the authority of a licence. An example here might be the administration of GIFT procedures (see supra for this debate) which, if not regulated by the statutory scheme, nonetheless are subject to the control of the common law and professional guidelines, including the recent advice issued by the Royal College of Obstetricians and Gynaecologists (supra).

Secondly, there are three sub-sections which relate to the broad issue of record-keeping. Section 13(3) provides that the records which a clinic must keep in pursuance of a licence must include information about the consents as provided for in sch. 3 and a number of other specified matters. These latter are specified in s. 13(2), which provides that HUFEA may require a licensed clinic to record information about the following:

(i) people treated at the clinic in pursuance of the treatment licence, s. 13(2)(a);
(ii) what services they were provided with s. 13(2)(b);
(iii) the providers of gametes (whether for donation or for one's own use) kept or used for providing services in pursuance of the licence, s. 13(2)(c);
(iv) the providers of gametes (whether by donation or for one's own use) from which embryos kept or used in pursuance of a licence derive, s. 13(2)(c);
(v) any child whom the person responsible (under s. 17(1)) believes to have been born following licensed treatment services, s. 13(2)(d);
(vi) any mixing of sperm and egg, s. 13(2)(e);
(vii) any taking of an embryo from a woman, s. 13(2)(e);
(viii) any other acquisition of an embryo (for example in pursuance of ss. 14(1)(a) or 12(f), s. 13(2)(e);
(ix) any other matter which HUFEA specifies in directions made under s. 23, s. 13(2)(f).

Additionally, s. 13(4) enables HUFEA to specify the period of time for which any information in a clinic's records must be preserved. Such information shall not be removed before the expiration of the period provided for records of the class in question. Where a treatment licence holder does not know whether a child has been born following the provision of treatment services, the information held under s. 13 shall be maintained for a period of not less than 50 years from when it was first recorded (s. 24(1)). The intent behind this provision is clear. It may arise that a person is born following treatment services, but initially have no reason to suspect that. If later in life, the person becomes aware of circumstances which suggest that she or he might have been born following the provision of treatment services to others, then she or he may wish to make enquiries to that effect under ss. 31(3)-(6). Section 24(1) attempts to ensure that in those cases where the person responsible under the licence does not know of the conception and birth of any child following licensed services, information is stored for a sufficiently lengthy period of time to anticipate most enquiries under section 31 (although, notice that a comparable Swedish provision requires the storage of information for 70 years; see Law on Insemination No 1140 of 20 December 1984, reprinted in Jan Stepan, *op.cit.*, pp. 169–70).

Thirdly, and most controversially, s. 13 details two grounds which seek to limit access to licensed treatment services. Section 13(6) requires that a woman, (or where she is being treated together with a man, both of them), is given access to a 'suitable opportunity' to receive 'proper counselling' about the implications of the services which she proposes to use. This applies where the services consist of the use of donated gametes where the donor's consent is required under sch. 3; the use of an embryo created *in vitro*; or the use of an embryo obtained from a woman by lavage. In each case, the woman or the couple must also have been provided with 'such information as is proper.' We return to consider these counselling requirements in more detail, infra, pp. 148–51. Here, we concentrate on the access to treatment condition laid out in s. 13(5).

Licensing Parents; section 13(5) and the Concept of Welfarism

Section 13(5) provides that:

> A woman shall not be provided with treatment services unless account has been taken of the welfare of any child who may be born as a result of the treatment (including the need of that child for a father), and of any other child who may be affected by the birth.

This section raises but does not address a fundamental question in respect of assisted conception. If all the financial and counselling hurdles are surmounted, does every one have a right to 'marry and found a family' (European Convention on Human Rights art. 12), such that they can either demand the provision of treatment services or not be excluded on spurious grounds? Recall that Warnock clearly thought that such a 'right' would be undesirable:

> many believe that the interests of the child dictate that it should be born into a home where there is a loving, stable, heterosexual relationship and that, therefore, the deliberate creation of a child for a woman who is not a partner in such a relationship is morally wrong . . . we believe that as a general rule it is better for children to be born into a two-parent family, with both father and mother, although we recognise that it is impossible to predict with any certainty how lasting such a relationship will be' (Warnock Report, para. 2.11).

Indeed before Warnock had reported, Diana Brahams, the legal correspondent for *The Lancet* had written:

> When a woman presents for treatment with IVF, the doctor should keep in mind the interests of the child he is helping to create. Thus either marriage or stable relationship is desirable, and particularly where there is donated ova or sperm, the character of the potential parents should be kept in mind (14 September 1983).

Not all official commissions and enquiries have reached this conclusion. For example the comprehensive report by the Ontario Law Reform Commission, *Report on Human Artificial Reproduction and Related Matters,* (1985, Ministry of the Attorney General, Toronto) considered the constitutionality of excluding single or unmarried people from access to assisted conception, and concluded that eligibility to participate in an artificial conception programme should be limited to 'stable single women and to stable men and stable women in stable marital or nonmarital unions' (Recommendation 5, p. 275, and see pp. 45 et. seq. and pp. 153 et. seq.). They conclude that criteria for participation in an assisted conception programme should be set out in provincial regulations. In the Australian State of Victoria, the Infertiltiy (Medical Procedures) Act 1984 (as amended) provides in respect of eligibility to treatment that a 'married woman' includes a woman who is living with a man as his wife 'on a bona fide basis' although not married to him, but it excludes single women for eligibility for treatment services (s. 3(2)(a)(i) and ss. 10(3)(a), 11(3)(a), 12(3)(a), 13(3)(a)). In what is habitually regarded as the 'liberal' jurisdiction of Sweden, the 'Screening' process discloses its most apparent possibilities. Article 3 of the Law on Insemination No 1140 of 20 December 1984 provides that:

> The physician shall determine if it is appropriate that insemination take place taking into consideration the medical, psychological and social circumstances of the couple. Insemination may take place only if it is probable that the child resulting therefrom will be brought up under favourable conditions.

An appeal from the physician's Assessment lies to the National Board of Health and Welfare (cf. Stepan, op.cit., pp. 168–67).

According to *Population Trends* (John Haskey and Kathleen Kiernan) in 1987, 900,000 couples were cohabiting and living together as families with 400,000 dependent children. Two thirds of those were single and had never married. A rough approximation based on infertility figures suggesting that around 1 in 8 — 1 in 10 couples are affected by involuntary childlessness suggests that some 100,000 unmarried couples may experience fertility problems. A House of Lords amendment to restrict the provision of services to married couples which would have made it an offence to provide treatment services (but not to receive them) for an unmarried couple, and hence, for a single woman, was defeated by 61 votes to 60. Lord Ashbourne had supported the amendment by arguing that the full impact of ss. 3 and 4 is that:

national resources may be used legally to encourage single parenthood and that children . . . would obviously have no statutory father (House of Lords, Official Report 6 February 1990, col. 757).

And in the House of Commons Standing Committee B, David Wilshire argued that the deliberate creation of one-parent families through assisted conception offends against the rights of the individual who will result from the treatment services, the values and standards of society and the 'biological facts of life'. He argued that:

> Science cannot stop us being social animals in the animal kingdom and . . . it cannot stop us reproducing by means of a mother and a father (House of Commons, Official Report Standing Committee B, 15 May 1990, cols. 145-46).

He appears here to make a common conflation between woman and mother and father and man; between social parenthood and biological parenthood. Lord Ennals had strongly argued the alternative view:

> Having children is a private area of human affairs. I believe that it is really not for the state to decide who should or should not be allowed to bear children . . . Parenting, in any case, is a high risk activity . . . The question of whether a couple has gone through a form of marriage vows is hardly relevant to the quality of parenthood (House of Lords, Official Report 6 February 1990, col. 789).

In the debates Lord Mackay, the Lord Chancellor, set out the cautionary note which the Government would sound throughout the debates. It would 'clearly be unfortunate', he said, if the Act was seen in any way to be conflicting with 'the importance which we attach to family values'. In particular he thought that HUFEA would want to give general guidance to clinics in the Code of Practice to be prepared and 'approved by Ministers' under s. 25 in respect of 'this sensitive aspect of their work' (House of Lords, Official Report 6 February 1990, col. 800)

The Government was determined to ensure that if it was to remain possible for unmarried couples to receive treatment services, then both should have the responsibility for any resulting child. This is achieved by s. 28(3). Accordingly, where an unmarried woman and her partner together undergo a treatment service using donor sperm (whether embryo transfer, IVF, GIFT or AID) he (and no other (s. 28(3), (4)) is to be treated as the father of any child. The provision extends the general scheme of s. 28 to treat an unmarried couple in a similar way to a married one. There is a saving in respect of 'any child who, by virtue of the rules of common law, is treated as the legitimate child of the parties to a marriage' (s. 28(2), (5)). There are some particular benefits for the child of this section, while conferring no automatic parental rights, only responsibilites, onto the father, unless he obtains a court order under the Family Law Reform Act 1987 s. 4 (or its successor under the Children Act 1989). First, if the woman dies, whether during childbirth or later, the child will have a legally recognised 'family' which may serve as an alternative to the child being taken into care. Secondly, it will enable the child to seek support from the man's estate following his death. It removes the spectre of large numbers of legally 'fatherless children' from the legislation, a possibility which had troubled commentators on the original draft of the Bill; it does not go the whole way and remove them altogether. Finally, according to Lord Mackay, the formal recognition of fatherhood may help to:

> cement and strengthen the relationship with the informal family and reduce the risks of breakdown with its consequences for the child and, indeed, the taxpayer (House of Lords, Official Report 20 March 1190, col. 210).

Clearly, the Government's concept of 'making the father pay' was a subsidiary motivation in the drafting of this clause.

Where an unmarried woman uses donated sperm for the purposes of self-insemination the donor will be treated as the father of the child, with all the legal responsibilities that that entails (see below, 'Self-insemination'). In a later debate, introducing a Government amendment which was to become s. 13(5), Lord Mackay spelt out clearly the Government's thinking behind the sub-section:

> It may be helpful if I begin by setting out the size of the group that may be involved. At present only a very small number of relevant treatments are made available outside marriage. The best and most recent estimate that can be made is that fewer than 100 out of some 3,500 patients who received the AID treatment in 1989 were single women, and some of those will have had permanent partners' (House of Lords, Official Report 6 March 1990, col. 1097-98).

It was in this context, he said, that the importance of the family was manifest; it is important that children are born into a stable and loving environment. The family is a concept whose health is fundamental to the health of society in general. Hence, the fundamental principle of law relating to children, that their welfare is the paramount consideration, had a necessary place in legislation dealing with assisted conception. The concept of the welfare of the child was, he said, very broad and all-embracing. A very wide range of factors would need to be taken into account when considering the future lives of children who may be born as a result of the licensed treatment services. He referred specifically to a discussion of the 'welfare concept' by Hardie Boyce J in *Walker* v *Harrison* [1981] 257 New Zealand Recent Law. There Hardie Boyce J had said that:

> 'Welfare' is an all-encompassing word. It includes material welfare, both in the sense of an adequacy of resources to provide a pleasant home and a comfortable standard of living and in the sense of an adequacy of care to ensure that good health and due personal pride are maintained. However, while material considerations have their place, they are secondary matters. More important are the stability and the security, the loving and understanding care and guidance, the warm and compassionate relationships, that are the

essential for the full development of the child's own character, personality and talents (House of Lords, Official Report 6 March 1990, col. 1097).

ord Mackay interpreted this to mean, among other things, that it would be ppropriate to take into account whether a guardian had been appointed for the hild in the event of the death(s) of its parent(s). But the Government's intentions ith s. 13(5) are more clearly identified. The wording of the sub-section gives rise a number of issues. First, it is not limited to the provision of donated gametes r to embryos created outside the body. It extends to any treatment service, as efined in the Act to mean 'medical, surgical or obstetric services provided to the ublic or a section of the public for the purpose of assisting women to carry hildren' (s. 2(1)).

Secondly, it clearly applies to surrogacy, for the welfare criterion is not limited any child who may be born as a result of the treatment for the woman to keep, ut merely provides for any child. In all cases, including perhaps most nportantly the surrogate-mother case, the welfare of 'any other child' who may e affected is to be accounted. Thus, the welfare of any existing child of the utative surrogate mother will fall to be considered, and this may pose an dditional obstacle to the provision of formal services to an intending surrogate nd the couple for whom she proposes to carry a child (we deal with further rovisions of the Act with respect to surrogacy, infra, in Chapter 6).

Thirdly, what does it mean to say that 'account has been taken' of the future hild's welfare and that of 'any child who may be affected by the birth'? What nust be shown in order to demonstrate that the statutory duty has been lischarged? This gives rise to the additional difficulty, not addressed in the Act, f who takes account, and what is to happen if services are provided in breach f the duty. Similarly, the Act itself is silent on who may have locus standi standing to bring proceedings) either to determine that 'account has [not] been aken' or to challenge the account which has been taken and the conclusions rrived at. The Government expressed the view that the ultimate decision of vhether to proceed with the treatment in accordance with the conditions laid lown by HUFEA will be made by the clinician, subject to such review by the Iigh Court as it is prepared to allow (see Chapter 4, supra). But what if, for xample, after taking account, the provider of a treatment service decides that it vould not be in the interests of a woman's daughter (or her sister's daughter) for reatment services to be employed? May the woman challenge this decision? And f so, on what public law principles? (see, supra, Chapter 4). Or suppose that Belinda's Aunt Mahala and Uncle Adam think that Belinda's daughter Katie Morag's interests have not been properly safeguarded now that Belinda lives vith Euan, who is impotent. Can they challenge Dr Amete's decision to rtifically inseminate Belinda with Phil Archer's donated sperm? Can they seek declaration that it would not be in the child's or Katie Morag's interests for the hild to be born? Suppose, additionally, that they argued that it would not be in Katie Morag's interests because she would only inherit a fraction of the estate hat she would otherwise have done because Dr Amete proposes to transfer up o five embryos and to ensure, to the best of her ability, that five foetuses are orn?

It is not difficult to conceive of other circumstances in which difficulties of interpretation and application of the section's requirement may arise. Here, we canvass six for the purposes of enquiry only. What account is to be taken of:

(a) a couple one of whom already has children but cannot reproduce as a couple (e.g., Lesley and John Brown);
(b) a woman who wants to become pregnant in order to produce an abortus which could provide foetal tissue for use in a therapeutic operation to save her husband's life (or the life of her three year old daughter);
(c) a woman (or a couple) who only wants a son;
(d) a woman who suffers from Munchenhausen's disease, in which sufferers present with imagined or induced medical problems (is the infertility such a problem?), and in whom the existence of 'Munchenhausen's by Proxy' is a real possibility. Here, sufferers may mutilate their children in order to attract medical care;
(e) a woman who has formerly worked as a prostitute;
(f) a woman whose partner has low sperm motility because of the excessive alcohol which he consumes?

The message from the Parliamentary discussions is not clear, but not surprisingly, it has all the hallmarks of a profamilist ideology. Assisted conception is to be, for the most part, for the married, mortgaged middle-classes; a conclusion which is entirely consonant with infertility services being unavailable on any scale through the National Health Service. One (defeated) amendment in the House of Lords sought to limit treatment services to married couples using their own gametes, i.e., to AIH and not AID. The Earl of Lauderdale described the former as embodying the ethics of the household, while the latter embodied the ethics of the farmyard (House of Lords, Official Report 6 February 1990, col. 762). This sort of argument makes the debates on the status of children born following assisted conception seeking to succeed to various hereditary titles at least comprehensible, if nonetheless anachronistic. (We review this extraordinary provision in Chapter 6.)

To read the speeches of Lord Mackay and Health Minister Bottomley, s. 13(5) would appear to be a relatively benign, even laudatory sentiment. For some, however, it did not go far enough. It speaks only of the child's welfare being 'taken account of' and not, as one amendment would have ensured, that the welfare of that child be considered as paramount. However, unless the section is devoted to a philosophical appreciation of existence against non-existence, which we suspect it is not, it effectively introduces a 'social' conscience clause, whereby consideration of the 'fitness to parent' of prospective applicants, (and the effect of the section will ensure that they are all usually couples), will be to apply a prospective licensing system for parenthood similar to that used in adoption. If this is coupled with the 'conscience clause' as formally stated, s. 38, and the exhortation to be issued in the Code of Practice (s. 25(2)) as rehearsed by Lord Mackay, an effective screening mechanism (similar to that approved by the High Court in *R* v *St Marys Hopital Ethics Committee ex parte Harriott* [1988] 1 FLR 512), has been introduced.

There will undoubtedly be some who think that is all and well to the good, and that indeed it is a concept which might with benefit be extended more widely to cover all prospective parents (see Hugh LaFollette, 'Licensing Parents' (1971) 2 *Philosophy and Public Affairs* 182 for such an argument; and Onora O'Neill 'Children's Rights and Children's Lives' (1988) *Ethics* 445 for a review). That we do indeed exercise an increasingly sophisticated and pervasive continuing licensing system of the fitness to continue parenting does not mean that we are thereby justified in extending that regime back before birth or into pregnancy (see Margot Somerville, 'Birth Technology, Parenting and "Deviance"' (1982) 5 *International J of Law and Psychiatry* 123).

In fact, it has been suggested that only 200 single or lone women have been knowingly treated at clinics in the past 12 years. It is possible to argue that lesbian couples who choose maternity and motherhood are those who have perhaps most clearly examined and rejected patriarchal notions of motherhood and the family with which western society is most totally suffused. For them, it is the lifestyle truly of choice rather than of convention and it is they who are most likely to be deprived by unsupported appeals to those conventions.

The extraordinary facet of this debate is that the evidence which would enable the negative conclusions to be drawn about single or lesbian couple parenting is in scant supply. While it is true that there is a high correlation between one parent families and emotional or behavioural deprivation, that does not lead straight to the conclusion that it is the single parenting which causes the poverty; rather it tells us about some of the priorities in social welfare spending. This way of framing the debates and the arguments has been powerfully challenged by a number of commentators, but perhaps most forcefully and to greatest effect by Susan Golombok, who has explored the assumptions on which these negative images are developed. With Ann Spencer and Michael Rutter she has argued that the expectation that a woman's lesbianism would in itself increase the likelihood of psychiatric disorder has arisen from the assumption that the children living in lesbian households would be teased, ostracised or disapproved of by their peers, and that they would be adversely affected by this. In fact, no such differences could be detected when comparing the children of women who were now lesbian with those living in a single parent household. If anything, the tendency towards behavioural and emotional problems was more the other way. The caveat in that important study, ('Children in Lesbian and Single Parent Households: Psychosexual and Psychiatric Appraisal' (1983) 24(4) *J Child Psychology and Psychiatry* 551) that the findings cannot be applied to exclusively and permanently homosexual women who have become pregnant by means of AID, has to be balanced with their conclusion. While it remains possible that there are effects on development of being brought up in a home that lacks any contact with men, and in which there is a negative attitude towards things masculine, they have not been shown. Indeed, these negative descriptions of lesbian households were not born out in their sample:

> We should cease regarding lesbian households as all the same. . . . Perhaps it is the quality of family relationships and the pattern of upbringing that matters for psychosexual development, and not the sexual orientation of the mother.

In a later essay with John Rust ('The Warnock Report and Single Women: What about the Children?' (1986) *J Medical Ethics* 182) Golombok returns to argue that while children in 'fatherless families' are more likely to have emotional and behavioural problems, this is not, as often assumed, because of the absence of a father but a direct consequence of the poverty and isolation that these families have to endure. Implicit in the view that children need fathers, they write, is the notion that the two parent heterosexual family is the norm and that any deviation from this ideal is bound to cause problems for the child. Around 1 in 8 families with children in Britain are one parent families. The large majority are headed by women and a growing percentage are unmarried. Is it really sensible, they ask, to suppose that one and a half million children will be damaged by this experience? In what way does it make sense to suppose that the social and emotional development of AID and IVF children in fatherless families would be different from children who find themselves in heterosexual one parent families or in lesbian families after they reach the age of two or three years? They caution that there is no empirical support for either psychoanalytic theories which posit that boys and girls would develop atypically because of the lack of clearly differentiated father and mother roles; nor for some social learning theorists who have suggested that lesbian mothers might use a different pattern of reinforcement for male behaviour in boys, and that girls might be influenced by an atypical role model and might experience different patterns of reinforcement for sex-typed behaviours. Of the Warnock Report's preference for the two partner heterosexual model they conclude that 'on the basis of two hundred words which amount to dogma rather than argument, some women are to be denied the right to have children' (p. 185).

Of course, the assumption that the legislation will have its intended effects, and only those, can be challenged. One of the arguments advanced in debate was that it was better to allow clinically supervised treatments with appropriate screening of donated gametes, than to encourage an unsupervised 'informal' system to flourish, with attendant risks of serious disease. Whether the adoption of this 'welfarist' notion will prove to be successful in regulating the use of assisted conception, and in whose interests it is seen to work remains to be seen.

'The Coloscopy Nurse at Margate': Counselling and Conception

The Harman Report (op.cit., p. 4) remarks that there is 'very little specific counselling for those who are embarking on infertility tests for treatment'. District Health Authorities responding to the questionnaire reported that most counselling is done informally by the consultant during the appointment, by Family Planning Clinics, or staff in out-patients departments. One authority reported that 'the coloscopy nurse at Margate is very good at talking to patients but she is not a fully trained counsellor'. South Manchester reported a reduction in the non-medical counselling, due to the curtailment of social work services, and the British Infertility Counselling Association has reported that in practice very few infertility clinics have professionally trained counsellors available. Those that do, offer such a limited service that only a small minority of patients can benefit from it. The RCOG is to set up a new clinical Audit Unit to monitor all infertility units which will ensure further monitoring of counselling, patient information and openness, and the Institute of Population Studies at the University of Exeter has been commissioned to produce a report on the current provision of counselling services available at IVF clinics in the United Kingdom. It is clear, however, that despite ILA Guideline 13(g) that centres should have 'appropriate counselling services with access to properly trained independent counselling staff,' much turns on the interpretation given to 'counselling' by individual centres. There is nothing to resemble the statutory requirement in the Infertility (Medical Procedures) Act 1984 ss. 10-13 in Victoria, Australia, which places upon the doctor providing treatment services a duty to ensure that both the woman and the man have been counselled, and (an important lacuna in the 1990 Act), that further counselling is available after the procedures have been performed (on this point see Stepan, op.cit., p. 68).

The ILA introduced in 1990 a new guideline which supplemented its Guideline 13(g) which provides that centres should have 'appropriate counselling facilities with access to properly trained independent counselling staff.' The new Guideline 15 provides that, when receiving donated oocytes from both those donating for purely altruistic reasons and those receiving free sterilisation or other operative procedures, skilled and independent counselling, by someone other than the medical practitioner involved in the procedure must be available to the donor to ensure that sufficient information has been given and understood. In particular, it is directed that the discomfort and the risk should be properly understood, and that if the woman consents to the donation, she should do so with her judgment unimpaired, with the counsellor looking for 'stability of purpose' so that neither consent nor withdrawal during treatment would be lightly undertaken. The guideline emphasises that the donor must know that she is free to withdraw consent from the egg donation at any time without threat of financial penalty or without impairment of her interest in the successful conduct of the primary operation. The donor must be told of the purpose for which her eggs are to be used, and where they are to be used. The eggs must not be sold, and the centre must be prepared to absorb the costs of a woman who withdraws from the donation. The donor must be given the ILA booklet and the consent form signed and retained in the centre's records. The local ethics committee of the centre, or under whose purview the work of the centre comes, must be satisfied that these conditions can and will be met.

In addition to these general requirements about counselling, a new Guideline 16 was issued in 1990 to respond to reports that some women had been offered fast track routes to surgery, including free sterilisations, if they would agree to act as an egg donor. The ILA was concerned that no undue pressure was exerted on a woman in this, or any other way. Accordingly, Guideline 16 provides that where a free sterilisation or other related surgery is to be offered to a woman in return for donated gametes, the centre must have the ILA's specific approval. The discussion of egg donation must be entirely separate from decisions taken concerning the clinical care of the patient for whom the sterilisation or other operation is intended, and only when those decisions have been finalised should the question of egg donation be raised. An accelerated route for operative treatment must not be used in relation to egg donations unless there is independent clinical justification for that. The fact of donation is not in itself adequate. These provisions are likely to form the basis of the requirements which HUFEA will issue in its Code of Practice under s. 25 dealing with, among other things, the counselling arrangements which licensed centres will have to observe as a condition of their licence.

The Act provides in s. 13(6) that treatment services which involve the use of donated gametes or a donated embryo obtained by lavage, or an embryo which was brought about *in vitro,* shall not be provided to a woman unless she has been given 'a suitable opportunity to receive counselling'. The Act envisages that the counselling will be directed towards the implications of the taking the proposed steps, and it requires that she is to have been provided with 'such relevant information as is proper'. Where a woman is being treated together with a man, the same facility must be made available to both of them. The Government announced that the independent King's Fund Centre had been asked to set up a working party to recommend to health departments the best way to proceed on this requirement.

The issue of counselling was recognised as important by the Warnock Committee, and throughout the debates, as a way of preparing for the emotional impact of treatment services, whether following failure or unlooked-for success, which the unpredictabilty of treatment services can bring. It was clearly envisaged that for some women and couples the counselling would be an opportunity to consider whether they should proceed with the treatment services, following which they would decide not to go ahead. (Lord Mackay, House of Lords, Official Report, 6 February 1990, col. 800.)

The Act does not on its face specify what the counselling is to consist of, nor when it is to be made available, nor whether an individual centre may do more by way of encouraging the use of the counselling services. The Minister, Virginia Bottomley, made it clear that it would be expected that the counselling would be non-directive, in the sense that the woman or couple would be exploring their own feelings and attitudes, and not those of the counsellor. Given that the Secretary of State must approve any Draft Code which HUFEA produces, it seems reasonable to assume that this will be the policy to be implemented. On other questions, too, the legislation is presently silent. For example, when should the opportunity for counselling be made available? Once counselling has been given at the outset of treatment services, does that satisfy the requirement to provide a 'suitable opportunity' or should this be made available each time a woman or couple come back into the Centre for treatment? On this question s. 13(6) is ambiguous; it speaks of being 'provided with any treatment services' and 'the woman being treated', implying a continuing availability of counselling. Elsewhere, however, it could be taken to imply a one-off session at the outset of treatment: 'unless [she or they] have been given a suitable opportunity'.

This is an important point. One opinion suggests that if after 4-6 IVF treatment cycles a pregnancy has not been established, it is not really worth proceeding further (Correspondence, *New England Journal of Medicine* 12 December 1989). Yet, in the UK, some clinics perform up to ten treatment cycles. This carries with it rising emotional and financial expense each time. It is possible that after many repeated, unsuccessful attempts to establish a pregnancy, counselling is more necessary than at the beginning. The issue to be faced by the woman or couple here is when or whether to stop, attempt to accept and begin to come to terms with the involuntary childlessness. There is concern that one of the deficits of assisted conception is that it raises hopes of overcoming or circumventing infertility only for those to be dashed at a later and heightened time.

This point is borne out by the *Third* VLA *Annual Report* (1986), where the Authority noted that some IVF clinics employ 'specially trained' counsellors, but only so that 'patients who fail to achieve a pregnancy have the opportunity to discuss their problems and decide on future treatment with either the medical or nursing staff' (at p. 16). There was also a late recognition that there may be a conflict of interest in the practitioner's control over counselling, where the counsellor is the prescribing doctor. They observed that:

> Proper counselling is possible only if space and time are available to the couple in a neutral atmosphere with a fully-trained counsellor, possibly a member of the team who is not the prescribing doctor (p. 15).

The Department of Health appears to have taken the question of counselling seriously during the Parliamentary debates. Whether the reality meets the aspiration remains to be seen.

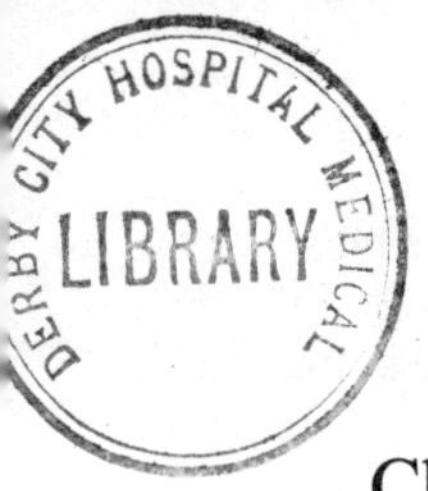

Chapter 6
Children of the Reproduction Revolution: Status Provisions

Status Provisions

The question of genetic status and personal identity is a complex intermeshing construct of psychological, philosophical, historical, cultural, ethical and legal matrices. That said, the reader may be relieved that we shall not attempt here to unravel them all. Suffice it to say that, in a society where an estimated 1 in 20, or 5%, of the population, have a genetic parent who is other than the one or two named on their birth certificate (Baroness Hooper, House of Lords, Official Report 7 December 1989, col. 1112), the problem of 'designer genes' raised by assisted conception is insignificant compared with the 'genetic passing off' which appears widespread. However, Susan Golombok and Tony Rutherford acknowledge that 'very little is known about the effects of [new reproductive technologies] on the families concerned' (Golombok and Rutherford, 'Psychological Development of Children of the New Reproductive Technologies: Issues and a Pilot Study of Children Conceived by IVF' (1990) 8 *Journal of Reproductive and Infant Psychology* 130). They do suggest, however, that:

> It may also be the case that when children conceived by the new reproductive technologies develop psychological problems the parents may attribute these problems to the children's origins and cope with them differently from parents who conceived their children normally. . . . It remains possible that the procedures involved in the new reproductive technologies have a direct effect on the child . . . [but] from the findings of this pilot study, it seems that children conceived by IVF are making good developmental progress. . . . With respect to behavioural and emotional problems, the IVF children showed a significantly higher incidence of such difficulties than a normal population sample of children . . . (Ibid.)

It will clearly remain necessary for longer term follow-up studies to be conducted to assess what, if any, social, psychological and psycho-sexual differences children of the reproduction revolution experience, and it may be that the way in which their formal status is recognised and characterised legally will have some direct or tangential effect on that. We now turn to an examination of the way in which the Act has dealt with these questions of status.

The Act contains four important sections on the status of the various participants in assisted conception procedures; s. 27 deals with mothers; s. 30 with the special position of children born to a surrogate mother; s. 28 deals with fatherhood and s. 29 states the effect of these provisions.

Mothers

Section 27 provides that a woman who has carried a child as a result of the placing in her of an embryo or sperm and eggs (GIFT or ZIFT procedures) shall be the mother of that child, whatever its genetic makeup. There is a saving in s. 27(2) for adoption. Section 30 also introduces a saving where a parental order may be made in respect of gamete donors. Section 27(3) provides that s. 27 applies whether the woman was within the UK or not when the embryo or sperm and eggs were placed within her.

Saving Surrogacy

Section 30 was a late amendment to the Bill. It provides limited circumstances in which a 'parental order' in respect of gamete donors can be sought. Where a woman, a 'surrogate mother', has carried a child on behalf of another couple who were either: (i) both that child's genetic parents (full surrogacy) or (ii) where one of the couple is the child's genetic parent, having donated sperm or an egg, they may apply for an order to be treated as legally the child's parents. The section can be used wherever the procedures effecting surrogacy arrangement was agreed (s. 30(11)). Section 30(2) provides that the application for the 'commissioning' parents to be treated as the child's lawful parents must be made within six months of the child's birth. In an extraordinary procedural manoeuvre, MP Michael Jopling secured a retrospective application of this section, almost literally at the last minute in the Parliamentary voting. The section is thus to be made to apply to the birth of children born before the Act comes into force. In order for this provision to operate, the parents must apply for the parental order within six months of the Act's commencement (30(2)).

Mr Jopling's specific concern had been with the case of constituents of his. They had been challenged by the local Social Services Department when they applied formally to adopt twin children who had been living with them since their birth following a 'full' surrogacy arrangement. They were the children's genetic parents, but the Department argued that they should be required to fulfil the full, legal criteria for adoption before the child was allowed to remain with them permanently. In a letter to *The Times,* their solicitor argued that:

> My client, the genetic mother, would appear to have no legal rights whatsoever in her own children. On the contrary, her husband, the genetic father, would have the right to apply under the guardianship legislation to have himself recognised as the father of illegitimate children and no doubt, custody, if he required; a truly anomalous situation in these days of the equality of the sexes.

> Parliament appears to be proposing to perpetuate a definition of motherhood which flies in the face of present genetic knowledge and medical technology . . . Surely genetic mothers, at the very least, should be accorded the same rights and privileges as genetic fathers? (D B Forrest, *The Times*, 28 February 1990.)

Clearly, there are a number of assumptions and controversial arguments which could be joined here, but the straightforward question is a relatively simple one; should surrogacy arrangements, generally disfavoured by the legislation, be given this apparent encouragement, even in the marginal case? That it is a simple question does not, of course, mean that it admits of a simple answer. Indeed, we would maintain that it is highly complex. But the answer to it, and the route by which we arrive at it, discloses much about our underlying approach to the field of reproductive technology more generally. We do not have space here to rehearse those arguments. Section 30 is itself a formal admission that there are no easy answers to the riddles of reproductive assistance. Almost every case is a hard case.

In order for the section to apply, the conditions of sub-sections (2)-(7) must be satisifed. Broadly, these require that:

(a) the child's home is with the applicant husband and wife (s. 30(3)(a)); the section applies only for the benefit of married couples (s. 30(1));

(b) the husband, the wife, or both of them must be domiciled in the United Kingdom, the Channel Islands or the Isle of Man (s. 30(3)(b));

(c) both husband and wife must be at least 18 years old (s. 30(4));

(d) the court must be satisfied that the child's father (where he is not the husband) and the surrogate mother freely agree to the making of the order; that agreement must be freely and unconditionally given with full understanding of what is involved (s. 30(5)), unless either the father or the surrogate mother cannot be found or is incapable of giving agreement (s. 30(6));

(e) there is a minimum 'thinking period' for the woman who gave birth to the child; hence, a surrogate mother's agreement is ineffective if given less than six weeks after the birth (s. 30(6));

(f) the court must be satisfied that no money or other benefit has changed hands in consideration of:

(i) the making of the parental order;
(ii) the agreement to relinquish the child to the 'parents';
(iii) the handing over of the child to the applicants;
(iv) the making of the arrangements prior to the making of the parental order (s. 30(7)). There are two exceptions to this prohibition; the court may authorise any such payments (30(7)(d)), and it does not prohibit the payment to the surrogate mother of reasonable expenses (s. 30(7)).

Fathers

Section 28 defines 'father' for the purposes of the Act. It is a complex and difficult provision, but one of great significance creating, as it does, a new class of child, the (legally) 'fatherless child' (see Robert Lee and Derek Morgan, 'Children of the Reproduction Revolution' (1990) 87(18) *Law Society Gazette* 2).

It proceeds by providing a saving in certain circumstances for any child treated as the legitimate child of the parties to a marriage or of any person, whether by virtue of statute or common law. So, where a woman is married, s. 28(2) provides that if she becomes pregnant following embryo transfer, or GIFT or ZIFT, or following artificial insemination, her husband is to be treated as the father of any resulting child. However, if he can show that he did not consent to the treatment service, he is not to be treated as father under s. 28(2), although he will remain the child's presumed father by virtue of s. 28(5). This saves the common law presumption of paternity that a child is the child of a marriage, unless the husband shows otherwise. It will also deal with the husband who changes his mind about accepting his wife's child as his own. Section 28(2) provides that the lack of consent must be shown to have been at the time of the treatment of his wife, and not at some later time. Thus, a man who has not consented to his wife's treatment (and there is no requirement in the Act that it be sought, although it is almost invariable practice) may later accept that the child is his. As s. 28(2) is drafted, his lack of consent at the time of treatment would have been enough for him later to disown the child. The common law presumption will operate to secure the continuing link between the child and its presumed father. The man could, if he so wished, then seek to rebut the common law presumption. This he would have to do by way of blood tests, or any other method of DNA testing. The scheme of s. 28(2) extends that introduced by the Family Law Reform Act s.27 for artificial insemination to the other treatments here discussed, and, by saving the common law presumption, refines the earlier provision, which had made the question of the husband's consent conclusive as to paternity.

Section 28(3) applies in a similar way to an unmarried woman who seeks infertility treatment together with a man who is not the sperm donor. That man, and no other person, is to be treated as the father of the child subject to the s. 28(5) presumptions. There was disquiet and confusion throughout the Parliamentary debates about access to treatment of what are sometimes called 'unconventional' families, despite the evidence that the 'conventional' family of the advertisements of the 1940s and 1950s has disappeared. Section 13(5) provides that before a woman is provided with treatment services regard is to be paid to the welfare of the child, including the need of that child for a father. It is thought that this will act as a major 'screening' device in respect of access to treatment services, although many clinics already refuse to provide assistance to single women, and only six or seven are known to accept single or lesbian women. But in truth, that section is an odd provision. *Ex hypothesi,* the child has a father; the section is not making special provision for parthenogenesis. What the section means to provide for, of course, is that the woman seeking treatment should have a man. That is rather different. Given this, it is extraordinary that, as we shall see, s. 28 goes on to create categories of 'legally fatherless' children and to prevent some children from ever discovering their genetic origins. However, as we have seen, the policy behind the legislation is actively to discourage treatment for those infertile people who live outside the umbrella of the nuclear family. This was made crystal clear in one contribution to the debate by Lord Chancellor Mackay:

> . . . if it is to remain possible for unmarried couples to receive the benefit of treatment to bring a child into being, both should have imposed upon them the responsibility for the child. I was most concerned that this proposal [to amend the Bill] should not be seen as encouraging unmarried people to use infertility treatments thus undermining marriage or leading to children having unsuitable fathers because of the difficulty in distinguishing partners to stable relationships from more transitory ones (House of Lords, Official Report, 20 March 1990, col. 1209-10).

Where a married woman seeks treatment services together with a man other than her husband, her husband will nonetheless be treated as, or be presumed to be the father, unless he can defeat both the statutory provision and the common law presumption.

Where a man is by virtue of s. 28(2) or 28(3) treated as a child's father, s.28(4) provides that no other man is to be so regarded. Section 28(6)(a) provides that where a donor's gametes are used in accordance with the consents required under sch. 3, para. 5, then the donor is not to be treated as the father of the child. An attempt to ensure that the birth certificate of a child born following treatment services should have this fact endorsed upon it was defeated in the House of Commons.

Section 28(6) is intended to provide 'protection' to a donor whose sperm is used in accordance with his consent to establish a pregnancy to which a married woman's husband has not consented. Two conclusions seem to follow. First, that a child born in such circumstances will be one of the new legally 'fatherless children'. Secondly, where sperm is used outwith the effective consents given under sch 3, para. 5, a donor may not be protected by s. 28(6)(a), and may indeed be treated as the father of a child produced without his consent.

Posthumous Children

The second category of legally 'fatherless child' is created by s. 28(6)(b). This provides that where an embryo is created with a man's sperm following his death, or where a woman is allowed access to frozen sperm (whether for the purposes of artificial insemination or for a procedure such as GIFT) after a man's death, then he is 'not [posthumously] to be treated as the father of the [resulting] child'. This will be the case whether the woman becoming pregnant is using her deceased husband's frozen sperm in accordance with his express consent given under sch. 3, para. 2(2)(b), or that of an unknown donor. Given that death ends the marriage, the child will be born not only legally fatherless, but also illegitimate, unless the woman has remarried prior to the insemination, in which case s. 28(5) and (2) and will operate, as above, to treat the new husband as the child's father.

This provision is inserted, as the Warnock report recommended, to ensure that estates can be administered with some degree of finality (see Warnock, paras 10.9 and 10.15) and to give effect to Warnock's expressed desire that fertilisation of a woman following the death of her partner (or husband as Warnock would have limited it) 'should be actively discouraged'. This they recommended because it may give rise to profound psychological problems for the child and the mother (para. 4.4). They did recommend, however, that where one of a couple who has stored an embryo dies, the right to use or dispose of that embryo should pass to the survivor. Whether that is to be the case will depend on the consent given under sch. 3, para. 2(2)(b) and whether the surviving spouse is seen to have a right to demand treatment with the stored sperm.

There is one case in which the section as drafted renders the position complex. This is where an embryo created legitimately becomes illegitimate on its use following its genetic father's death. Where during a man's lifetime his sperm is used to create an embryo which is then frozen, the embryo is clearly then the legitimate offspring of the marriage. He subsequently dies, and his widow later uses the frozen embryo to establish a pregnancy. The created embryo is 'used after his death' within s. 28(6)(b) and is legally fatherless and illegitimate. This assumes, of course, that the woman has not remarried, for the s. 28 presumptions would apply so that the husband of her remarriage would again be treated as the father of the child.

The policy behind these sections is clearly to discourage posthumous pregnancies. But the instrument which is used is that of punishing the child for what are seen as 'the sins of its mother'. This is an odd, not to say indefensible, way of proceeding. First, it seems inconsistent with the general legislative mood of recent years which has sought to minimise or mitigate the differential statuses of children (and the adults they will become) based solely on the conduct of their parents (e.g. Family Law Reform Act 1987, s. 1). Indeed, it offends against the judgment of the European Court of Human Rights in *Johnston* v *Ireland* (1987) 9 ECHR 203, which condemned such distinctions between children.

And secondly, it seems to fly in the face of the approach taken under legislation such as the Surrogacy Arrangements Act 1985. The specific reason why the surrogate and the intending parents were exempted from the criminal provisions of that Act was to give effect to Warnock's anxiety to 'avoid children being born to mothers subject to the taint of criminality' (para. 8.19). It seems unfortunate, to say the least, that that philosophy has not informed the drafting of these important status provisions.

In relation to the post-mortem inseminations of s. 28(6)(b), clearly, the 'legitimacy' and paternity of the child are not protected by the common law presumptions which are specifically saved by s. 28(5). The effect of those rules of common law is: (i) a child conceived before marriage but born after her father's death would be presumed to be and be treated as legitimate; (ii) a child born to a married woman during the subsistence of her marriage is presumed also to be the child of her husband — this presumption is given a very wide scope and can be shifted only by discharging a heavy burden of rebuttal. It arises even though the child must have been conceived before marriage, because in marriage the man is prima facie taken to have acknowledged the child as his own.

To rebut the presumption, it must be shown either that blood tests establish no genetic link or that no sexual intercourse took place between the spouses during the possible time when the child must have been conceived, which can be achieved by showing that, (i) sexual intercourse was impossible because the parties were physically absent from one another — which presumably includes the fact that one of them was dead — or that at least one of them was impotent, or, (ii) that the circumstances were such as to render it highly improbable that sexual intercourse took place. The litigation which these grounds, and especially the second, have spawned need not detain us here. In the case of a man who has died, the death terminates the marriage and reliance on the common law presumption will be insufficient to 'save' the paternity and the legitimacy of the child of the marriage. However, the possibility arises that s. 1(1) of the Legitimacy Act 1976 (as amended by the Family Law Reform Act 1987, s. 28(1)), which creates a form of statutory legitimacy, might apply. Section 1(1), which is derived from s. 2 of the Legitimacy Act 1959, applies to the children of a void marriage. (Section 28(7)(b) of the 1990 Act 'saves' void marriages if one of the parties reasonably believed that the marriage was valid.) It provides for the legitimacy of the child of a void marriage if at the time of insemination resulting in the birth, or at the time of the child's conception, or at the time of the celebration of the marriage if later, both or either of the partners reasonably believed that the marriage was valid. The debates on the Family Law Reform Act 1987 made it clear that for the purposes of conception *in vitro,* conception takes place when the ovum is fertilised and not when the resulting zygote or embryo is replaced in the uterus. (House of Lords, Official Report, 10 February 1987, cols. 519-22). As the leading commentator Bevan observes, this raises the possibility that:

> if at the time of *in vitro* fertilisation, both or either of the parties reasonably believe that the marriage is valid, but the fertilised egg is then frozen and later inserted into the woman, even some years later (perhaps after the man has died), the child would be legitimate. (Bevan, *Child Law* (1987) p. 67.)

If this is correct (and some commentators dispute this) in respect of void marriages, and s. 28(7)(b) and sch. 3 gives no indication that that provision is to be repealed or amended in any way, then it appears to place the child born posthumously following conception during a void marriage in a better position than one of a marriage where all the formalities had properly been attended to. But then it means generally that children of marriages declared void are consistently advantaged in the legitimacy stakes as against children of the post-mortem births which we have described.

Under s. 28(2), the husband of the marriage will not be treated as father at all (subject to s. 28(5)) if he can show that he did not consent to the infertility treatment. However, in the case of a void marriage not 'saved' by s. 28(7)(b), arguably the Legitimacy Act 1976 provisions prevail. In such a case, the provisions of the 1976 Act would mean that it would avail the man nothing to plead an absence of consent, for the legitimacy of the child would be preserved.

Returning to post-mortem births, the presumption under s. 28(5) applies where the child is born within the possible period of gestation after the marriage has been terminated by the husband's death. (For the modern authorities, see *Re Leman's Will Trusts* (1945) 115 LJ Ch 89 and *Knowles* v *Knowles* [1962] P 161; although Cohen J in *Re Heath, Stacey* v *Baird* [1945] Ch 417 declined to decide definitely whether the presumption applied to the posthumous child.) This might raise the distasteful possibility of the bereaved woman seeking the thawing and implantation of the frozen embryo at the earliest opportunity after her deceased husband's death, in order to save the legitimacy and parentage of the child under the common law presumption. However, the statutory language militates against this course of action. The language of s. 28(6) is too unambiguous to allow the common law presumption to arise; unlike s. 28(2), s. 28(6) is not made subject to the common law presumption, as it was on the first draft of the Bill published in November 1989.

But, suppose that, if the man and woman were not married, while the man was still alive and the embryos were frozen he declared himself as father of the child, and the woman later applied to register the parentage under the Family Law Reform Act. Section 22 of the Family Law Reform Act 1987 (replacing s. 56, Family Law Act 1986) enables a county court or the High Court to grant declarations of parentage, legitimacy or legitimation. A new kind of declaration, introduced by the 1987 Act, enables a person to apply for a declaration that a person named in the application is or was his or her parent. Difficult questions arise as to whether a child born posthumously could use this section for a declaration of parentage. Section 28(6) seems to preclude this, although there must be some doubt about the meaning of 'not to be treated' in that section. Where the embryo was brought about before his death, the man is not being *treated as* the child's father, because he *was* the child's father at conception, and is now her *deceased* father. It might be argued that no question of 'treating' him as such arises. As we have seen, however, the policy of the Act is that the genetic father is not necessarily to be taken as the father. A parallel question arises under s. 24, Family Law Reform Act 1987, which substitutes a new s. 10 in the Births and Deaths Registration Act 1953. This provides that an unmarried father can obtain registration of his name as the father on the child's birth certificate at the joint request of the mother and him; at the request of the mother and on production of declarations by her and him to the effect that he is the father; at his own request and on production of similar declarations; or at the written request of either himself or the mother and on production of a paternal parental rights order made under various provisions. The entry of a man's name in the register as the father of a child is prima facie evidence that he is the father (s. 34, Births and Deaths Registration Act 1953). Could the father make the request and produce the declaration before his death and the child's birth, or must the evidence supporting the acquisition of the declaration necessary to found the mother's request for registration be adduced only after the child's birth?

On this particular point, the Law Commission Report *Family Law: Illegitimacy* (Law Com. No.118, 20 December 1982) observed that, where the father dies before the child's birth, a declaration of parentage will be available for the child once born:

> doubtless any statement made by the man alleged to be the father would be relevant as evidence for a future declaration of parentage. There is, in our view, no need to provide specially for this type of case because once a declaration of parentage has been made the birth could . . . be registered so as to show the father's name (para. 10.75).

In other words, the answer to this conundrum, as before, turns on the meaning to be given to the phrase 'is not to be treated' in s. 28(6).

These questions are vital since they surround the possible creation of a new category of child: those *prohibited by law* from establishing their paternity. The late addition of what is now s. 31(5) manufactures a similar difficulty for children born following anonymous donation; short of primary legislation they too are hostages to the 'reproduction revolution'. One lesson is clear from this benighted policy and complex mesh of statute and common law. Any married couple contemplating the freezing of the gametes before the man undergoes major surgery with a risk of death (which occurs in almost any operative procedure under general anaesthetic) or treatment which may render him sterile, such as chemotheraphy, and where there is in any case a real risk of early death, must be advised that if they wish to have any possibility of circumventing these rules on posthumously conceived children they must have fertilised ovum — embryos — frozen, and not just their unmixed gametes. Statutory legitimacy may apply to save the former, but could not operate on the latter.

General Provisions

Section 28(8) applies the provisions of the section wherever the treatments took place. For example, if an English couple domiciled in the UK live abroad for a while where they obtain infertility treatment and later return to the UK, where the child is born, then, by virtue of s. 27(1) and 28(2), they are treated as that child's parents. In the absence of the section, the donor of sperm would have been the child's father. In more than one sense, the Act gives us the opportunity to determine what sort of children we want.

Section 29 provides that the legal effect of ss. 27 and 28 is to apply for all purposes, such as incest and prohibited degrees of marriage (s. 29(1), (2)), except succession to and transmission of succession rights to dignities or titles of honour (s. 29(4) and 29(5)). The effect of s. 29(1) and (2) in respect of inheritance is that children born following assisted conception will take under a will, a trust or deed as would a blood relative. A donor child whom, for example, the testator (maybe long ago) could not have had in contemplation and of whose existence she or he may have even disapproved, will take, perhaps to the exclusion of others. But that is much how life is. Where trusts or deeds are made after this Act, of course, they can be framed so as to give effect to a contrary intention and exclude donor children. If the testator is still alive, they can be redrawn. But where the testator is dead, there is no chance to vary the trust. It will, of course, remain open to any person to demonstrate that the terms of a past or future will, trust or deed show a contrary intention to s. 29(3), so as to exclude children born following treatment services.

Sections 29(4) and (5) reintroduce provisions which occupied a great deal of time and emotional energy in the House of Lords' debates. They represent a major derogation from the scheme of the provisions which we have just been considering. When the Bill passed to the Commons, the clauses as they then were, were thrown out almost peremptorily (House of Commons, Standing Committee B, 15 May 1990, cols. 187-91):

> . . . I heard on the radio the debates in another place about the inheritance of clan chieftainships and titles. I could not believe that such a debate was taking place in the late twentieth century (*per* Mrs Fyfe MP, at col. 187).

It was always clear, however, that this could provoke a major clash between the two Houses, and when Government ministers and business managers were working hard to get the Act passed before the summer recess in 1990, this was one of the hostages which the Lords were able to liberate. Accordingly, these provisions were reinserted in the Bill in an attempt to ensure that it reached the statute book in July.

The effect of the sections is that succession in England, Wales and Northern Ireland to any dignity or title of honour and property limited to devolve with it will remain through the blood line only. In other words, donor children will not be able to succeed to such titles and property as though they were children conceived 'in the usual manner'. The law of arms, with which we are here concerned, comes under the jurisdiction of the High Court of Chivalry, a civilian court, which last sat in 1954 (see *Manchester Corporation* v *The Manchester Palace of Varieties* [1955] P 133). There was much discussion in the House of Lords' debates on the present legislation of whether a coat of arms is included within a dignity or title of honour (and hence was not a property right), which are matters of common law. Earlier statutes referring to dignities, such as the Adoption and Legitimacy Acts of 1976 and the Family Law Reform Act 1987, have adopted the wording preferred here, relying on the dictum of Lord Goddard (sitting as the surrogate for the Earl Marshall) in the *Manchester Corporation* case that a coat of arms was so protected. But as Lord Mackay confessed, this is a point 'not free from difficulty' (House of Lords, Official Report, 6 March 1990, col. 1156). The College of Arms and the Lord Lyon King of Arms are already charged with the problems of succession in disputed parentage cases, including ones in which assisted conception is alleged. The Act does not affect that present position.

The law of arms in Scotland is quite different, with the Scottish law of peerages, dignities and offices having its own difficulties and niceties. In that jurisdiction, it is taken as settled that a title, honour or dignity does not include a coat of arms (Succession (Scotland) Act 1964 s. 37(1)). A separate Scottish provision had originally been included in the Bill only on amendment, when it was disclosed that the original draft, of November 1989, had not taken account of these differences. Of particular concern to the Scottish peers and peeresses was that, as drafted, the Bill appeared to be separating Clan Chieftainships and Hereditary Offices from associated peerages, dignities or other titles. The reason for this concern is that such 'hereditary offices' are viewed as incorporeal heritable property like land, rather than as a title or dignity, and are often closely linked to the landed estate which is granted with them and with which they descend. The rights to these offices can be and are recorded in the General Register of Sasines or Land Register of Scotland.

In Scotland, there are five heritable offices (England has only two) and each is associated with a specific peerage carrying with it associated lands. The offices are those of the Lord High Constable (attached to the Earl of Errol); Hereditary

Banner Bearer (the Earl of Dundee); Hereditary Bearer of St Andrew's Flag (the Earl of Lauderdale); Hereditary Master of the Household (the Duke of Argyll) and Hereditary Keeper of the Palace of Holyrood House (the Duke of Hamilton). The effect of ss. 29(4) and 29(5) is that these nobles can rest once again peacefully in their beds, thanks to the efforts of Lady Saltoun of Abernathy, a Scottish chief and member of the Standing Council of Scottish Chiefs (see, House of Lords, Official Report, 7 December 1990, cols. 1089-91 for her most belligerent intervention).

Sections 27–29 will apply only to births after the coming into force of the sections, and s. 27 of the Family Law Reform Act 1987, which deals with status questions of children born following AID only, will cease to have effect after the commencement of those sections.

Access to Information

In *Gaskin* v *United Kingdom* [1990] 1 FLR 167, the European Court of Human Rights held that art. 8 of the European Convention on Human Rights, demanding respect for the private life of an individual, requires that 'everyone should be able to establish details of their identity as individual human beings'. This judgment was relied upon in debate as the source of a right to know information about the genetic and personal identity of donors whose gametes were used in the provision of treatment services.

In respect of treatment licences, s. 13 provides that by directions issued under s. 23 or 24, the Authority may direct licence holders to record information about the recipients of treatment, the services provided, the identity of gamete donors and of any child apparently born following treatment services. (A gamete donor may be paid for his or her donation in accordance with directions made by HUFEA (s. 12(e).)

If the licensee does not know whether a child has been born following treatment, all this information must be stored for at least 50 years (s. 24(1)). Section 31 requires the Authority to keep a register of information acquired from licensed centres, and s. 31(3) gives an applicant aged over 18 the power to obtain specified and limited information. That information is predicated upon HUFEA's register showing that the applicant was born following the use of donated gametes. If, from the information held by HUFEA it appears that the applicant was or may have been born following treatment services, as defined, and the applicant has been given a 'suitable' opportunity for counselling, the Authority must comply with the request to provide the applicant with information. Precisely what form that information will take is to be specified in regulations, but it is clear that while presently only non-identifying information is likely to be disclosed, the position will be kept under review, and may even indeed be made retroactive (*Human Fertilisation and Embryology: A Framework for Legislation,* Cm 259, 1987, paras. 79-86, which also make it clear that the provisions for disclosure may be made retroactive). A late safeguard was written into the Act by s. 31(5). That provides that HUFEA can not be required to give information about the *identity* of a donor if acquired by a licence holder before or at any other time when HUFEA could not have been required to give the information. Of course, this could later be repealed; but the section was inserted to ensure that a full Parliamentary debate and primary legislation would be necessary to achieve that result.

There are four positions with regard to releasing information; that no identifying information be provided, that identification may be made with the consent of the donor, and that all identifying information be given. A fourth possibility, that adopted by the Act, is that some non-identifying information should be provided. An amendment during the Report stage of the House of Commons to add to s. 13(2)(c) that HUFEA should require information to be stored about the physical characteristics, family background, education, skills and interests and the health history of donors, was defeated. Additionally, the regulations will provide that the applicant may require the Authority to disclose if she or he is genetically related to a person whom they propose to marry. A minor who intends to marry may acquire similar information about their intended partner, but not the more widely ranging information available from the age of 18.

A limited survey conducted at the King's College Hospital Unit in London and quoted by Peter Thurnham (in House of Commons, Official Report 20 June 1990, col. 985) revealed that only one third of donors there were opposed to identification, while the other two thirds were in favour or reserved their position. Similarly, the British Association of Adoption and Fostering, the British Association of Social Workers, the Association of Directors of Social Services and the British Infertility Counselling Association are all in favour of moving away from anonymity and in favour of counselling. Counsellors working with infertile couples receiving infertility treatment have found that a lack of information about the donors is frequently the cause of much disquiet and distress.

It is of interest to observe here that the Glover Report, *Fertility and the Family* (supra,–. p. 1), concludes that there should be a presumption that children born through semen donation should have access to knowledge of the identity of their biological fathers when they reach adulthood. Because of worries about a resulting reduction in the supply of donors, the Report advocates a trial period of experiment following Swedish law (p. 150, discussed ibid at pp. 35-8). The Swedish experience is illuminating, because there are many forceful opponents of anonymity who argue for the child's or later adult's right to know of their genetic heritage. Following the abolition of anonymity in Sweden, there was an initial decline not only in donors, but also in couples seeking AID and physicians prepared to continue AID practice under the new decree. (See, 'Law on Insemination' No 1140 of 20 December 1984, art. 4, in Stepan, op.cit., p. 64 at 65.) Since then, in centres continuing to offer assistance (before the law was introduced there were 12, whereas there are now 9, with others starting up continuously), the numbers of donors have returned to their previous levels, although with two marked changes. The donors now tend to be older men, and also more often to be married men (see Glover, p. 36). The general experience, shared even by those who were most forceful in their opposition to the law, is that it has been and is working most successfully, and that the experience with adopted children seeking to discover their genetic identity is so strong that the denial of that interest to children of reproductive technology would be mistaken (see Erica Haimes 'Recreating the Family? Policy Considerations Relating to the 'New' Reproductive Technologies' in Maureen McNeil, Ian Varcoe and Steven Yearley, *The New Reproductive Technologies,* (1990) p. 154 at 158-59; for a contrary argument and view see Braude et al, 'Editorial' (1990) 330 *British Medical Journal* 1410).

The best report of the Swedish experience is given by Alexina McWhinnie, following a study visit in March 1990 (see, 'Visit to Sweden', unpublished manuscript 1990, Department of Social Work, Dundee University). In this report McWhinnie confirms the observations of Glover and remarks that the donors:

> . . . understand that the child in later life could come and see them. They are reported as saying they find this understandable, a 'human right to know the biological parents'. Those who volunteer accept the need to give name, address and details about themselves. Many clinics take a photograph of them for the file (op. cit., p. 2).

Information about the donors, who are asked to obtain the verbal consent of their partner, is kept in hospital files for 70 years. Those couples who want secrecy, or who fear possible competition from the donor figure, and who can afford to do so, travel to Finland, Denmark (where there are few controls on clinical practice and some practices which cause medical concern), or come to clinics in the United Kingdom. Although not all clinicians who opposed the introduction of the law in 1985 are persuaded, McWhinnie reports a favourable response now, even from some of those who were the most forceful critics. The number of births from assisted conception has, however, fallen back from around 200-250 p.a. to 50 p.a., although this is reportedly picking up again (op. cit., p. 2).

Those who look to Glover or elsewhere for a similar recommendation in respect of egg donation will be disappointed. The Report does not make any general statement about access to the identity of the biological mother; nor does it distinguish between biological parents by providing, for example, that gestation is what is important in the child/mother relationship. (The Human Fertilisation and Embryology Act does contain such a provision, s. 27 supra.) Rather, it fails to discuss this issue and addresses itself instead to the question of whether egg donors should be related to the recipient or unknown. The UK Interim Licensing Authority has insisted that egg donation remain anonymous and that donation by relatives is to be avoided. (Guideline 13(j), discussed in the *ILA Fourth Annual Report,* pp. 15-16.) Glover questions whether there are sufficient reasons for the exclusion of relative donors. Arguments about identity problems are conjectural. However, to avoid family pressure, the conclusion is that daughters should not normally donate eggs to their mothers. (This may be contrasted with the position adopted under the Human Organ Transplant Act 1989 which favours familial relationship donation.) There appears to be no restriction of egg donation in the Human Fertilisation and Embryology Act, but it is possible that this may be dealt with by the Secretary of State in regulations to be made under s. 45 or in HUFEA's Code of Practice, to be issued under the authority of s. 25. In the case of a related donor, Glover maintains that a child should not be deceived about the relationship (p. 41).

The decision of what to tell the children born of assisted conception has long stood as one of the most problematic aspects of technological creation. The balance between preserving the identity of the donor and fracturing the identity of the resulting child has produced one of the deepest of philosophical and pragmatic tensions. With artificial insemination and gamete donation there arises not just the possibility of anonymity for the donor, but of secrecy surrounding the circumstances of the person's conception. In a parallel case, that of adoption, the law in England and Wales has moved hesitantly towards that of Scotland where, since the inception of adoption regulation in 1930, adoptees have had access to their original birth certificate from the age of 17. Section 26 of the Children Act 1975 introduced the entitlement of a person of the age of 18 to a copy of their original birth certificate (see now Adoption Act 1976 s. 51; for a brief discussion of comparative approaches to donor identification see Rona Achilles, 'Donor Insemination: The Future of a Public Secret' in Christine Overall, ed., *The Future of Human Reproduction,* (1989), p. 105 at 113-17).

Katherine O'Donovan has argued that the need to know one's genetic ancestry is socially induced, and that we should concentrate on changing society's attitude to the importance of the blood relationship rather than undermining the anonymity protection presently given to gamete donors. She has further questioned the notion of a 'search for identity' said to characterise people who have been adopted; the empirical evidence is lacking which would substantiate the claim that there is an overwhelming urge on the part of adoptees to seek out their genitors (Katherine O'Donovan, 'What Shall We Tell The Children?' in Robert Lee and Derek Morgan, *Birthrights, Law and Ethics at the Beginnings of Life* (eds), (1989); and see Erica Haimes, 'Secrecy: What Can Artificial Insemination Learn From Adoption?' (1988) *International Journal of Law and the Family* 46-61). In reply, Don Evans has questioned whether the need of the infertile person or couple, and the accompanying demands for secrecy expressed by many, should require the deployment of medicine at the price of denying another need, that of any resulting child to know its genetic parents. And of the 'constructed' need to know one's genetic parentage, he has argued that the 'needs' of the infertile, for treatment or for secrecy, may themselves be thought of as socially constructed. If the importance of socially induced needs for the provision of medical treatment are to be denied, he writes, then we shall have to deny treatments of longevity, physical grace and beauty and the avoidance of, or palliation of, pain ('Government Legislation and Medical Practice', (1990) 55 *Bulletin of the Institute of Medical Ethics* 13).

The Act makes limited provision for rights of access to genetic information for those born of assisted conception or for those who think they may have been. Section 31 provides that HUFEA shall maintain a register of information supplied to it by clinics providing treatment services within the Act. On attaining the age of 18 an applicant may require HUFEA to furnish certain information. If HUFEA's information shows that the applicant was or may have been born following assisted conception, and the applicant has been given the opportunity to receive suitable counselling about the implications of receiving the information, then the Authority is placed under a duty to furnish it. It is the Government's stated intention that, for the moment, this information will not enable the applicant to identify any gamete or embryo donor involved, i.e., the applicant will not be able to trace her or his genetic parent unless they have already been told of their identity. The Act in making provision for an extraordinary case may require reconsideration. An applicant may require HUFEA to disclose if she or he is genetically related to a person whom they propose to marry. It is submitted that this provision should be amended, such that it is only on the application of both intending marriage partners that HUFEA will be able to disclose if the joint applicants are genetically related.

Section 31 makes provision for a register of information relating to the provision of treatment services, the keeping or use of gametes or embryos and births resulting from treatment services. There are then a number of procedures (outlined above) allowing access to that information. Section 33 then limits the disclosure of both registered information under s. 31 and also of any other information obtained in confidence by HUFEA and its staff. This is achieved by a strict prima facie rule against disclosure by HUFEA members and employees of such information. There are exemptions from this rule. One allows for such obvious purposes as disclosure to another member or to the Registrar General or a court who, by virtue of ss. 32 or 34 of the Act, may demand the assistance of HUFEA in determining paternity claims. Registered information may also be disclosed:

(i) to members and staff of HUFEA, acting as such;
(ii) to licence holders where necessary to discharge relevant functions (s. 33(3)(b));
(iii) to the Registrar General (s. 33(3)(e));
(iv) for stastical or other purposes where no individual can be identified (s. 33(3)(c));
(v) as allowed for in section 31 (above) (s. 33(3)(f));
(vi) on the order of a court in favour of a child seeking to bring an action under the Congenital Disabilities (Civil Liability) Act 1976 (s. 33(3)(d)); or a child in Scotland seeking to pursue an action for damages consisting of or including damages or soliatum for personal injury (s. 33(3)(d));
(vii) on the order of a court (usually in camera) in the interests of justice during any proceedings before that court (s. 33(3)(d)); this will accommodate orders such as those which may be made for example, on an application for a maintenance order for a child where paternity is disputed. In both cases (vi) and (vii), the court is enjoined strictly in the way it must determine whether or not to make the orders requested.

Non-registered information of a nonetheless confidential nature may be disclosed (s. 33(4)):

(i) to members and staff of HUFEA acting as such;
(ii) with the consent of the person whose confidence would otherwise be protected;
(iii) where lawful public disclosure has previously been made.

In the latter category, it is possible to argue that the information has already lost the necessary quality of confidence anyway.

Existing and previous licence holders are also bound by non-disclosure rules similar to those under s. 33(3). However, they can be required to disclose if directed to do so under s. 24(5) or (6) (see s. 33(6)(e)).

In addition to the above rules, information under s. 31(2)(a) and (b), namely information about the provision of treatment services or the keeping or use of gametes of any identifiable individual or of an embryo taken from an identifiable woman, can be disclosed if it relates only to that individual, or, if they are being treated with another, if it relates only to that person and that other. Notice that s. 33(7)(b) excludes the provision of information to a person who was, or might have been born, as a result of treatment services by providing that only information falling within s. 31(2)(a) or (b) is protected by the relaxation of the prohibition on disclosure. Difficulty surrounds the interpretation of the phrase 'and that other' which occurs at the end of s. 33(7)(b). It would have been clearer if the section had provided that information about A and B could have been disclosed to A or B. But that is not what it says. The difficulty which this creates can be illustrated in the following example:

> A and B are being provided with treatment services. In the course of so doing, the clinic discovers that B has recently come under suspicion by the local social services department of child abuse, or chronic alcohol abuse, such that the clinic now fear for the welfare of any child to be born as a result of the treatment service. Taking such factors into account under s. 13(5), the clinic decide to suspend the provision of the treatment services provided to A and B. May they lawfully disclose the reason for their discontinuance to A?

It is necessary to consider the disclosure provisions in conjunction with those of the Data Protection Act 1984. That Act is aimed at the prevention of holding inaccurate information in computerised records and at disclosing the existence of such records where they exist. It affords a right to see the records and ensure their accuracy. Note that the Act only applies to computerised records. Under s.29(1) of that Act, the Secretary of State is empowered to exempt certain categories of data, one of which is personal data concerning physical or mental health of the data subject. The power is one of either granting total exemption or modifying the operation of the access provisions. In general, this is subject to the Secretary of State being satisfied that, given the nature of the information, confidentiality ought to prevent the availability of subject access.

From an early stage in the life of the Data Protection Act it was made known that these powers would be used to restrict the disclosure of certain personal health data. This has been done in the Data Protection (Subject Access Modification) (Health) Order 1987 (SI 1987, No. 1903). Under this statutory instrument, permission is given to withhold data which might otherwise have to be disclosed in line with the current Act. In consequence, it has been possible to refuse to disclose personal data on the physical and/or mental health of the data subject which is held by a health professional. This exemption also applies to any other person, provided that the information constituting the data was first recorded by, or on behalf of, a health professional.

However, it must be noted that the withholding of information under this order is permissible only on two grounds. These are that the data will be likely to:

1. cause serious harm to the physical or mental health of the data subject; or
2. lead the data subject to identify another person (other than a health professional who has been involved in the care of the data subject) who has not consented to the disclosure of his or her identity.

This latter ground, which does not apply to health professionals involved in the care of the particular patient, will presumably mean that a data subject cannot, by searching their own health records, discover information relating to the health records of any other person (e.g., as to whether serious harm is likely to result). In each case the decision on disclosure is that of the health professional, a non-health professional being required under the order to consult the medical practitioner responsible for the clinical data ('an appropriate health professional') before deciding whether or not to supply the health data required. Similar categories of non-disclosure are likely to pertain when the Access to Health Records Act comes into force on 1 November 1991 (see ss. 4 and 5 of that Act).

These subject access provisions are generally exempted by s. 33(8) of the Act, except in so far as disclosure accords with the s. 31 rules. However, it seems that the data protection access provisions will apply to two categories of information held either by HUFEA or individual clinics or hospitals in computerised form. The first concerns 'personal data' relating to gamete donors (s. 13(2)(c)). A donor whose gametes are stored, or used in providing treatment services, or used in creating an embryo which is stored or used, may require HUFEA to furnish a copy of the information which the Authority directs a treatment centre to keep by virtue of ss. 13(2), 22 and 23. Secondly, 'personal information' held by virtue of s. 14(1)(d) also attracts access of the specific data subject. Section 14(1)(d) requires any clinic holding a licence enabling it to store frozen gametes or embryos to hold, in respect of any person whose consent is necessary under sch. 3 for continued storage of those gametes or embryos, such information as HUFEA may specify in directions. This information, which will include the terms on which consent to storage has been given and the circumstances of the storage, is preserved within the subject access provisions of the 1984 Act.

Conclusion

The information which a treatment licence holder granted by HUFEA under s. 13 and sch. 2 is to assemble will include information about any child who appears to have been born as a result of treatment services provided by the licensee. This falls short of obliging recipients of treatment to report the birth of any children either to the licence holder or to HUFEA, a condition which the Government White Paper thought would constitute 'an unacceptable intrusion on the privacy of couples' (para. 86). While this issue cannot be considered fully here, it goes to the heart of the question of secrecy canvassed earlier. It constitutes a regrettable omission from the attempts to provide for any resultant child access to information concerning its conception.

HUFEA will specify in directions how long this information, which will be held in the records maintained in pursuance of the licence, (s. 13(3)), must be maintained (s. 13(4)). In any case where the provider of treatment services does not know whether a birth subsequently took place, that information must be held for at least 50 years from its first registration (s. 24(1)). This again underlines a point made earlier about the regulation of GIFT; the lack of any parental obligation to inform may produce circumstances in which GIFT is not clinically indicated as the fertility treatment of choice, but where the greater degree of secrecy with which it can be practised make it appear an easier and more acceptable option, with attendant risks to the pregnant woman and perhaps to the foetuses which she will carry.

Chapter 7
Miscellaneous Provisions

In this final chapter we look at a number of miscellaneous issues to which assisted conception gives rise. We consider here:

(i) the question of civil liability to a child born with disability following infertility treatment;
(ii) surrogacy;
(iii) some legal issues of self-insemination, which although outside the statutory scheme, discloses at least two issues of particular difficulty;
(iv) the conscience clause provision which enables health care practitioners to dissociate themselves from any of the activities with which the Act is concerned;
(v) the scheme of offences created by the Act and the powers given to police and enforce regulated activities;
(vi) finally, provisions as to territoriality and commencement in the Act.

Civil Liability: Congenital Disability

The Congenital Disabilities (Civil Liability) Act 1976 provides for civil liability in the case of children born disabled in consequence of the intentional act, negligence, or breach of statutory duty of some person prior to the birth of the child. In so doing, it implemented the Law Commission's recommendation (*Report on Injuries to Unborn Children,* Law Com. No. 60 (1974)). The Act covers liability for children born alive; 'born' here meaning reaching the point at which the child has life separate from its mother (s. 4(2), 1976 Act and lives for 48 hours; and see *Rance,* supra). The defendant is answerable to the child if that defendant was liable in tort to one or both of the parents in respect of the matters which gave rise to the disability at birth. Such matters could arise either before conception, or during the pregnancy of the mother or the process of childbirth. In relation to matters arising before conception, this would clearly cover an injury to the parent which, at the time of conception, was transmitted to the child. And in *B* v *Islington Health Authority, The Times,* 15 November 1990, Potts J held that pre-natal tortious liability to a child subsequently born alive existed prior to the 1976 Act at common law. Such a claim was 'potential' or 'contingent', and crystallised on the child's live birth. It could not be defeated on public policy grounds that many similar claims might be generated. Note that under the 1976 Act, liability on the part of the mother to her own child is excluded, but the liability of the father is not. Such preconception or preimplantation liability is now additionally provided for in s. 44 of the 1990 Act.

The 1976 Act provides a number of defences to an action. A significant one is that if the parents, or either of them, knew the risk of the child being born disabled and accepted that risk, then the creator of the occurrence carrying that risk is excused liability. Clearly, this applies only to matters which precede conception (s. 1(4)). This defence is not available to the father where he is the defendant, and where he but not the mother had knowledge of the risk. For present purposes, however, s. 1(5) also provides a significant defence. Section 1(5) states that:

> The defendant is not answerable to the child, for anything he did or omitted to do when responsible in a professional capacity for treating or advising the parent, if he took reasonable care having due regard to then received professional opinion applicable to the particular class of case; but this does not mean that he is answerable only because he departed from received opinion.

This implements para. 96 of the Law Commission Report, but probably does little more than to enshrine, within the statute, standards which would be applicable in the law of negligence under the principles laid down in *Bolam* v *Friern Hospital Management Committee* [1957] 2 All ER 118 (see discussion above in relation to consent to treatment; Chapter 5).

The 1990 Act, by s. 44(1) introduces a new s. 1A to the 1976 Act specifically to provide for actions which might arise in the course of providing assisted conception. It follows the scheme of the 1976 Act, and introduces for children born as a result of assisted conception the same sort of regime in respect of statutory conditions for liability as that Act did for natural conception. It applies to any case where:

(i) a child has been born disabled following the placing in a woman of an embryo, or sperm and eggs, or following her artificial insemination;

(ii) the disability results from an act or omission in the course of the selection of the embryo or the gametes used to bring about the embryo; or

(iii) the disability results from some act or omission in the keeping or use of the embryo or gametes outside the body;

(iv) the defendant is (or would if sued in time have been) liable for negligence or breach of statutory duty to one or both of the parents, irrespective of whether they suffered actionable injury as long as there was a breach of duty which if injury had occurred would have given rise to liability (s. 44(1)(1A(1)(a)-(c))).

Section 44(1)(1A(3)) provides a defence to an action by a child where at the time of the treatment either or both of the parents knew the risk created by the particular act or omission of their child being born disabled (we discuss this infra). The other defences available under the 1976 act are also available in this extended action (s. 44(1)(1A(4))).

This section clearly covers damage caused by the keeping or storage of the embryos or gametes, whether they have been frozen or not. It also applies to the procedure of selection of the embryos for implantation, although so little is known about this process that it is more of a morphological check than a scientific screening procedure. There are on the face of the section some difficulties. For example, it is not clear that it applies to an act or omission which causes damage to an embryo being recovered from a woman by lavage for subsequent implantation in another woman who gestates the child subsequently born injured. It is arguable that the recovery of the embryo could be regarded as a 'selection', but it is probable that that wording would be more strictly confined to the selection of one rather than another embryo for transfer to the woman's uterus.

Where a surrogacy arrangement within the provisions of s. 30 (parental orders section) has taken place and the genetic parent(s) apply for an order, the provisions of the Congenital Disabilities Act will still apply for the benefit of the child. Subsection 44(1A)(2) provides that it is a condition of a successful action that the defendant was liable in tort to one or both of the 'parents'. Prima facie, where a parental order in favour of the gamete donors is later made, they are not the parents referred to in that section and hence the basis for the child's claim fails. Section 30(1) refers to 'a child to be treated in law as the child of the parties to a marriage . . .' If this is applied in the same way as, say, s. 29(1) and 29(2) (person to be treated in law as the mother or father of a child '. . . for all purposes') then this may give rise to difficulty in this one case of surrogacy. This argument can be assailed, however, in that s. 30(1) speaks not of the parental order ensuring that that person or couple is to be regarded as the child's parents for all purposes, as does s. 29(1) and (2), but of 'an order providing for a child to be treated in law as the child of the parties to a marriage . . .' It might be argued that the difference in wording is significant, and that it should be interpreted so as to save, rather than defeat the introduction of a scheme for the benefit of that child.

Section 44(1)(1A)(3) provides the same defence in respect of parental knowledge as in the 1976 Act. Thus, where at the time the embryo, or sperm and eggs were placed in the woman, or at the time she was inseminated, either or both of the parents knew the particular risk created by the act or omission of their child being born disabled, then the defendant (a 'person answerable to the child' under s. 44(1)(1A)(2)) is not answerable to the child. It will be interesting to monitor the way in which infertility clinics attempt to discharge their liability under this section. It has been suggested by some clinicians that a blanket warning as to risks of handicap as a result of infertility treatment would be sufficient to exculpate from liability. It will probably develop as practice to include some such provision in the consents form which the woman or the couple will sign at the outset of the treatment. The Draft Agreement for *In Vitro* Fertilisation produced by the ILA (and reproduced here as Appendix 6) suggests the adoption of the following:

> We understand and accept that there is no certainty that a pregnancy will result from these procedures, since the success rate is uncertain even where an egg is recovered and replacement carried out. We further understand and accept that the medical and scientific staff can give no assurance that pregnancy will result in the delivery of a normal living child.

In the light of the speeches of Lords Bridge and Keith in *Sidaway* [1985] 1 All ER 643 about the disclosures of risk it may well be that such a blanket attempt to provide 'information' would be insufficient for the parents to be satisfactorily appraised, as a matter of law, of the 'particular risk created by the act or omission' of which s. 44(1)(1A)(3) speaks. Recall that Lord Bridge had said:

> . . . even where, as here, no expert witness in the relevant medical field condemns the practice of non-disclosure as being in conflict with accepted and responsible medical practice, I am of the opinion that the judge might in certain circumstances come to the conclusion that disclosure of a particular risk was so obviously necessary to an informed choice on the part of the patient that no reasonably prudent medical man would fail to make it. The kind of case I have in mind would be an operation involving substantial risk of grave adverse consequences . . . (at p. 663).

When this is coupled with Lord Diplock's assertion that this general duty

> is not subject to dissection into a number of component parts to which different criteria of what satisfy the duty of care apply, such as diagnosis, treatment and advice (including warning of risks of something going wrong however skillfully the treatment has been carried out . . .) (at p. 657).

then the basis for understanding s. 44(1)(1A)(3) in a more comprehensive light is laid out. There will be some risks of congenital disability which are so grave and adverse, that specific disclosure of them and the consequences to which they may give rise if they materialise, will be necessary to escape liability under s. 44.

It is clear that, in a number of instances, for the purpose of instituting proceedings under s. 1 of the 1976 Act, it would be necessary to identify the genetic father or mother of the child. Suppose, for example, a complete failure of genetic screening at a treatment centre resulted in the birth of a child disabled within the meaning of the 1976 Act. If a mother were then to make a claim that the failure of genetic screening at the centre 'affected . . . her ability to have a normal, healthy child' since she was introduced to a donor whose sperm was always likely to give rise to a disabled child, it might be necessary for evidential purposes to trace that donor. Similarly, we speculate below (see p. 177) that the donor himself might be liable where, knowing that he was HIV positive, he nonetheless allowed his sperm to be used for infertility treatment. As the Act places liability upon 'a person (other than the child's own mother)', it is clear that there is nothing in the 1976 Act itself which would exempt the donor, even if considered as father, from liability (on the effect of s. 1(4) of the 1976 Act, see infra p. 177; this possibility was canvassed several times during the Commons debate; see House of Commons, Official Report, 20 June 1990, cols. 993 et.seq.). However, the problem would be identifying the donor. Finally, the state of the father's knowledge may be relevant to the s. 1(4) defence considered above. But who is the 'father' for these purposes?

A new s. 4(4A) of the Congenital Disabilities Act is included to provide that where, as the result of assisted conception, a child carried by a woman is born disabled, then references within the 1976 Act to a 'parent' will include a reference to a person who would be a parent but for ss. 27–29 of the 1990 Act (s. 35(4)). Also, in an attempt to resolve some of the difficulties of identifying parents, s. 35(1) states that where for the purposes of initiating proceedings under the 1976 Act, it is necessary to identify a person who would or might be the parent of a child (cf. the wording in s. 35(1)) but for ss. 27–29 of this Act, then the court may, on the application of the child, make an order requiring HUFEA to disclose registered information under s. 31 of the Act such that the person could be identified. Most importantly, this will include sections such as 29(1) and 29(2) which provide that donors are not ordinarily to be treated as either the mother or the father of the child in question. Note that this is only available on a court order which requires the Authority to disclose such information.

Congenital Disability: Product Liability

In the Introduction (pp. 28–32) we considered a number of areas which it seems the Government have chosen not to regulate through this Act. As we have already discussed, that the Act does not regulate these areas does not mean that they are not subject to sanction through the common law, let alone the wider jurisprudential point which would consider non-legal regulation. We pointed in that Introduction to the outstanding problem of whether gametes or embryos could ever amount to a 'product' within the meaning of the Consumer Protection Act 1987. Although there will be some who regard the asking of the question as itself evidence of the moral bankruptcy of this whole area, it is one to which we now return.

The 1987 Act places upon producers strict liability for products which prove to be defective and which cause damage or personal injury. 'Producer' in this context generally means the manufacturer of the product, but it can also encompass a person who is responsible for extracting a non-manufactured product. Liability may attach to a person who is not a producer if that person imports a product into the European Community. The Act gives a very broad meaning to the word products; it includes 'goods' (s. 1(2)), which is itself deemed to include substances. 'Substances', for the purposes of the Act 'means any natural or artificial solid, vaporous or liquid substance' (s. 45(1)). A product is considered to contain a 'defect' when 'the safety of the product is not such as persons are generally entitled to expect' (s. 3(1); and see also Art. 6, Directive of the Council of the European Community on Product Liability, 85/374/EEC; adopted July 1985). In determining whether or not a product has lived up to its expectations of safety, regard must be paid to the manner of the marketing of he product, including any instructions or warnings provided at the time of its supply.

Providing causation can be shown, then physical damage, including personal njury, is recoverable. Physical injury here includes disease, and the impairment of mental as well as physical health (s. 45(1)). Section 6(3) of the 1987 Act gives effect to s. 1 of the Congenital Disabilities Act 1976, thereby incorporating the provisions of this legislation into the strict liability regime. This is done by providing that where a parent has a right to sue for an occurrence arising out of a defect in a product, the defendant faces the same liability towards a child suffering from disability following the parent's exposure to that occurrence. This provision clearly has regard to matters such as the Thalidomide litigation which in part has given rise to the implementation of this form of product liability measure. There are a number of defences under the Consumer Protection Act, but the most significant one is that at the time of supply, the state of scientific knowledge was not such that a producer of products of the same description might be expected to have discovered the defect if it had existed in his products whilst they were under his control (the 'state of the art' defence, s. 49(1)(e); cf. Art. 7(e) of the Directive, supra). Looking at the operation of the product liability law under the 1987 Act, there is no reason in principle why gametes and embryos may not be 'products' within the meaning of the 1987 Act. They are clearly 'substances', and it is interesting to recall that the Pearson Commission on *Civil Liability and Compensation for Personal Injury* (Cmnd 7054 (1978) para. 1276) recommended that 'human blood and organs should be regarded as "products" and authorities responsible for distributing them as their "producers" for the purposes of product liability'. The argument against this might be that the provision of infertility treatment is the provision of services which ought not to be encompassed within the Act (see Whittaker (1989) 105 *Law Quarterly Review* 125, who argues that professional liability should remain fault-based).

Although s. 6(3) of the 1987 Act specifically incorporates claims for congenital disability, it is likely that it had in mind claims based on pharmaceutical products. It is a rather different matter to consider claims where the 'product' which was alleged to be defective is the very stuff which gave rise to the life of the litigant herself or himself. Courts might prove highly reluctant to allow such claims, especially in view of the rejection of such matters as wrongful life claims (see *McKay* v *Essex Area Health Authority* [1982] QB 1166 and Lee, 'To Be or Not to Be: Is That the Question?' in Robert Lee and Derek Morgan, (eds.), *Birthrights*, supra). Issues of liability might also founder on the question of 'damage'. 'Damage' means 'death or personal injury or any loss of or damage to property' (s. 5(1)), but liability is excluded when the defect in the product causes loss of or damage to the product itself or to 'the whole or any part of any product which has been supplied with the product in question comprised in it' (s. 5(2)). It is a difficult question of British jurisprudence whether a person could properly be described as a 'product supplied', even where she comprises the gametes or embryos from which she is derived. On the other hand, would the courts find it so difficult if, in the course of offering infertility treatment, the embryo which was implanted into the woman caused the woman to become seriously ill?

In many ways the whole tone of the 1987 Act seems inappropriate for this body of law. Consider the defence under s. 4(1)(f). This applies where the product was a component in some other product, and the defect causing damage is wholly attributable either to the design of the other product or to specifications given by the designer of the other product to the producer of the component, or to inadequate installation. One can see arguments arising as to whether the sperm was a defective component or whether the actual problem was the adequate installation of the fertilised egg. It seems to make genetic engineering a most appropriate term. On the other hand, are there reasons in principle why, if persons are engaged in such activities, they ought not to be liable for the damage which may result?

Surrogacy

We have already examined one of the two provisions in the Act which make specific provision for surrogacy. The first is that contained in s. 30, and which provides for the making of a parental order following a surrogacy arrangement in favour of the intending parents (see, supra, pp. 153–54). The second provision amends s. 1 of the Surrogacy Arrangements Act 1985. By s. 36(1) the common law position adopted in *A* v *C* (1978, [1985] FLR 445), that a surrogacy arrangement is unenforceable, is put on a statutory footing. Section 36(2) extends the meaning of a surrogacy arrangement, by providing that an arrangement under the Act relates not only to embryo transfer, but also placing in the surrogate mother an egg in the process of fertilisation or of sperm and eggs. In other words, the Surrogacy Arrangements Act is now drawn even wider in the types of medical assistance which it seeks to discourage and takes into account new techniques of fertility treatment not available in 1985.

Self-insemination; Some Legal Issues

> If a donor wilfully donates what he knows to be contaminated or genetically defective sperm, such an action could possibly arise, but that is to go into the realm of fantasy (Secretary of State for Health Kenneth Clarke, House of Commons Official Report, 20 June 1990, col. 994).

AI is a relatively straightforward procedure, and do-it-yourself kits, which have been available on the market for many years, represent the white-heat state of the technology. As the Act was originally presented to Parliament, however, it was unclear whether it was the intention to render self-insemination unlawful, as in Victoria, where the Infertility (Medical Procedures) Act 1984 makes it a criminal offence subject to a maximum of two years' imprisonment to undertake unlicensed self-insemination. The original definition of treatment services was amended to include the present formulation. This now defines a treatment service as 'medical, surgical or obstetrical services provided to the public *or a section of the public* for the purposes of assisting women to carry children' (s. 2(1)). The emphasised words were included to make it clear that the Government did not intend to include such a draconian provision as Victoria.

However, those who are using donated sperm, whether through a known donor or anonymously, should be aware of the hazards of a negligence action. In particular, given the risks of transmitted disease such as HIV and hepatitus B attached to donor semen which has not been screened, a real question of a negligence suit at the instance of any child born following an affected donation must arise. Would it be negligent to donate sperm for the purposes of insemination knowing oneself to be HIV antibody positive? The answer would probably be 'yes' (see Law Commission *Report on Injuries to Unborn Children* (supra), para. 76; 'the negligent supply of male sperm for artificial insemination would seem to be another possible source of pre-natal injury'). Indeed, the defence in s. 1(4) of the Congenital Disabilities (Civil Liability) Act 1976 in respects of risks of disability to the child known to one or both parents is specifically avoided where the risk (as here, for example, of infection) is known to the father but not to the mother. It might also amount to a criminal battery or causing a noxious substance to be taken contrary to s. 23 of the Offences Against the Person Act 1861, but on these questions it is more difficult to express a definite opinion here (see Smith and Hogan, *Criminal Law,* (1988), Butterworths 6th. ed., p. 382, discussing *Clarence* (1888) 22 QBD 23, a case of inflicting grevious bodily harm by having intercourse while affected with a venereal disease).

A further, more difficult question arises. Could it amount to negligence to donate sperm knowing the specific purpose to which it was to be put, and knowing that a specific and identifiable class of persons might be affected by your act or omission, for a man to donate sperm without knowing whether or not he was antibody positive? What are the grounds on which such liability could be avoided? That the party suffering the harm, the child, was not yet in being at the time of the negligent act or omission; i.e., that the act or omission occurred not while the child was *en ventre sa mere,* but before that. As we have seen in the discussion of congenital disability, that is not a ground upon which liability may be avoided, a point now confirmed at common law by *B* v *Islington Health Authority,* (supra).

Conscience Clauses

Section 4 of the Abortion Act 1967 provides that:

> No person shall be under a duty, whether by contract or by statutory or other legal requirement, to participate in any treatment authorised by this Act to which he has a conscientious objection.

The remainder of s. 4 goes on to state that, in legal proceedings, the burden of proof in conscientious objection shall rest upon the person claiming to rely on it. It is also made clear that the section is not intended to affect any duty of practitioners to participate in treatment which will be necessary to save life or prevent grave permanent injury to the physical and mental health of a pregnant woman.

Surrounding this statutory requirement is a long-standing agreement between the Department of Health and the medical profession to the effect that no reference to termination duties will be included in the advertisement of hospital posts, but that if posts involved such duties, mention of them should be made in job descriptions so that doctors who do not want to be involved in termination duties are aware of the position. This agreement is encompassed in a series of letters sent to regional medical officers from the Chief Medical Officer at the Department of Health. The latest of these is dated 11 October 1989. This letter followed a breach of the guidelines by Trent Regional Health Authority who placed advertisements in *The Lancet* in April 1989 in breach of the CMO's guideline. All these posts were subsequently readvertised, but the CMO took the opportunity to reiterate earlier guidelines (PL/CMO (89)(8)). Amongst other things, the guidelines state that unless the job description specifies that there are likely to be termination duties, candidates should not be asked whether they would be prepared to undertake such duties. Even where job descriptions do state that termination duties are necessary, questions should be confined to professional intentions, and not to candidates' personal beliefs. It should be noted, however, that in the case of junior medical staff it is thought inappropriate for termination responsibilities to be included in the job description. This is because it is thought unnecessary for training purposes to require all junior staff in training grades to undertake such duties.

As regards nursing staff, the requirements of s. 4 obviously apply equally to both nurses and midwives. It is important to note also that the statute applies both to the NHS and to the private sector. This is of particular importance in considering the equivalent conscience clause in the 1990 Act, section 38.

The provisions in relation to nursing staff are similar to those as to doctors; there may be no mention of the duties in the advertisement, but the job description may include reference to terminations. In the House of Commons, before the Social Services Committee in Hearings on the Abortion Act 1967 'Conscience Clause' (1989-90, 10 January 1990), the Department of Health disclosed that they had had only five enquiries relating to the operation of the 'Conscience Clause' in the three years 1986 to 1988 inclusive. On the other hand, in the Second Committee Hearing (21 March 1990), the Committee heard from five doctors all of whom claimed to have some evidence of discrimination against medical staff, indicating that to some degree moral views were not fully honoured. Their view might be adequately summed up as follows:

> there is no doubt at all in my mind that the 'Conscience Clause' is vital to the protection of doctors who do have a conscience about these matters, [and] that at the moment it is not adequately operating, it is operating by default (21 March 1990, at p. 54).

Similarly, it was asserted in written evidence that:

> the tendency is for many doctors who hold pro-life views deliberately not to choose to do gynaecology. There are enough career uncertainties anyway in hospital medicine without adding this one (21 March 1990, at p. 50).

These remarks have to be contrasted with the views of doctors who also attended the same hearing and gave evidence to the opposite effect. The thrust of these is neatly summarised as follows:

> I have no evidence at all that people who have a conscientious objection to doing terminations, or those who are willing to do them, have any hurdles put in their way in terms of promotion (21 March 1990, at p. 37).

It would seem to follow that, thus far, in spite of the original concerns of discrimination that led to the Select Committee reviewing the 'Conscience Clause' in the 1967 Act, evidence seems inconclusive as to whether or not the operation of this clause causes practical difficulties. One path along which the Select Committee was urged to travel, however, was to remove the provision of abortion services from alongside other gynaecological services by the provision of separate abortion units within the NHS. Some of the doctors who gave evidence before the Committee later wrote to state that in spite of their initially favourable reaction to this suggestion, they were concerned that it might increase the overall level of abortions (21 March 1990, pp. 61-2). In the event, the Committee did not recommend such a drastic reorganisation of service provision (see Social Services Committee, Tenth Report, HC 123 (17 October 1990) 'Abortion Act: The Conscience Clause').

One question which was put to the Department of Health representatives before the Committee was whether it was reasonable to reproduce the 'Conscience Clause' in s. 4 of the 1967 Act within the Human Fertilisation and Embryology Bill. The answer received was that, because certain people would clearly have conscientious objections to some of the treatments for infertility which the Act would license, it would be appropriate to include a 'Conscience Clause'. Moreover, in the Department's view there was 'no evidence to suggest that "Conscience Clauses" were causing sufficient problems' to the point that it would be unwise to include one within the Human Fertilisation and Embryology Bill. Section 38 of the Act now contains a provision on conscientious objection. This is phrased rather differently from the one contained in the Abortion Act, for whilst it retains the burden of proof on the objector, (a matter which the Social Services Committee thought should be reformed by the Department of Health) it simply says that no person who has a conscientious objection to participating in any activity governed by the Act shall be under any duty howsoever arising to do so. It does not repeat s. 4(2) of the Abortion Act to the effect that a duty to participate in life saving treatment is retained. This may be because it is assumed that participation in the activities governed by the 1990 Act will not generally give rise to life threatening or seriously disabling conditions. This of course was frustrated, at the point where abortion was included as an activity governed by the 1990 Act, and indeed, there is now an implicit conflict between s. 38 of the Act and s. 4 of the Abortion Act. To the extent that any activity governed by the Act might give rise to a life threatening condition, it might be stated that, in spite of the absence of any proviso relating to this within the statute, at common law once a doctor had commenced treatment on a patient, the doctor would be under a duty to intervene in order to arrest conditions which are life threatening or causing grave physical injury (see *Re F; F* v *Berkshire Health Authority* [1990] 2 All ER 545). Such duty may arise both out of negligence and the criminal law.

There is also a body of law on the scope of the conscience objection allowed by s. 4, which may be relevant here. This concerns the question of what might amount to participating in treatment (see *Royal College of Nursing* v *Department of Health & Social Security* [1981] AC 800.) This case concerned a circular dated 21 February 1980 from the Department of Health & Social Security which purported to explain the law relating to abortion in connection with the termination of pregnancy by medical induction. The Royal College of Nursing sought a declaration that the circular was wrong in law in so far as it allowed that important parts of this process would be performed not by a registered medical practitioner, but by a nurse acting under instruction. The issue arose as to whether the actions of the nurse were unlawful, and it was held that they were not. The grounds given were that what was authorised by the Act was the whole medical process which would result in the termination of pregnancy, and providing that process was carried out by a registered medical practitioner, then procedures done under her or his supervision and in accordance with those instructions could be lawful. The declaration was refused. In the course of the judgment in the House of Lords, Lord Roskill considered the application of s. 4 and the words 'participate in treatment'. The importance of the provision, in Lord Roskill's view, for the purposes of the case, was that unless it was anticipated that nursing staff would from time to time become involved in the treatment procedures for terminating pregnancy, then it was difficult to see why conscientious objection might be permitted.

A case more directly in point is *Janaway* v *Salford Health Authority* [1988] 3 All ER 1079. In this case the applicant was employed by the local Health Authority as a doctor's receptionist and secretary. She refused to type a letter of referral for an abortion on conscientious grounds. She was then dismissed by the Authority. The applicant sought judicial review of this decision, contending that she was entitled to refuse by virtue of s. 4(1) of the 1967 Act. The House of Lords, however, applied the ordinary and natural meaning of the word 'participate' to mean that the objector had to be required actually to take part in administering treatment in a hospital or other approved centre for the purpose of terminating a pregnancy. Consequently, arrangements preliminary to the termination, such as typing letters of referral would not be included. Unfortunately, this does not resolve all the questions concerning what amounts to 'participating.'

Under the Abortion Act, it is usual for a form of certification (the Green Form) to be signed by two registered medical practitioners in pursuance of s. 1(1)(a) of the 1967 Act. It is well known that certain medical practitioners will not sign the Green Form as a matter of practice, and request that other practitioners be found. In *Janaway,* Lord Keith in the House of Lords considered the question as to whether or not in the light of their decision, s. 4(1) would extend to practitioner refusals to sign the Green Form. Unfortunately, he then concluded that:

> The fact that during the twenty years that the 1967 Act has been in force no problem seems to have surfaced in this connection may indicate that in practice none exists. So I do not think it appropriate to express any opinion on the matter (at p. 1083).

In view of the extension of the abortion section of the 1967 Act to the present Act, it is unfortunate that the House of Lords did not take the opportunity presented in *Janaway* to express a clearer view upon the operation of the conscience clause. There is apparent uncertainty as to the extent of the clause in relation to participating in treatment. In written evidence to the Social Services Committee it was averred that 'the status of others such as anaesthetists who help the practitioner provide the treatment is uncertain' (supra, 21 March 1990, p. 22). In the nature of things, it would seem that if the anaesthetists help to provide the treatment, then by definition, they participate in it, and must be covered by the 'Conscience Clause'. A good deal of discussion within the Social Services Committee concerned the extent to which nurses may be required to treat patients who are attending hospital for an abortion. In fact, however, a broad consensus has emerged. It was agreed that a patient haemorrhaging on a ward would be treated by a nurse whatever her convictions (evidence to Social Services Committee, 10 January 1990, p. 13). It was also accepted that in general staff would not be so frivolous as to wish to refuse such a patient a cup of tea (ibid). This still leaves the difficult middle ground unexplored, although significantly all doctors appear to show great respect for the limits of the individual nurse's conscience. Wendy Savage at one point interrupted the questioning of the Committee to point out that in her view; 'the nurse should not be asked to top up prostaglandin infusion if she has a conscientious objection to that.'

One final point of interest that emerged within the Committee (10 January 1990, p. 15) is that in the process of inspecting and approving facilities for abortion in the private sector, it is regular practice on the part of the Department of Health, when dealing with an application for approval to provide abortion facilities, to talk with the proprietors and senior staff of the centre. Included in the subjects always discussed is the 'Conscience Clause' and the provision made within the establishment for the operation of that clause. Therefore, by analogy, it could be that one issue to be considered by licensing committees considering applications for grant or renewal of licences in relation to HUFEA functions is the operation of s. 38 of the Act.

Criminal Offences: Powers and Penalties

The Act creates a variety of offences which have been considered in the appropriate chapters. Here, however, we provide a brief résumé. The penalties for these offences are set out in s. 41, and the powers of enforcement given to members and employees in ss. 39 and 40.

No proceedings under these sections may be instituted without the consent of the Director of Public Prosecutions or, in Northern Ireland, the Director of Public Prosecutions for Northern Ireland (s. 42).

There are four categories of offence under the Act:

1. Acting in contravention of s. 3(2) or s. 4(1)(c) by placing in a woman a live embryo other than a human embryo, or live gametes other than human gametes or mixing human gametes with live animal gametes without a licence: these are offences punishable on indictment with up to 10 years' imprisonment or an unlimited fine or both (s. 41(1)(a)). Similarly, anyone who keeps or uses an embryo after the appearance of the primitive streak; places a human embryo in an animal; keeps or uses an embryo in contravention of regulations; engages in nucleus substitution, commits an offence (s. 41(1)(b)) punishable with the same sentences. Section 41(11) provides a statutory defence to all offences charged under this Act, in favour of a person to whom a licence applies or a person to whom statutory directions had been given. Where they show that they took all such steps as were reasonable, and exercised all due diligence to avoid committing an offence, they will be entitled to acquittal. Section 41(10) provides for an additional defence in respect of the offence under ss. 3(1) and 4(1) of unlicensed creation, keeping or use of an embryo or unlicensed mixing of gametes. Where the defendant can show that she or he was acting under the direction of another whom they believed on reasonable grounds (i) to be the person responsible under a licence, a person designated as one to whom a licence applies under s. 17(2)(b) or a person to whom statutory directions had been given under s. 24(9) and (ii) that she or he was authorised by virtue of the licence or directions to do the activity now complained of.

2. The unlicensed keeping, using or bringing about the creation of an embryo, (but falling short of either keeping or using it after the appearance of the primitive streak, placing it in an animal, keeping or using it in contravention of regulations or practising nucleus substitution with it) contrary to s. 3(1); or unlicensed storage of gametes or provision of treatment services involving the use of donated gametes contrary to s. 4(1)(a) and (b); or unlicensed placing of sperm and eggs in a woman in any circumstances specified in regulations (s. 4(3)); or failure to comply with directions given by HUFEA under s. 24(7)(a) to provide information when a licence committee proposes to take certain specified action; each of these four activities is an offence (s. 41(2)) triable either way and punishable on conviction on indictment with a maximum of two years' imprisonment or an unlimited fine or both; or on a summary conviction, to a maximum of six months' imprisonment and a fine not in excess of the statutory maximum (presently £2,000; the Criminal Justice Bill 1990 seeks to raise this to £5,000) or both (s. 41(4)). In addition to the statutory defence of s. 41(11) which applies to all these offences, a person tried in respect of an offence under s. 3(1) or 4(1) (keeping or using gametes or embryos in contravention of the Act) may seek to avail themselves of the additional statutory defence under s. 41(10), discussed above. The same penalties are provided by s. 41(4) for offences under s. 41(3) of knowingly or recklessly providing information for the purposes of the grant of a licence which is false or misleading in a material particular. A misstatement of the experience and qualifications of a laboratory technician employed to prepare culture fluid might not be material for these purposes, whereas a similar misstatement in respect of the person to be the 'person responsible' under the licence would be.

3. The unauthorised disclosure of information by a member, employee, former member or former employee of HUFEA in contravention of s. 33 of the Act is an offence punishable following conviction on indictment with up to two years' imprisonment or an unlimited fine or both, and following summary conviction to imprisonment for up to six months or a fine not exceeding the statutory maximum or both (s. 41(5)). The s. 41(11) defence is available.

4. Section 41(9) provides a similar scale of penalties for six offences under sections 41(6), (7) and (8). These offences may only be tried before a magistrates' court and on conviction a person is liable to imprisonment for up to six months or a fine not exceeding level 5 on the standard scale, or both. In respect of each of the six offences, s. 41(11) applies. The offences are:

(i) failure to comply with a requirement made under s. 39(1)(b) (for reasonable assistance to be rendered to any member or employee of HUFEA entering and inspecting premises and seeking to preserve or prevent interference with anything which may be necessary as evidence for an offence under the Act or in connection with the grant, variation, suspension or revocation of a licence) (s. 41(6));

(ii) failure to comply with a requirement made under s. 39(2)(b) (request to produce copy of information to member or employee of HUFEA) (s. 41(6));

(iii) failure to comply with a requirement made under ss. 40(2)(b)(ii) or 40(5)(b) (request to produce copy of information to someone entering premises under warrant) (s. 41(6));

(iv) intentional obstruction of the exercise of rights conferred by a warrant issued under s. 40 (s. 41(7));

(v) failing, without reasonable excuse to comply with requirement imposed by regulations made under s. 10(2)(a) (requiring persons to produce documents or give evidence) (s. 41(7));

(vi) the unauthorised receipt or making by the person to whom a licence applies or the nominal licensee, of any payment, whether money or other benefit, in respect of the supply of gametes or embryos (s. 41(8)).

Powers of policing and enforcement of the provisions of the Act are given in ss. 39 and 40. Any member of HUFEA or any employee entering and inspecting licensed premises may take possession of anything which she or he has reasonable grounds to believe may be required as evidence of an offence or may be necessary in HUFEA's discharge of its licensing functions (s. 39(1)(a)). Such a person is given power to take such steps as appear to be necessary to prevent interference with the evidence or to preserve it (s. 39(1)(b)), and may request any one having the power to do so to provide assistance with the preservation or prevention of interference. Anything taken may be kept for as long as necessary for the purpose in question (s. 39(1)).

The 'things' referred to in this section clearly contemplate embryos kept beyond the appearance of the primitive streak, the creation of hybrids, nucleus substitution and so on; but it also extends to cover information kept at licensed clinics. There is a saving in s. 39(3) to protect members or employees of HUFEA;

nothing in the Act makes it unlawful for them to keep embryos or gametes in pursuance of their functions.

Section 40(1) provides for the issuance to a member or employee of HUFEA of a warrant to enter and inspect premises and to search premises. The usual allied powers of calling on the assistance of constables and the use of reasonable force is also granted (s. 40(2)). Anything taken under authority of a warrant must be returned within six months, unless proceedings for an offence are instituted, in which case the evidence may be retained until the conclusion of the proceedings.

Territorial Extent and Commencement

The Act extends to England, Wales, Scotland, and, except the provision in relation to abortion law reform, Northern Ireland (s. 48). Orders in Council may be used to provide that the Act should extend to any of the Channel Islands and with such adaptations or modifications as may be there specified (s. 49(7)).

An interesting parallel provision, the Family Law Bill 1990, presently before the House of Keyes in the Tynwald, makes some provision for dealing with assisted conception matters in the Isle of Man (one of the British Islands but not a part of the United Kingdom). Clause 33 of that Bill is in terms similar to s. 27 of the Family Law Reform Act 1987 in England and Wales. It deals only with the case of artificial insemination of a married woman. It provides that any child born of artificial insemination after the passing of the legislation shall be deemed to be the child of the marriage, unless:

> . . . it is proved to the satisfaction of any court by which the matter has to be determined that the other party to that marriage did not consent to the insemination . . .

There is a similar saving in clause 33(3) of that Bill to s. 29(4) and (5) in the 1990 Act, that nothing in that Act affects succession to any dignity or title of honour or renders any person capable of succeeding to or transmitting a right to succeed to any such dignity or title.

The Human Fertilisation and Embryology Act comes into force on days to be appointed by the Secretary of State for Health (s. 49(2)). Different days may be appointed for different sections, and those constituting HUFEA were be among the earliest to be introduced. The Human Fertilisation and Embryology Act 1990 (Commencement No 1) Order 1990 (SI 1990 No 2165) was made on 2 November 1990. It brought into force on 7 November 1990 some of the foundational provisions of the Act. These include s. 2(1) (where it defines 'the Authority'); s. 5 and sch. 1 establishing HUFEA; ss. 6–7 dealing with accounts and audit and HUFEA's report to the Secretary of State; s. 26, the procedure for approval of the Code of Practice; s. 33(1), (2)(b) and (4) which implement restrictions on disclosure of information and s. 40 which gives power to enter premises and s. 41(5), the section constituting various offences, so far as it relates to those provisions of s. 33 seeking to safeguard information, and 41(6) and (9) so far as they create offences relating to the power to enter premises under s. 40. That

Commencement Order also introduced on 7 November s. 42, requiring the consent of the DPP to any prosecution under the Act; s. 48(1), so far as that extends to Northern Ireland the provisions brought into force by the Order and s. 49(1), (2), (6) and (7): the short title and commencement provisions. Finally, the Order also brought into force s. 36 which introduces amendments to the Surrogacy Arrangements Act 1985. Section 49(6) contains arrangements for making transitional provisions; this is particularly important in the respect of ss. 3 and 4, which provide that some activities may only be done under licence from HUFEA. Orders made under s. 49(6) may make such transitional provisions as the Secretary of State considers necessary or desirable. In particular, an order made under that section may provide that activities already being carried on by a person shall be regarded as authorised by licence for such transitional period as is specified in the order. The order may also impose conditions on the exercise of the licence in addition to those specified in the Act.

Sections 27–29 will have effect in respect of the matters with which they deal only after they have been brought into effect (s. 49(3)), and after that time, s. 27 of the Family Law Reform Act 1987, dealing with the status of children born following artificial insemination, will cease to have effect (s. 49(4)).

Appendix 1
Human Fertilisation and Embryology Act 1990

CHAPTER 37

ARRANGEMENT OF SECTIONS

SCHEDULES

Schedule 1 — The Authority: supplementary provisions.
Schedule 2 — Activities for which licences may be granted.
Schedule 3 — Consents to use of gametes or embryos.
Schedule 4 — Status: amendments of enactments.

Human Fertilisation and Embryology Act 1990

1990 Chapter 37. An Act to make provision in connection with human embryos and any subsequent development of such embryos; to prohibit certain practices in connection with embryos and gametes; to establish a Human Fertilisation and Embryology Authority; to make provision about the persons who in certain circumstances are to be treated in law as the parents of a child; and to amend the Surrogacy Arrangements Act 1985. [1 November 1990]

BE IT ENACTED by the Queen's most Excellent Majesty, by and with the advice and consent of the Lords Spiritual and Temporal, and Commons, in this present Parliament assembled, and by the authority of the same, as follows:—

Principal terms used

Meaning of "embryo", "gamete" and associated expressions.

1.—(1) In this Act, except where otherwise stated—

(a) embryo means a live human embryo where fertilisation is complete, and

(b) references to an embryo include an egg in the process of fertilisation, and, for this purpose, fertilisation is not complete until the appearance of a two cell zygote.

(2) This Act, so far as it governs bringing about the creation of an embryo, applies only to bringing about the creation of an embryo outside the human body; and in this Act—

(a) references to embryos the creation of which was brought about *in vitro* (in their application to those where fertilisation is complete) are to those where fertilisation began outside the human body whether or not it was completed there, and

(b) references to embryos taken from a woman do not include embryos whose creation was brought about *in vitro*.

(3) This Act, so far as it governs the keeping or use of an embryo, applies only to keeping or using an embryo outside the human body.

(4) References in this Act to gametes, eggs or sperm, except where otherwise stated, are to live human gametes, eggs or sperm but references below in this Act to gametes or eggs do not include eggs in the process of fertilisation.

Other terms.
2.—(1) In this Act—
"the Authority" means the Human Fertilisation and Embryology Authority established under section 5 of this Act,
"directions" means directions under section 23 of this Act,
"licence" means a licence under Schedule 2 to this Act and, in relation to a licence, "the person responsible" has the meaning given by section 17 of this Act, and
"treatment services" means medical, surgical or obstetric services provided to the public or a section of the public for the purpose of assisting women to carry children.

(2) Reference in this Act to keeping, in relation to embryos or gametes, include keeping while preserved, whether preserved by cryopreservation or in any other way; and embryos or gametes so kept are referred to in this Act as "stored" (and "store" and "storage" are to be interpreted accordingly).

(3) For the purposes of this Act, a woman is not to be treated as carrying a child until the embryo has become implanted.

Activities governed by the Act

Prohibitions in connection with embryos.
3.—(1) No person shall—
(a) bring about the creation of an embryo, or
(b) keep or use an embryo,
except in pursuance of a licence.

(2) No person shall place in a woman—
(a) a live embryo other than a human embryo, or
(b) any live gametes other than human gametes.

(3) A licence cannot authorise—
(a) keeping or using an embryo after the appearance of the primitive streak,
(b) placing an embryo in any animal,
(c) keeping or using an embryo in any circumstances in which regulations prohibit its keeping or use, or
(d) replacing a nucleus of a cell of an embryo with a nucleus taken from a cell of any person, embryo or subsequent development of an embryo.

(4) For the purposes of subsection (3)(a) above, the primitive streak is to be taken to have appeared in an embryo not later than the end of the period of 14 days beginning with the day when the gametes are mixed, not counting any time during which the embryo is stored.

Prohibitions in connection with gametes.
4.—(1) No person shall—
(a) store any gametes, or

(b) in the course of providing treatment services for any woman, use the sperm of any man unless the services are being provided for the woman and the man together or use the eggs of any other woman, or

(c) mix gametes with the live gametes of any animal,

except in pursuance of a licence.

(2) A licence cannot authorise storing or using gametes in any circumstances in which regulations prohibit their storage or use.

(3) No person shall place sperm and eggs in a woman in any circumstances specified in regulations except in pursuance of a licence.

(4) Regulations made by virtue of subsection (3) above may provide that, in relation to licences only to place sperm and eggs in a woman in such circumstances, sections 12 to 22 of this Act shall have effect with such modifications as may be specified in the regulations.

(5) Activities regulated by this section or section 3 of this Act are referred to in this Act as "activities governed by this Act".

The Human Fertilisation and Embryology Authority, its functions and procedure

The Human Fertilisation and Embryology Authority.

5.—(1) There shall be a body corporate called the Human Fertilisation and Embryology Authority.

(2) The Authority shall consist of—

(a) a chairman and deputy chairman, and

(b) such number of other members as the Secretary of State appoints.

(3) Schedule 1 to this Act (which deals with the membership of the Authority, etc.) shall have effect.

Accounts and audit.

6.—(1) The Authority shall keep proper accounts and proper records in relation to the accounts and shall prepare for each accounting year a statement of accounts.

(2) The annual statement of accounts shall comply with any direction given by the Secretary of State, with the approval of the Treasury, as to the information to be contained in the statement, the way in which the information is to be presented or the methods and principles according to which the statement is to be prepared.

(3) Not later than five months after the end of an accounting year, the Authority shall send a copy of the statement of accounts for that year to the Secretary of State and to the Comptroller and Auditor General.

(4) The Comptroller and Auditor General shall examine, certify and report on every statement of accounts received by him under subsection (3) above and shall lay a copy of the statement and of his report before each House of Parliament.

(5) The Secretary of State and the Comptroller and Auditor General may inspect any records relating to the accounts.

(6) In this section "accounting year" means the period beginning with the day when the Authority is established and ending with the following 31st March, or any later period of twelve months ending with the 31st March.

Reports to Secretary of State.

7.—(1) The Authority shall prepare a report for the first twelve months of its existence, and a report for each succeeding period of twelve months, and shall send each report to the Secretary of State as soon as praticable after the end of the period for which it is prepared.

(2) A report prepared under this section for any period shall deal with the activities of the Authority in the period and the activities the Authority proposes to undertake in the succeeding period of twelve months.

(3) The Secretary of State shall lay before each House of Parliament a copy of every report received by him under this section.

General functions of the Authority.

8. The Authority shall—

(a) keep under review information about embryos and any subsequent development of embryos and about the provision of treatment services and activities governed by this Act, and advise the Secretary of State, if he asks it to do so, about those matters,

(b) publicise the services provided to the public by the Authority or provided in pursuance of licences,

(c) provide, to such extent as it considers appropriate, advice and information for persons to whom licences apply or who are receiving treatment services or providing gametes or embryos for use for the purposes of activities governed by this Act, or may wish to do so, and

(d) perform such other functions as may be specified in regulations.

Licence committees and other committees.

9.—(1) The Authority shall maintain one or more committees to discharge the Authority's functions relating to the grant, variation, suspension and revocation of licences, and a committee discharging those functions is referred to in this Act as a "licence committee".

(2) The Authority may provide for the discharge of any of its other functions by committees or by members or employees of the Authority.

(3) A committee (other than a licence committee) may appoint sub-committees.

(4) Persons, committees or sub-committees discharging functions of the Authority shall do so in accordance with any general directions of the Authority.

(5) A licence committee shall consist of such number of persons as may be specified in or determined in accordance with regulations, all being members of the Authority, and shall include at least one person who is not authorised to carry on or participate in any activity under the authority of a licence and would not be so authorised if outstanding applications were granted.

(6) A committee (other than a licence committee) or a sub-committee may include a minority of persons who are not members of the Authority.

(7) Subject to subsection (10) below, a licence committee, before considering an application for authority—

(a) for a person to carry on an activity governed by this Act which he is not then authorised to carry on, or

(b) for a person to carry on any such activity on premises where he is not then authorised to carry it on,

shall arrange for the premises where the activity is to be carried on to be inspected on its behalf, and for a report on the inspection to be made to it.

(8) Subject to subsection (9) below, a licence committee shall arrange for any premises to which a licence relates to be inspected on its behalf once in each calendar year, and for a report on the inspection to be made to it.

(9) Any particular premises need not be inspected in any particular year if the licence committee considers an inspection in that year unnecessary.

(10) A licence committee need not comply with subsection (7) above where the premises in question have been inspected in pursuance of that subsection or subsection (8) above at some time during the period of one year ending with the date of the application, and the licence committee considers that a further inspection is not necessary.

(11) An inspection in pursuance of subsection (7) or (8) above may be carried out by a person who is not a member of a licence committee.

Licensing procedure.

10.—(1) Regulations may make such provision as appears to the Secretary of State to be necessary or desirable about the proceedings of licence committees and of the Authority on any appeal from such a committee.

(2) The regulations may in particular include provision—

(a) for requiring persons to give evidence or to produce documents, and

(b) about the admissibility of evidence.

Scope of licences

Licences for treatment, storage and research.

11.—(1) The Authority may grant the following and no other licences—

(a) licences under paragraph 1 of Schedule 2 to this Act authorising activities in the course of providing treatment services,

(b) licences under that Schedule authorising the storage of gametes and embryos, and

(c) licences under paragraph 3 of that Schedule authorising activities for the purpose of a project of research.

(2) Paragraph 4 of that Schedule has effect in the case of all licences.

Licence conditions

General conditions.

12. The following shall be conditions of every licence granted under this Act—

(a) that the activities authorised by the licence shall be carried on only on the premises to which the licence relates and under the supervision of the person responsible,

(b) that any member or employee of the Authority, on production, if so required, of a document identifying the person as such, shall at all reasonable times be permitted to enter those premises and inspect them (which includes inspecting any equipment or records and observing any activity),

(c) that the provisions of Schedule 3 to this Act shall be complied with,

(d) that proper records shall be maintained in such form as the Authority may specify in directions,

(e) that no money or other benefit shall be given or received in respect of any supply of gametes or embryos unless authorised by directions,

(f) that, where gametes or embryos are supplied to a person to whom another licence applies, that person shall also be provided with such information as the Authority may specify in directions, and

(g) that the Authority shall be provided, in such form and at such intervals as it may specify in directions, with such copies of or extracts from the records, or such other information, as the directions may specify.

Conditions of licences for treatment.

13.—(1) The following shall be conditions of every licence under paragraph 1 of Schedule 2 to this Act.

(2) Such information shall be recorded as the Authority may specify in directions about the following—

(a) the persons for whom services are provided in pursuance of the licence,

(b) the services provided for them,

(c) the persons whose gametes are kept or used for the purposes of services provided in pursuance of the licence or whose gametes have been used in bringing about the creation of embryos so kept or used,

(d) any child appearing to the person responsible to have been born as a result of treatment in pursuance of the licence,

(e) any mixing of egg and sperm and any taking of an embryo from a woman or other acquisition of an embryo, and

(f) such other matters as the Authority may specify in directions.

(3) The records maintained in pursuance of the licence shall include any information recorded in pursuance of subsection (2) above and any consent of a person whose consent is required under Schedule 3 to this Act.

(4) No information shall be removed from any records maintained in pursuance of the licence before the expiry of such period as may be specified in directions for records of the class in question.

(5) A woman shall not be provided with treatment services unless account has been taken of the welfare of any child who may be born as a result of the treatment (including the need of that child for a father), and of any other child who may be affected by the birth.

(6) A woman shall not be provided with any treatment services involving—

(a) the use of any gametes of any person, if that person's consent is required under paragraph 5 of Schedule 3 to this Act for the use in question,

(b) the use of any embryo the creation of which was brought about *in vitro*, or

(c) the use of any embryo taken from a woman, if the consent of the woman from whom it was taken is required under paragraph 7 of that Schedule for the use in question,

unless the woman being treated and, where she is being treated together with a man, the man have been given a suitable opportunity to receive proper counselling about the implications of taking the proposed steps, and have been provided with such relevant information as is proper.

(7) Suitable procedures shall be maintained—

(a) for determining the persons providing gametes or from whom embryos are taken for use in pursuance of the licence, and

(b) for the purpose of securing that consideration is given to the use of practices not requiring the authority of a licence as well as those requiring such authority.

Conditions of storage licences.

14.—(1) The following shall be conditions of every licence authorising the storage of gametes or embryos—

(a) that gametes of a person or an embryo taken from a woman shall be placed in storage only if received from that person or woman or acquired from a person to whom a licence applies and that an embryo the creation of which has been brought about *in vitro* otherwise than in pursuance of that licence shall be placed in storage only if acquired from a person to whom a licence applies,

(b) that gametes or embryos which are or have been stored shall not be supplied to a person otherwise than in the course of providing treatment services unless that person is a person to whom a licence applies,

(c) that no gametes or embryos shall be kept in storage for longer than the statutory storage period and, if stored at the end of the period, shall be allowed to perish, and

(d) that such information as the Authority may specify in directions as to the persons whose consent is required under Schedule 3 to this Act, the terms of their consent and the circumstances of the storage and as to such other matters as the Authority may specify in directions shall be included in the records maintained in pursuance of the licence.

(2) No information shall be removed from any record maintained in pursuance of such a licence before the expiry of such period as may be specified in directions for records of the class in question.

(3) The statutory storage period in respect of gametes is such period not exceeding ten years as the licence may specify.

(4) The statutory storage period in respect of embryos is such period not exceeding five years as the licence may specify.

(5) Regulations may provide that subsection (3) or (4) above shall have effect as if for ten years or, as the case may be, five years there were substituted—

(a) such shorter period, or

(b) in such circumstances as may be specified in the regulations, such longer period,

as may be specified in the regulations.

Conditions of research licences.

15.—(1) The following shall be conditions of every licence under paragraph 3 of Schedule 2 to this Act.

(2) The records maintained in pursuance of the licence shall include such information as the Authority may specify in directions about such matters as the Authority may so specify.

(3) No information shall be removed from any records maintained in

pursuance of the licence before the expiry of such period as may be specified in directions for records of the class in question.

(4) No embryo appropriated for the purposes of any project of research shall be kept or used otherwise than for the purposes of such a project.

Grant, revocation and suspension of licences

Grant of licence.

16.—(1) Where application is made to the Authority in a form approved for the purpose by it accompanied by the initial fee, a licence may be granted to any person by a licence committee if the requirements of subsection (2) below are met and any additional fee is paid.

(2) The requirements mentioned in subsection (1) above are—

(a) that the application is for a licence designating an individual as the person under whose supervision the activities to be authorised by the licence are to be carried on,

(b) that either that individual is the applicant or—

(i) the application is made with the consent of that individual, and

(ii) the licence committee is satisfied that the applicant is a suitable person to hold a licence,

(c) that the licence committee is satisfied that the character, qualifications and experience of that individual are such as are required for the supervision of the activities and that the individual will discharge the duty under section 17 of this Act,

(d) that the licence committee is satisfied that the premises in respect of which the licence is to be granted are suitable for the activities, and

(e) that all the other requirements of this Act in relation to the granting of the licence are satisfied.

(3) The grant of a licence to any person may be by way of renewal of a licence granted to that person, whether on the same or different terms.

(4) Where the licence committee is of the opinion that the information provided in the application is insufficient to enable it to determine the application, it need not consider the application until the applicant has provided it with such further information as it may require him to provide.

(5) The licence committee shall not grant a licence unless a copy of the conditions to be imposed by the licence has been shown to, and acknowledged in writing by, the applicant and (where different) the person under whose supervision the activities are to be carried on.

(6) In subsection (1) above "initial fee" and "additional fee" mean a fee of such amount as may be fixed from time to time by the Authority with the approval of the Secretary of State and the Treasury, and in determining any such amount, the Authority may have regard to the costs of performing all its functions.

(7) Different fees may be fixed for different circumstances and fees paid under this section are not repayable.

The person responsible.

17.—(1) It shall be the duty of the individual under whose supervision the activities authorised by a licence are carried on (referred to in this Act as the "person responsible") to secure—

(a) that the other persons to whom the licence applies are of such character, and are so qualified by training and experience, as to be suitable persons to participate in the activities authorised by the licence,

(b) that proper equipment is used,

(c) that proper arrangements are made for the keeping of gametes and embryos and for the disposal of gametes or embryos that have been allowed to perish,

(d) that suitable practices are used in the course of the activities, and

(e) that the conditions of the licence are complied with.

(2) References in this Act to the persons to whom a licence applies are to—

(a) the person responsible,

(b) any person designated in the licence, or in a notice given to the Authority by the person who holds the licence or the person responsible, as a person to whom the licence applies, and

(c) any person acting under the direction of the person responsible or of any person so designated.

(3) References below in this Act to the nominal licensee are to a person who holds a licence under which a different person is the person responsible.

Revocation and variation of licence.

18.—(1) A licence committee may revoke a licence if it is satisfied—

(a) that any information given for the purposes of the application for the grant of the licence was in any material respect false or misleading,

(b) that the premises to which the licence relates are no longer suitable for the activities authorised by the licence,

(c) that the person responsible has failed to discharge, or is unable because of incapacity to discharge, the duty under section 17 of this Act or has failed to comply with directions given in connection with any licence, or

(d) that there has been any other material change of circumstances since the licence was granted.

(2) A licence committee may also revoke a licence if—

(a) it ceases to be satisfied that the character of the person responsible is such as is required for the supervision of those activities or that the nominal licensee is a suitable person to hold a licence, or

(b) the person responsible dies or is convicted of an offence under this Act.

(3) Where a licence committee has power to revoke a licence under subsection (1) above it may instead vary any terms of the licence.

(4) A licence committee may, on an application by the person responsible or the nominal licensee, vary or revoke a licence.

(5) A licence committee may, on an application by the nominal licensee, vary the licence so as to designate another individual in place of the person responsible if—

(a) the committee is satisfied that the character, qualifications and experience of the other individual are such as are required for the supervision of the activities authorised by the licence and that the individual will discharge the duty under section 17 of this Act, and

(b) the application is made with the consent of the other individual.

(6) Except on an application under subsection (5) above, a licence can only be varied under this section—

(a) so far as it relates to the activities authorised by the licence, the manner in which they are conducted or the conditions of the licence, or

(b) so as to extend or restrict the premises to which the licence relates.

Procedure for refusal, variation or revocation of licence.

19.—(1) Where a licence committee proposes to refuse a licence or to refuse to vary a licence so as to designate another individual in place of the person responsible, the committee shall give notice of the proposal, the reasons for it and the effect of subsection (3) below to the applicant.

(2) Where a licence committee proposes to vary or revoke a licence, the committee shall give notice of the proposal, the reasons for it and the effect of subsection (3) below to the person responsible and the nominal licensee (but not to any person who has applied for the variation or revocation).

(3) If, within the period of twenty-eight days beginning with the day on which notice of the proposal is given, any person to whom notice was given under subsection (1) or (2) above gives notice to the committee of a wish to make to the committee representations about the proposal in any way mentioned in subsection (4) below, the committee shall, before making its determination, give the person an opportunity to make representations in that way.

(4) The representations may be—

(a) oral representations made by the person, or another acting on behalf of the person, at a meeting of the committee, and

(b) written representations made by the person.

(5) A licence committee shall—

(a) in the case of a determination to grant a licence, give notice of the determination to the person responsible and the nominal licensee,

(b) in the case of a determination to refuse a licence, or to refuse to vary a licence so as to designate another individual in place of the person responsible, give such notice to the applicant, and

(c) in the case of a determination to vary or revoke a licence, give such notice to the person responsible and the nominal licensee.

(6) A licence committee giving notice of a determination to refuse a licence or to refuse to vary a licence so as to designate another individual in place of the person responsible, or of a determination to vary or revoke a licence otherwise than on an application by the person responsible or the nominal licensee, shall give in the notice the reasons for its decision.

Appeal to Authority against determinations of licence committee.

20.—(1) Where a licence committee determines to refuse a licence or to refuse to vary a licence so as to designate another individual in place of the person responsible, the applicant may appeal to the Authority if notice has been given to the committee and to the Authority before the end of the period of twenty-eight days beginning with the date on which notice of the committee's determination was served on the applicant.

(2) Where a licence committee determines to vary or revoke a licence, any person on whom notice of the determination was served (other than a person who applied for the variation or revocation) may appeal to the Authority if notice has been given to the committee and to the Authority before the end of the period of twenty-eight days beginning with the date on which notice of the committee's determination was served.

(3) An appeal under this section shall be by way of rehearing by the Authority and no member of the Authority who took any part in the proceedings resulting in the determination appealed against shall take any part in the proceedings on appeal.

(4) On the appeal—

(a) the appellant shall be entitled to appear or be represented,

(b) the members of the licence committee shall be entitled to appear, or the committee shall be entitled to be represented, and

(c) the Authority shall consider any written representations received from the appellant or any member of the committee and may take into account any matter that could be taken into account by a licence committee,

and the Authority may make such determination on the appeal as it thinks fit.

(5) The Authority shall give notice of its determination to the appellant and, if it is a determination to refuse a licence or to refuse to vary a licence so as to designate another individual in place of the person responsible or a determination to vary or revoke a licence, shall include in the notice the reasons for the decision.

(6) The functions of the Authority on an appeal under this section cannot be discharged by any committee, member or employee of the Authority and, for the purposes of the appeal, the quorum shall not be less than five.

Appeals to High Court or Court of Session.

21. Where the Authority determines under section 20 of this Act—

(a) to refuse a licence or to refuse to vary a licence so as to designate another individual in place of the person responsible, or

(b) to vary or revoke a licence,

any person on whom notice of the determination was served may appeal to the High Court or, in Scotland, the Court of Session on a point of law.

Temporary suspension of licence.

22.—(1) Where a licence committee—

(a) has reasonable grounds to suspect that there are grounds for revoking the licence under section 18 of this Act, and

(b) is of the opinion that the licence should immediately be suspended,

it may by notice suspend the licence for such period not exceeding three months as may be specified in the notice.

(2) Notice under subsection (1) above shall be given to the person responsible or, where the person responsible has died or appears to the licence committee to be unable because of incapacity to discharge the duty under section 17 of this Act, to some other person to whom the licence applies or the nominal licensee and a licence committee may, by a further notice to that person, renew or further renew the notice under subsection (1) above for such further period not exceeding

three months as may be specified in the renewal notice.

(3) While suspended under this section a licence shall be of no effect, but application may be made under section 18(5) of this Act by the nominal licensee to designate another individual as the person responsible.

Directions and guidance

Directions: general.

23.—(1) The Authority may from time to time give directions for any purpose for which directions may be given under this Act or directions varying or revoking such directions.

(2) A person to whom any requirement contained in directions is applicable shall comply with the requirement.

(3) Anything done by a person in pursuance of directions is to be treated for the purposes of this Act as done in pursuance of a licence.

(4) Where directions are to be given to a particular person, they shall be given by serving notice of the directions on the person.

(5) In any other case, directions may be given—

(a) in respect of any licence (including a licence which has ceased to have effect), by serving notice of the directions on the person who is or was the person responsible or the nominal licensee, or

(b) if the directions appear to the Authority to be general directions or it appears to the Authority that it is not practicable to give notice in pursuance of paragraph (a) above, by publishing the directions in such way as, in the opinion of the Authority, is likely to bring the directions to the attention of the persons to whom they are applicable.

(6) This section does not apply to directions under section 9(4) of this Act.

Directions as to particular matters.

24.—(1) If, in the case of any information about persons for whom treatment services were provided, the person responsible does not know that any child was born following the treatment, the period specified in directions by virtue of section 13(4) of this Act shall not expire less than 50 years after the information was first recorded.

(2) In the case of every licence under paragraph 1 of Schedule 2 to this Act, directions shall require information to be recorded and given to the Authority about each of the matters referred to in section 13(2)(a) to (e) of this Act.

(3) Directions may authorise, in such circumstances and subject to such conditions as may be specified in the directions, the keeping, by or on behalf of a person to whom a licence applies, of gametes or embryos in the course of their carriage to or from any premises.

(4) Directions may authorise any person to whom a licence applies to receive gametes or embryos from outside the United Kingdom or to send gametes or embryos outside the United Kingdom in such circumstances and subject to such conditions as may be specified in the directions, and directions made by virtue of this subsection may provide for sections 12 to 14 of this Act to have effect with such modifications as may be specified in the directions.

(5) A licence committee may from time to time give such directions as are

mentioned in subsection (7) below where a licence has been varied or has ceased to have effect (whether by expiry, suspension, revocation or otherwise).

(6) A licence committee proposing to suspend, revoke or vary a licence may give such directions as are mentioned in subsection (7) below.

(7) The directions referred to in subsections (5) and (6) above are directions given for the purpose of securing the continued discharge of the duties of the person responsible under the licence concerned ("the old licence"), and such directions may, in particular—

(a) require anything kept or information held in pursuance of the old licence to be transferred to the Authority or any other person, or

(b) provide for the discharge of the duties in question by any individual, being an individual whose character, qualifications and experience are, in the opinion of the committee, such as are required for the supervision of the activities authorised by the old licence, and authorise those activities to be carried on under the supervision of that individual,

but cannot require any individual to discharge any of those duties unless the individual has consented in writing to do so.

(8) Directions for the purpose referred to in subsection (7)(a) above shall be given to the person responsible under the old licence or, where that person has died or appears to the licence committee to have become unable because of incapacity to discharge the duties in question, to some other person to whom the old licence applies or applied or to the nominal licensee.

(9) Directions for the purpose referred to in subsection (7)(b) above shall be given to the individual who under the directions is to discharge the duty.

(10) Where a person who holds a licence dies, anything done subsequently by an individual which that individual would have been authorised to do if the licence had continued in force shall, until directions are given by virtue of this section, be treated as authorised by a licence.

(11) Where the Authority proposes to give directions specifying any animal for the purposes of paragraph 1(1)(f) or 3(5) of Schedule 2 to this Act, it shall report the proposal to the Secretary of State; and the directions shall not be given until the Secretary of State has laid a copy of the report before each House of Parliament.

Code of practice.

25.—(1) The Authority shall maintain a code of practice giving guidance about the proper conduct of activities carried on in pursuance of a licence under this Act and the proper discharge of the functions of the person responsible and other persons to whom the licence applies.

(2) The guidance given by the code shall include guidance for those providing treatment services about the account to be taken of the welfare of children who may be born as a result of treatment services (including a child's need for a father), and of other children who may be affected by such births.

(3) The code may also give guidance about the use of any technique involving the placing of sperm and eggs in a woman.

(4) The Authority may from time to time revise the whole or any part of the code.

(5) The Authority shall publish the code as for the time being in force.

(6) A failure on the part of any person to observe any provision of the code shall not of itself render the person liable to any proceedings, but—

(a) a licence committee shall, in considering whether there has been any failure to comply with any conditions of a licence and, in particular, conditions requiring anything to be "proper" or "suitable", take account of any relevant provision of the code, and

(b) a licence committee may, in considering, where it has power to do so, whether or not to vary or revoke a licence, take into account any observance of or failure to observe the provisions of the code.

Procedure for approval of code.

26.—(1) The Authority shall send a draft of the proposed first code of practice under section 25 of this Act to the Secretary of State within twelve months of the commencement of section 5 of this Act.

(2) If the Authority proposes to revise the code or, if the Secretary of State does not approve a draft of the proposed first code, to submit a further draft, the Authority shall send a draft of the revised code or, as the case may be, a further draft of the proposed first code to the Secretary of State.

(3) Before preparing any draft, the Authority shall consult such persons as the Secretary of State may require it to consult and such other persons (if any) as it considers appropriate.

(4) If the Secretary of State approves a draft, he shall lay it before Parliament and, if he does not approve it, he shall give reasons to the Authority.

(5) A draft approved by the Secretary of State shall come into force in accordance with directions.

Status

Meaning of "mother".

27.—(1) The woman who is carrying or has carried a child as a result of the placing in her of an embryo or of sperm and eggs, and no other woman, is to be treated as the mother of the child.

(2) Subsection (1) above does not apply to any child to the extent that the child is treated by virtue of adoption as not being the child of any person other than the adopter or adopters.

(3) Subsection (1) above applies whether the woman was in the United Kingdom or elsewhere at the time of the placing in her of the embryo or the sperm and eggs.

Meaning of "father".

28.—(1) This section applies in the case of a child who is being or has been carried by a woman as the result of the placing in her of an embryo or of sperm and eggs or her artificial insemination.

(2) If—

(a) at the time of the placing in her of the embryo or the sperm and eggs or of her insemination, the woman was a party to a marriage, and

(b) the creation of the embryo carried by her was not brought about with the sperm of the other party to the marriage, then, subject to subsection (5) below, the other party to the marriage shall be treated as the father of the child unless it is shown that he did not consent to the placing in her of the embryo or the sperm and eggs or to her insemination (as the case may be).

(3) If no man is treated, by virtue of subsection (2) above, as the father of the child but—

(a) the embryo or the sperm and eggs were placed in the woman, or she was artificially inseminated, in the course of treatment services provided for her and a man together by a person to whom a licence applies, and

(b) the creation of the embryo carried by her was not brought about with the sperm of that man,

then, subject to subsection (5) below, that man shall be treated as the father of the child.

(4) Where a person is treated as the father of the child by virtue of subsection (2) or (3) above, no other person is to be treated as the father of the child.

(5) Subsections (2) and (3) above do not apply—

(a) in relation to England and Wales and Northern Ireland, to any child who, by virtue of the rules of common law, is treated as the legitimate child of the parties to a marriage,

(b) in relation to Scotland, to any child who, by virtue of any enactment or other rule of law, is treated as the child of the parties to a marriage, or

(c) to any child to the extent that the child is treated by virtue of adoption as not being the child of any person other than the adopter or adopters.

(6) Where—

(a) the sperm of a man who had given such consent as is required by paragraph 5 of Schedule 3 to this Act was used for a purpose for which such consent was required, or

(b) the sperm of a man, or any embryo the creation of which was brought about with his sperm, was used after his death,

he is not to be treated as the father of the child.

(7) The references in subsection (2) above to the parties to a marriage at the time there referred to—

(a) are to the parties to a marriage subsisting at that time, unless a judicial separation was then in force, but

(b) include the parties to a void marriage if either or both of them reasonably believed at that time that the marriage was valid; and for the purposes of this subsection it shall be presumed, unless the contrary is shown, that one of them reasonably believed at the time that the marriage was valid.

(8) This section applies whether the woman was in the United Kingdom or elsewhere at the time of the placing in her of the embryo or the sperm and eggs or her artificial insemination.

(9) In subsection (7)(a) above, "judicial separation" includes a legal separation obtained in a country outside the British Islands and recognised in the United Kingdom.

Effect of sections 27 and 28.

29.—(1) Where by virtue of section 27 or 28 of this Act a person is to be treated as the mother or father of a child, that person is to be treated in law as the mother or, as the case may be, father of the child for all purposes.

(2) Where by virtue of section 27 or 28 of this Act a person is not be be treated as the mother or father of a child, that person is to be treated in law as not being the mother or, as the case may be, father of the child for any purpose.

(3) Where subsection (1) or (2) above has effect, references to any relationship between two people in any enactment, deed or other instrument or document (whenever passed or made) are to be read accordingly.

(4) In relation to England and Wales and Northern Ireland, nothing in the provisions of section 27(1) or 28(2) to (4), read with this section, affects—

(a) the succession to any dignity or title of honour or renders any person capable of succeeding to or transmitting a right to succeed to any such dignity or title, or

(b) the devolution of any property limited (expressly or not) to devolve (as nearly as the law permits) along with any dignity or title of honour.

(5) In relation to Scotland—

(a) those provisions do not apply to any title, coat of arms, honour or dignity transmissible on the death of the holder thereof or affect the succession thereto or the devolution thereof, and

(b) where the terms of any deed provide that any property or interest in property shall devolve along with a title, coat of arms, honour or dignity, nothing in those provisions shall prevent that property or interest from so devolving.

Parental orders in favour of gamete donors.

30.—(1) The court may make an order providing for a child to be treated in law as the child of the parties to a marriage (referred to in this section as "the husband" and "the wife") if—

(a) the child has been carried by a woman other than the wife as the result of the placing in her of an embryo or sperm and eggs or her artificial insemination,

(b) the gametes of the husband or the wife, or both, were used to bring about the creation of the embryo, and

(c) the conditions in subsections (2) to (7) below are satisfied.

(2) The husband and the wife must apply for the order within six months of the birth of the child or, in the case of a child born before the coming into force of this Act, within six months of such coming into force.

(3) At the time of the application and of the making of the order—

(a) the child's home must be with the husband and the wife, and

(b) the husband or the wife, or both of them, must be domiciled in a part of the United Kingdom or in the Channel Islands or the Isle of Man.

(4) At the time of the making of the order both the husband and the wife must have attained the age of eighteen.

(5) The court must be satisfied that both the father of the child (including a person who is the father by virtue of section 28 of this Act), where he is not the husband, and the woman who carried the child have freely, and with full understanding of what is involved, agreed unconditionally to the making of the order.

(6) Subsection (5) above does not require the agreement of a person who cannot be found or is incapable of giving agreement and the agreement of the woman who carried the child is ineffective for the purposes of that subsection if given by her less than six weeks after the child's birth.

(7) The court must be satisfied that no money or other benefit (other than for expenses reasonably incurred) has been given or received by the husband or the wife for or in consideration of—

(a) the making of the order,

(b) any agreement required by subsection (5) above,

(c) the handing over of the child to the husband and the wife, or

(d) the making of any arrangements with a view to the making of the order,

unless authorised by the court.

(8) For the purposes of an application under this section—

(a) in relation to England and Wales, section 92(7) to (10) of, and Part I of Schedule 11 to, the Children Act 1989 (jurisdiction of courts) shall apply for the purposes of this section to determine the meaning of "the court" as they apply for the purposes of that Act and proceedings on the application shall be "family proceedings" for the purposes of that Act,

(b) in relation to Scotland, "the court" means the Court of Session or the sheriff court of the sheriffdom within which the child is, and

(c) in relation to Northern Ireland, "the court" means the High Court or any county court within whose division the child is.

(9) Regulations may provide—

(a) for any provision of the enactments about adoption to have effect, with such modifications (if any) as may be specified in the regulations, in relation to orders under this section, and applications for such orders, as it has effect in relation to adoption, and applications for adoption orders, and

(b) for references in any enactment to adoption, an adopted child or an adoptive relationship to be read (respectively) as references to the effect of an order under this section, a child to whom such an order applies and a relationship arising by virtue of the enactments about adoption, as applied by the regulations, and for similar expressions in connection with adoption to be read accordingly,

and the regulations may include such incidental or supplemental provision as appears to the Secretary of State necessary or desirable in consequence of any provision made by virtue of paragraph (a) or (b) above.

(10) In this section "the enactments about adoption" means the Adoption Act 1976, the Adoption (Scotland) Act 1978 and the Adoption (Northern Ireland) Order 1987.

(11) Subsection (1)(a) above applies whether the woman was in the United Kingdom or elsewhere at the time of the placing in her of the embryo or the sperm and eggs or her artificial insemination.

Information

The Authority's register of information.

31.—(1) The Authority shall keep a register which shall contain any information obtained by the Authority which falls within subsection (2) below.

(2) Information falls within this subsection if it relates to—

(a) the provision of treatment services for any identifiable individual, or

(b) the keeping or use of the gametes of any identifiable individual or of an embryo taken from any identifiable woman,

or if it shows that any identifiable individual was, or may have been, born in consequence of treatment services.

(3) A person who has attained the age of eighteen ("the applicant") may by notice to the Authority require the Authority to comply with a request under subsection (4) below, and the Authority shall do so if—

(a) the information contained in the register shows that the applicant was, or may have been, born in consequence of treatment services, and

(b) the applicant has been given a suitable opportunity to receive proper counselling about the implications of compliance with the request.

(4) The applicant may request the Authority to give the applicant notice stating whether or not the information contained in the register shows that a person other than a parent of the applicant would or might, but for sections 27 to 29 of this Act, be a parent of the applicant and, if it does show that—

(a) giving the applicant so much of that information as relates to the person concerned as the Authority is required by regulations to give (but no other information), or

(b) stating whether or not that information shows that, but for sections 27 to 29 of this Act, the applicant, and a person specified in the request as a person whom the applicant proposes to marry, would or might be related.

(5) Regulations cannot require the Authority to give any information as to the identity of a person whose gametes have been used or from whom an embryo has been taken if a person to whom a licence applied was provided with the information at a time when the Authority could not have been required to give information of the kind in question.

(6) A person who has not attained the age of eighteen ("the minor") may by notice to the Authority specifying another person ("the intended spouse") as a person whom the minor proposes to marry require the Authority to comply with a request under subsection (7) below, and the Authority shall do so if—

(a) the information contained in the register shows that the minor was, or may have been, born in consequence of treatment services, and

(b) the minor has been given a suitable opportunity to receive proper counselling about the implications of compliance with the request.

(7) The minor may request the Authority to give the minor notice stating whether or not the information contained in the register shows that, but for sections 27 to 29 of this Act, the minor and the intended spouse would or might be related.

Information to be provided to Registrar General.

32.—(1) This section applies where a claim is made before the Registrar General that a man is or is not the father of a child and it is necessary or desirable for the purpose of any function of the Registrar General to determine whether the claim is or may be well-founded.

(2) The Authority shall comply with any request made by the Registrar

General by notice to the Authority to disclose whether any information on the register kept in pursuance of section 31 of this Act tends to show that the man may be the father of the child by virtue of section 28 of this Act and, if it does, disclose that information.

(3) In this section and section 33 of this Act, "the Registrar General" means the Registrar General for England and Wales, the Registrar General of Births, Deaths and Marriages for Scotland or the Registrar General for Northern Ireland, as the case may be.

Restrictions on disclosure of information.

33.—(1) No person who is or has been a member or employee of the Authority shall disclose any information mentioned in subsection (2) below which he holds or has held as such a member or employee.

(2) The information referred to in subsection (1) above is—

(a) any information contained or required to be contained in the register kept in pursuance of section 31 of this Act, and

(b) any other information obtained by any member or employee of the Authority on terms or in circumstances requiring it to be held in confidence.

(3) Subsection (1) above does not apply to any disclosure of information mentioned in subsection (2)(a) above made—

(a) to a person as a member or employee of the Authority,

(b) to a person to whom a licence applies for the purposes of his functions as such,

(c) so that no individual to whom the information relates can be identified,

(d) in pursuance of an order of a court under section 34 or 35 of this Act,

(e) to the Registrar General in pursuance of a request under section 32 of this Act, or

(f) in accordance with section 31 of this Act.

(4) Subsection (1) above does not apply to any disclosure of information mentioned in subsection (2)(b) above—

(a) made to a person as a member or employee of the Authority,

(b) made with the consent of the person or persons whose confidence would otherwise be protected, or

(c) which has been lawfully made available to the public before the disclosure is made.

(5) No person who is or has been a person to whom a licence applies and no person to whom directions have been given shall disclose any information falling within section 31(2) of this Act which he holds or has held as such a person.

(6) Subsection (5) above does not apply to any disclosure of information made—

(a) to a person as a member or employee of the Authority,

(b) to a person to whom a licence applies for the purposes of his functions as such,

(c) so far as it identifies a person who, but for sections 27 to 29 of this Act, would or might be a parent of a person who instituted proceedings under section 1A of the Congenital Disabilities (Civil Liability) Act 1976, but only for the purpose of defending such proceedings, or instituting connected proceedings for compensation against that parent,

(d) so that no individual to whom the information relates can be identified, or

(e) in pursuance of directions given by virtue of section 24(5) or (6) of this Act.

(7) This section does not apply to the disclosure to any individual of information which—

(a) falls within section 31(2) of this Act by virtue of paragraph (a) or (b) of that subsection, and

(b) relates only to that individual or, in the case of an individual treated together with another, only to that individual and that other.

(8) At the end of Part IV of the Data Protection Act 1984 (Exemptions) there is inserted—

> "*Information about human embryos, etc.*
>
> 35A. Personal data consisting of information showing that an identifiable individual was, or may have been born in consequence of treatment services (within the meaning of the Human Fertilisation and Embryology Act 1990) are exempt from the subject access provisions except so far as their disclosure under those provisions is made in accordance with section 31 of that Act (the Authority's register of information)."

Disclosure in interests of justice.

34.—(1) Where in any proceedings before a court the question whether a person is or is not the parent of a child by virtue of sections 27 to 29 of this Act falls to be determined, the court may on the application of any party to the proceedings make an order requiring the Authority—

(a) to disclose whether or not any information relevant to that question is contained in the register kept in pursuance of section 31 of this Act, and

(b) if it is, to disclose so much of it as is specified in the order,

but such an order may not require the Authority to disclose any information falling within section 31(2)(b) of this Act.

(2) The court must not make an order under subsection (1) above unless it is satisfied that the interests of justice require it to do so, taking into account—

(a) any representations made by any individual who may be affected by the disclosure, and

(b) the welfare of the child, if under 18 years old, and of any other person under that age who may be affected by the disclosure.

(3) If the proceedings before the court are civil proceedings, it—

(a) may direct that the whole or any part of the proceedings on the application for an order under subsection (2) above shall be heard in camera, and

(b) if it makes such an order, may then or later direct that the whole or any part of any later stage of the proceedings shall be heard in camera.

(4) An application for a direction under subsection (3) above shall be heard in camera unless the court otherwise directs.

Disclosure in interests of justice: congenital disabilities, etc.

35.—(1) Where for the purpose of instituting proceedings under section 1 of the Congenital Disabilities (Civil Liability) Act 1976 (civil liability to child born disabled) it is necessary to identify a person who would or might be the parent of a child but for sections 27 to 29 of this Act, the court may, on the application of the child, make an order requiring the Authority to disclose any information contained in the register kept in pursuance of section 31 of this Act identifying that person.

(2) Where, for the purposes of any action for damages in Scotland (including any such action which is likely to be brought) in which the damages claimed consist of or include damages or solatium in respect of personal injury (including any disease and any impairment of physical or mental condition), it is necessary to identify a person who would or might be the parent of a child but for sections 27 to 29 of this Act, the court may, on the application of any party to the action or, if the proceedings have not been commenced, the prospective pursuer, make an order requiring the Authority to disclose any information contained in the register kept in pursuance of section 31 of this Act identifying that person.

(3) Subsections (2) to (4) of section 34 of this Act apply for the purposes of this section as they apply for the purposes of that.

(4) After section 4(4) of the Congenital Disabilities (Civil Liability) Act 1976 there is inserted—

> "(4A) In any case where a child carried by a woman as the result of the placing in her of an embryo or of sperm and eggs or her artificial insemination is born disabled, any reference in section 1 of this Act to a parent includes a reference to a person who would be a parent but for sections 27 to 29 of the Human Fertilisation and Embryology Act 1990.".

Surrogacy

Amendment of Surrogacy Arrangements Act 1985.

36.—(1) After section 1 of the Surrogacy Arrangements Act 1985 there is inserted—

> "*Surrogacy arrangements unenforceable.*
>
> 1A. No surrogacy arrangement is enforceable by or against any of the persons making it."

(2) In section 1 of that Act (meaning of "surrogate mother", etc.)—

(a) in subsection (6), for "or, as the case may be, embryo insertion" there is substituted "or of the placing in her of an embryo, of an egg in the process of fertilisation or of sperm and eggs, as the case may be,", and

(b) in subsection (9), the words from "and whether" to the end are repealed.

Abortion

Amendment of law relating to termination of pregnancy.

37.—(1) For paragraphs (a) and (b) of section 1(1) of the Abortion Act 1967 (grounds for medical termination of pregnancy) there is substituted—

> "(a) that the pregnancy has not exceeded its twenty-fourth week and that the continuance of the pregnancy would involve risk, greater than if the pregnancy were terminated, of injury to the physical or mental health of the pregnant woman or any existing children of her family; or

(b) that the termination is necessary to prevent grave permanent injury to the physical or mental health of the pregnant woman; or

(c) that the continuance of the pregnancy would involve risk to the life of the pregnant woman, greater than if the pregnancy were terminated; or

(d) that there is a substantial risk that if the child were born it would suffer from such physical or mental abnormalities as to be seriously handicapped."

(2) In section 1(2) of that Act, after "(a)" there is inserted "or (b)".

(3) After section 1(3) of that Act there is inserted—

"(3A) The power under subsection (3) of this section to approve a place includes power, in relation to treatment consisting primarily in the use of such medicines as may be specified in the approval and carried out in such manner as may be so specified, to approve a class of places."

(4) For section 5(1) of that Act (effect on Infant Life (Preservation) Act 1929) there is substituted—

"(1) No offence under the Infant Life (Preservation) Act 1929 shall be committed by a registered medical practitioner who terminates a pregnancy in accordance with the provisions of this Act."

(5) In section 5(2) of that Act, for the words from "the miscarriage" to the end there is substituted "a woman's miscarriage (or, in the case of a woman carrying more than one foetus, her miscarriage of any foetus) is unlawfully done unless authorised by section 1 of this Act and, in the case of a woman carrying more than one foetus, anything done with intent to procure her miscarriage of any foetus is authorised by that section if—

(a) the ground for termination of the pregnancy specified in subsection (1)(d) of that section applies in relation to any foetus and the thing is done for the purpose of procuring the miscarriage of that foetus, or

(b) any of the other grounds for termination of the pregnancy specified in that section applies".

Conscientious objection

Conscientious objection.

38.—(1) No person who has a conscientious objection to participating in any activity governed by this Act shall be under any duty, however arising, to do so.

(2) In any legal proceedings the burden of proof of conscientious objection shall rest on the person claiming to rely on it.

(3) In any proceedings before a court in Scotland, a statement on oath by any person to the effect that he has a conscientious objection to participating in a particular activity governed by this Act shall be sufficient evidence of that fact for the purpose of discharging the burden of proof imposed by subsection (2) above.

Enforcement

Powers of members and employees of Authority.

39.—(1) Any member or employee of the Authority entering and inspecting premises to which a licence relates may—

(a) take possession of anything which he has reasonable grounds to believe may be required—

(i) for the purpose of the functions of the Authority relating to the grant, variation, suspension and revocation of licences, or

(ii) for the purpose of being used in evidence in any proceedings for an offence under this Act,

and retain it for so long as it may be required for the purpose in question, and

(b) for the purpose in question, take such steps as appear to be necessary for preserving any such thing or preventing interference with it, including requiring any person having the power to do so to give such assistance as may reasonably be required.

(2) In subsection (1) above—

(a) the references to things include information recorded in any form, and

(b) the reference to taking possession of anything includes, in the case of information recorded otherwise than in legible form, requiring any person having the power to do so to produce a copy of the information in legible form and taking possession of the copy.

(3) Nothing in this Act makes it unlawful for a member or employee of the Authority to keep any embryo or gametes in pursuance of that person's functions as such.

Power to enter premises.

40.—(1) A justice of the peace (including, in Scotland, a sheriff) may issue a warrant under this section if satisfied by the evidence on oath of a member or employee of the Authority that there are reasonable grounds for suspecting that an offence under this Act is being, or has been, committed on any premises.

(2) A warrant under this section shall authorise any named member or employee of the Authority (who must, if so required, produce a document identifying himself), together with any constables—

(a) to enter the premises specified in the warrant, using such force as is reasonably necessary for the purpose, and

(b) to search the premises and—

(i) take possession of anything which he has reasonable grounds to believe may be required to be used in evidence in any proceedings for an offence under this Act, or

(ii) take such steps as appear to be necessary for preserving any such thing or preventing interference with it, including requiring any person having the power to do so to give such assistance as may reasonably be required.

(3) A warrant under this section shall continue in force until the end of the period of one month beginning with the day on which it is issued.

(4) Anything of which possession is taken under this section may be retained—

(a) for a period of six months, or

(b) if within that period proceedings to which the thing is relevant are commenced against any person for an offence under this Act, until the conclusion of those proceedings.

(5) In this section—

(a) the references to things include information recorded in any form, and

(b) the reference in subsection (2)(b)(i) above to taking possession of anything includes, in the case of information recorded otherwise than in legible form, requiring any person having the power to do so to produce a copy of the information in legible form and taking possession of the copy.

Offences

Offences.

41.—(1) A person who—

(a) contravenes section 3(2) or 4(1)(c) of this Act, or

(b) does anything which, by virtue of section 3(3) of this Act, cannot be authorised by a licence,

is guilty of an offence and liable on conviction on indictment to imprisonment for a term not exceeding ten years or a fine or both.

(2) A person who—

(a) contravenes section 3(1) of this Act, otherwise than by doing something which, by virtue of section 3(3) of this Act, cannot be authorised by a licence,

(b) keeps or uses any gametes in contravention of section 4(1)(a) or (b) of this Act,

(c) contravenes section 4(3) of this Act, or

(d) fails to comply with any directions given by virtue of section 24(7)(a) of this Act,

is guilty of an offence.

(3) If a person—

(a) provides any information for the purposes of the grant of a licence, being information which is false or misleading in a material particular, and

(b) either he knows the information to be false or misleading in a material particular or he provides the information recklessly,

he is guilty of an offence.

(4) A person guilty of an offence under subsection (2) or (3) above is liable—

(a) on conviction on indictment, to imprisonment for a term not exceeding two years or a fine or both, and

(b) on summary conviction, to imprisonment for a term not exceeding six months or a fine not exceeding the statutory maximum or both.

(5) A person who discloses any information in contravention of section 33 of this Act is guilty of an offence and liable—

(a) on conviction on indictment, to imprisonment for a term not exceeding two years or a fine or both, and

(b) on summary conviction, to imprisonment for a term not exceeding six months or a fine not exceeding the statutory maximum or both.

(6) A person who—

(a) fails to comply with a requirement made by virtue of section 39(1)(b) or (2)(b) or 40(2)(b)(ii) or (5)(b) of this Act, or

(b) intentionally obstructs the exercise of any rights conferred by a warrant issued under section 40 of this Act, is guilty of an offence.

(7) A person who without reasonable excuse fails to comply with a requirement imposed by regulations made by virtue of section 10(2)(a) of this Act is guilty of an offence.

(8) Where a person to whom a licence applies or the nominal licensee gives or receives any money or other benefit, not authorised by directions, in respect of any supply of gametes or embryos, he is guilty of an offence.

(9) A person guilty of an offence under subsection (6), (7) or (8) above is liable on summary conviction to imprisonment for a term not exceeding six months or a fine not exceeding level five on the standard scale or both.

(10) It is a defence for a person ("the defendant") charged with an offence of doing anything which, under section 3(1) or 4(1) of this Act, cannot be done except in pursuance of a licence to prove—

(a) that the defendant was acting under the direction of another, and

(b) that the defendant believed on reasonable grounds—

(i) that the other person was at the material time the person responsible under a licence, a person designated by virtue of section 17(2)(b) of this Act as a person to whom a licence applied, or a person to whom directions had been given by virtue of section 24(9) of this Act, and

(ii) that the defendant was authorised by virtue of the licence or directions to do the thing in question.

(11) It is a defence for a person charged with an offence under this Act to prove—

(a) that at the material time he was a person to whom a licence applied or to whom directions had been given, and

(b) that he took all such steps as were reasonable and exercised all due diligence to avoid committing the offence.

Consent to prosecution.

42. No proceedings for an offence under this Act shall be instituted—

(a) in England and Wales, except by or with the consent of the Director of Public Prosecutions, and

(b) in Northern Ireland, except by or with the consent of the Director of Public Prosecutions for Northern Ireland.

Miscellaneous and General

Keeping and examining gametes and embryos in connection with crime, etc.

43.—(1) Regulations may provide—

(a) for the keeping and examination of gametes or embryos, in such manner and on such conditions (if any) as may be specified in regulations, in connection with the investigation of, or proceedings for, an offence (wherever committed), or

(b) for the storage of gametes, in such manner and on such conditions (if any) as may be specified in regulations, where they are to be used only for such purposes, other than treatment services, as may be specified in regulations.

(2) Nothing in this Act makes unlawful the keeping or examination of any gametes or embryos in pursuance of regulations made by virtue of this section.

(3) In this section "examination" includes use for the purposes of any test.

Civil liability to child with disability.
44.—(1) After section 1 of the Congenital Disabilities (Civil Liability) Act 1976 (civil liability to child born disabled) there is inserted—

"Extension of section 1 to cover infertility treatments.

1A.—(1) In any case where—

(a) a child carried by a woman as the result of the placing in her of an embryo or of sperm and eggs or her artificial insemination is born disabled,

(b) the disability results from an act or omission in the course of the selection, or the keeping or use outside the body, of the embryo carried by her or of the gametes used to bring about the creation of the embryo, and

(c) a person is under this section answerable to the child in respect of the act or omission,

the child's disabilities are to be regarded as damage resulting from the wrongful act of that person and actionable accordingly at the suit of the child.

(2) Subject to subsection (3) below and the applied provisions of section 1 of this Act, a person (here referred to as "the defendant") is answerable to the child if he was liable in tort to one or both of the parents (here referred to as "the parent or parents concerned") or would, if sued in due time, have been so; and it is no answer that there could not have been such liability because the parent or parents concerned suffered no actionable injury, if there was a breach of legal duty which, accompanied by injury, would have given rise to the liability.

(3) The defendant is not under this section answerable to the child if at the time the embryo, or the sperm and eggs, are placed in the woman or the time of her insemination (as the case may be) either or both of the parents knew the risk of their child being born disabled (that is to say, the particular risk created by the act or omission).

(4) Subsections (5) to (7) of section 1 of this Act apply for the purposes of this section as they apply for the purposes of that but as if references to the parent or the parent affected were references to the parent or parents concerned."

(2) In section 4 of that Act (interpretation, etc)—

(a) at the end of subsection (2) there is inserted—

"and references to embryos shall be construed in accordance with section 1 of the Human Fertilisation and Embryology Act 1990",

(b) in subsection (3), after "section 1" there is inserted "1A", and

(c) in subsection (4), for "either" there is substituted "any".

Regulations.
45.—(1) The Secretary of State may make regulations for any purpose for which regulations may be made under this Act.

(2) The power to make regulations shall be exercisable by statutory instrument.

(3) Regulations may make different provision for different cases.

(4) The Secretary of State shall not make regulations by virtue of section 3(3)(c), 4(2) or (3), 30, 31(4)(a), or 43 of this Act or paragraph 1(1)(g) or 3 of Schedule 2 to this Act unless a draft has been laid before and approved by resolution of each House of Parliament.

(5) A statutory instrument containing regulations shall, if made without a draft having been approved by resolution of each House of Parliament, be subject to annulment in pursuance of a resolution of either House of Parliament.

(6) In this Act "regulations" means regulations under this section.

Notices.

46.—(1) This section has effect in relation to any notice required or authorised by this Act to be given to or served on any person.

(2) The notice may be given to or served on the person—

(a) by delivering it to the person,

(b) by leaving it at the person's proper address, or

(c) by sending it by post to the person at that address.

(3) The notice may—

(a) in the case of a body corporate, be given to or served on the secretary or clerk of the body,

(b) in the case of a partnership, be given to or served on any partner, and

(c) in the case of an unincorporated association other than a partnership, be given to or served on any member of the governing body of the association.

(4) For the purposes of this section and section 7 of the Interpretation Act 1978 (service of documents by post) in its application to this section, the proper address of any person is the person's last known address and also—

(a) in the case of a body corporate, its secretary or its clerk, the address of its registered or principal office, and

(b) in the case of an unincorporated association or a member of its governing body, its principal office.

(5) Where a person has notified the Authority of an address or a new address at which notices may be given to or served on him under this Act, that address shall also be his proper address for the purposes mentioned in subsection (4) above or, as the case may be, his proper address for those purposes in substitution for that previously notified.

47. The expressions listed in the left-hand column below are respectively defined or (as the case may be) are to be interpreted in accordance with the provisions of this Act listed in the right-hand column in relation to those expressions.

Expression	*Relevant provision*
Activities governed by this Act	Section 4(5)
Authority	Section 2(1)
Carry, in relation to a child	Section 2(3)
Directions	Section 2(1)
Embryo	Section 1

Expression	*Relevant provision*
Gametes, eggs or sperm	Section 1
Keeping, in relation to embryos or gametes	Section 2(2)
Licence	Section 2(1)
Licence committee	Section 9(1)
Nominal licensee	Section 17(3)
Person responsible	Section 17(1)
Person to whom a licence applies	Section 17(2)
Statutory storage period	Section 14(3) to (5)
Store, and similar expressions, in relation to embryos or gametes	Section 2(2)
Treatment services	Section 2(1)

Northern Ireland.

48.—(1) This Act (except section 37) extends to Northern Ireland.

(2) Subject to any Order made after the passing of this Act by virtue of subsection (1)(a) of section 3 of the Northern Ireland Constitution Act 1973, the activities governed by this Act shall not be transferred matters for the purposes of that Act, but shall for the purposes of subsection (2) of that section be treated as specified in Schedule 3 to that Act.

Short title, commencement, etc.

49.—(1) This Act may be cited as the Human Fertilisation and Embryology Act 1990.

(2) This Act shall come into force on such day as the Secretary of State may by order made by statutory instrument appoint and different days may be appointed for different provisions and for different purposes.

(3) Section 27 to 29 of this Act shall have effect only in relation to children carried by women as a result of the placing in them of embryos or of sperm and eggs, or of their artificial insemination (as the case may be), after the commencement of those sections.

(4) Section 27 of the Family Law Reform Act 1987 (artificial insemination) does not have effect in relation to children carried by women as the result of their artificial insemination after the commencement of sections 27 to 29 of this Act.

(5) Schedule 4 to this Act (which makes minor and consequential amendments) shall have effect.

(6) An order under this section may make such transitional provision as the Secretary of State considers necessary or desirable and, in particular, may provide that where activities are carried on under the supervision of a particular individual, being activities which are carried on under the supervision of that individual at the commencement of sections 3 and 4 of this Act, those activities are to be treated, during such period as may be specified in or determined in accordance with the order, as authorised by a licence (having, in addition to the conditions required by this Act, such conditions as may be so specified or determined) under which that individual is the person responsible.

(7) Her Majesty may by Order in Council direct that any of the provisions of this Act shall extend, with such exceptions, adaptations and modifications (if any) as may be specified in the Order, to any of the Channel Islands.

SCHEDULES

Section 5.

SCHEDULE 1
THE AUTHORITY: SUPPLEMENTARY PROVISIONS

Status and capacity

1. The Authority shall not be regarded as the servant or agent of the Crown, or as enjoying any status, privilege or immunity of the Crown; and its property shall not be regarded as property of, or property held on behalf of, the Crown.

2. The Authority shall have power to do anything which is calculated to facilitate the discharge of its functions, or is incidental or conducive to their discharge, except the power to borrow money.

Expenses

3. The Secretary of State may, with the consent of the Treasury, pay the Authority out of money provided by Parliament such sums as he thinks fit towards its expenses.

Appointment of members

4—(1) All the members of the Authority (including the chairman and deputy chairman who shall be appointed as such) shall be appointed by the Secretary of State.

(2) In making appointments the Secretary of State shall have regard to the desirability of ensuring that the proceedings of the Authority, and the discharge of its functions, are informed by the views of both men and women.

(3) The following persons are disqualified from being appointed as chairman or deputy chairman of the Authority—

(a) any person who is, or has been, a medical practitioner registered under the Medical Act 1983 (whether fully, provisionally or with limited registration), or under any repealed enactment from which a provision of that Act is derived,

(b) any person who is, or has been, concerned with keeping or using gametes or embryos outside the body, and

(c) any person who is, or has been, directly concerned with commissioning or funding any research involving such keeping or use, or who has actively participated in any decision to do so.

(4) The Secretary of State shall secure that at least one-third but fewer than half of the other members of the Authority fall within sub-paragraph (3)(a), (b) or (c) above, and that at least one member falls within each of paragraphs (a) and (b).

Tenure of office

5.—(1) Subject to the following provisions of this paragraph, a person shall hold and vacate office as a member of the Authority in accordance with the terms of his appointment.

(2) A person shall not be appointed as a member of the Authority for more than three years at a time.

(3) A member may at any time resign his office by giving notice to the Secretary of State.

(4) A person who ceases to be a member of the Authority shall be eligible for re-appointment (whether or not in the same capacity).

(5) If the Secretary of State is satisfied that a member of the Authority—

(a) has been absent from meetings of the Authority for six consecutive months or longer without the permission of the Authority, or

(b) has become bankrupt or made an arrangement with his creditors, or, in Scotland, has had his estate sequestrated or has granted a trust deed for or entered into an arrangement with his creditors, or

(c) is unable or unfit to discharge the functions of a member,

the Secretary of State may declare his office as a member of the Authority vacant, and notify the declaration in such manner as he thinks fit; and thereupon the office shall become vacant.

Disqualification of members of Authority for House of Commons and Northern Ireland Assembly

6. In Part II of Schedule 1 to the House of Commons Disqualification Act 1975 and in Part II of Schedule 1 to the Northern Ireland Assembly Disqualification Act 1975 (bodies of which all members are disqualified) the following entry shall be inserted at the appropriate place in alphabetical order—

"The Human Fertilisation and Embryology Authority".

Remuneration and pensions of members

7.—(1) The Authority may—

(a) pay to the chairman such remuneration, and

(b) pay or make provision for paying to or in respect of the chairman or any other member such pensions, allowances, fees, expenses or gratuities,

as the Secretary of State may, with the approval of the Treasury, determine.

(2) Where a person ceases to be a member of the Authority otherwise than on the expiry of his term of office and it appears to the Secretary of State that there are special circumstances which make it right for him to receive compensation, the Authority may make to him a payment of such amount as the Secretary of State may, with the consent of the Treasury, determine.

Staff

8.—(1) The Authority may appoint such employees as it thinks fit, upon such terms and conditions as the Authority, with the approval of the Secretary of State and the consent of the Treasury, may determine.

(2) The Authority shall secure that any employee whose function is, or whose functions include, the inspection of premises is of such character, and is so qualified by training and experience, as to be a suitable person to perform that function.

(3) The Authority shall, as regards such of its employees as with the approval of the Secretary of State it may determine, pay to or in respect of them such pensions, allowances or gratuities (including pensions, allowances or gratuities by way of compensation for loss of employment), or provide and maintain for them such pension schemes (whether contributory or not), as may be so determined.

(4) If an employee of the Authority—

(a) is a participant in any pension scheme applicable to that employment, and

(b) becomes a member of the Authority,

he may, if the Secretary of State so determines, be treated for the purposes of the pension scheme as if his service as a member of the Authority were service as employee of the Authority, whether or not any benefits are to be payable to or in respect of him by virtue of paragraph 7 above.

Proceedings

9.—(1) The Authority may regulate its own proceedings, and make such arrangements as it thinks appropriate for the discharge of its functions.

(2) The Authority may pay to the members of any committee or sub-committee such fees and allowances as the Secretary of State may, with the consent of the Treasury, determine.

10.—(1) A member of the Authority who is any way directly or indirectly interested in a licence granted or proposed to be granted by the Authority shall, as soon as possible after the relevant circumstances have come to his knowledge, disclose the nature of his interest to the Authority.

(2) Any disclosure under sub-paragraph (1) above shall be recorded by the Authority.

(3) Except in such circumstances (if any) as may be determined by the Authority under paragraph 9(1) above, the member shall not participate after the disclosure in any deliberation or decision of the Authority or any licence committee with respect to the licence, and if he does so the deliberation or decision shall be of no effect.

11. The validity of any proceedings of the Authority, or of any committee or sub-committee, shall not be affected by any vacancy among the members or by any defect in the appointment of a member.

Instruments

12. The fixing of the seal of the Authority shall be authenticated by the signature of the chairman or deputy chairman of the Authority or some other member of the Authority authorised by the Authority to act for that purpose.

13. A document purporting to be duly executed under the seal of the Authority, or to be signed on the Authority's behalf, shall be received in evidence and shall be deemed to be so executed or signed unless the contrary is proved.

Investigation by Parliamentary Commissioner

14. The Authority shall be subject to investigation by the Parliamentary Commissioner and accordingly, in Schedule 2 to the Parliamentary Commissioner Act 1967 (which lists the authorities subject to investigation under that Act), the following entry shall be inserted at the appropriate place in alphabetical order—

"Human Fertilisation and Embryology Authority".

Section 11 etc.

SCHEDULE 2

ACTIVITIES FOR WHICH LICENCES MAY BE GRANTED

Licences for treatment

1.—(1) A licence under this paragraph may authorise any of the following in the course of providing treatment services—

(a) bringing about the creation of embryos *in vitro*,

(b) keeping embryos,

(c) using gametes,

(d) practices designed to secure that embryos are in a suitable condition to be placed in a woman or to determine whether embryos are suitable for that purpose,

(e) placing any embryo in a woman,

(f) mixing sperm with the egg of a hamster, or other animal specified in directions, for the purpose of testing the fertility or normality of the sperm, but only where anything which forms is destroyed when the test is complete and, in any event, not later than the two cell stage, and

(g) such other practices as may be specified in, or determined in accordance with, regulations.

(2) Subject to the provisions of this Act, a licence under this paragraph may be granted subject to such conditions as may be specified in the licence and may authorise the performance of any of the activities referred to in sub-paragraph (1) above in such manner as may be so specified.

(3) A licence under this paragraph cannot authorise any activity unless it appears to the Authority to be necessary or desirable for the purpose of providing treatment services.

(4) A licence under this paragraph cannot authorise altering the genetic structure of any cell while it forms part of an embryo.

(5) A licence under this paragraph shall be granted for such period not exceeding five years as may be specified in the licence.

Licences for storage

2.—(1) A licence under this paragraph or paragraph 1 or 3 of this Schedule may authorise the storage of gametes or embryos or both.

(2) Subject to the provisions of this Act, a licence authorising such storage may be granted subject to such conditions as may be specified in the licence and may authorise storage in such manner as may be so specified.

(3) A licence under this paragraph shall be granted for such period not exceeding five years as may be specified in the licence.

Licences for research

3.—(1) A licence under this paragraph may authorise any of the following—

(a) bringing about the creation of embryos *in vitro,* and

(b) keeping or using embryos,

for the purposes of a project of research specified in the licence.

(2) A licence under this paragraph cannot authorise any activity unless it appears to the Authority to be necessary or desirable for the purpose of—

(a) promoting advances in the treatment of infertility,

(b) increasing knowledge about the causes of congenital disease,

(c) increasing knowledge about the causes of miscarriages,

(d) developing more effective techniques of contraception, or

(e) developing methods for detecting the presence of gene or chromosome abnormalities in embryos before implantation,

or for such other purposes as may be specified in regulations.

(3) Purposes may only be so specified with a view to the authorisation of projects of research which increase knowledge about the creation and development of embryos, or about disease, or enable such knowledge to be applied.

(4) A licence under this paragraph cannot authorise altering the genetic structure of any cell while it forms part of an embryo, except in such circumstances (if any) as may be specified in or determined in pursuance of regulations.

(5) A licence under this paragraph may authorise mixing sperm with the egg of a hamster, or other animal specified in directions, for the purpose of developing more effective techniques for determining the fertility or normality of sperm, but only where anything which forms is destroyed when the research is complete and, in any event, not later than the two cell stage.

(6) No licence under this paragraph shall be granted unless the Authority is satisfied that any proposed use of embryos is necessary for the purposes of the research.

(7) Subject to the provisions of this Act, a licence under this paragraph may be granted subject to such conditions as may be specified in the licence.

(8) A licence under this paragraph may authorise the performance of any of the activities referred to in sub-paragraph (1) or (5) above in such manner as may be so specified.

(9) A licence under this paragraph shall be granted for such period not exceeding three years as may be specified in the licence.

General

4.—(1) A licence under this Schedule can only authorise activities to be carried on on premises specified in the licence and under the supervision of an individual designated in the licence.

(2) A licence cannot—

(a) authorise activities falling within both paragraph 1 and paragraph 3 above,

(b) apply to more than one project of research,

(c) authorise activities to be carried on under the supervision of more than one individual, or

(d) apply to premises in different places.

Section 12 etc.

SCHEDULE 3
CONSENTS TO USE OF GAMETES OR EMBRYOS

Consent

1. A consent under this Schedule must be given in writing and, in this Schedule, "effective consent" means a consent under this Schedule which has not been withdrawn.

2.—(1) A consent to the use of any embryo must specify one or more of the following purposes—

(a) use in providing treatment services to the person giving consent, or that person and another specified person together,

(b) use in providing treatment services to persons not including the person giving consent, or

(c) use for the purposes of any project of research,

and may specify conditions subject to which the embryo may be so used.

(2) A consent to the storage of any gametes or any embryo must—

(a) specify the maximum period of storage (if less than the statutory storage period), and

(b) state what is to be done with the gametes or embryo if the person who gave the consent dies or is unable because of incapacity to vary the terms of the consent or to revoke it,

and may specify conditions subject to which the gametes or embryo may remain in storage.

(3) A consent under this Schedule must provide for such other matters as the Authority may specify in directions.

(4) A consent under this Schedule may apply—

(a) to the use or storage of a particular embryo, or

(b) in the case of a person providing gametes, to the use or storage of any embryo whose creation may be brought about using those gametes,

and in the paragraph (b) case the terms of the consent may be varied, or the consent may be withdrawn, in accordance with this Schedule either generally or in relation to a particular embryo or particular embryos.

Procedure for giving consent

3.—(1) Before a person gives consent under this Schedule—

(a) he must be given a suitable opportunity to receive proper counselling about the implications of taking the proposed steps, and

(b) he must be provided with such relevant information as is proper.

(2) Before a person gives consent under this Schedule he must be informed of the effect of paragraph 4 below.

Variation and withdrawal of consent

4.—(1) The terms of any consent under this Schedule may from time to time be varied, and the consent may be withdrawn, by notice given by the person who gave the consent to the person keeping the gametes or embryo to which the consent is relevant.

(2) The terms of any consent to the use of any embryo cannot be varied, and such consent cannot be withdrawn, once the embryo has been used—

(a) in providing treatment services, or

(b) for the purposes of any project of research.

Use of gametes for treatment of others

5.—(1) A person's gametes must not be used for the purposes of treatment services unless there is an effective consent by that person to their being so used and they are used in accordance with the terms of the consent.

(2) A person's gametes must not be received for use for those purposes unless there is an effective consent by that person to their being so used.

(3) This paragraph does not apply to the use of a person's gametes for the purpose of that person, or that person and another together, receiving treatment services.

In vitro fertilisation and subsequent use of embryo

6.—(1) A person's gametes must not be used to bring about the creation of any embryo *in vitro* unless there is an effective consent by that person to any embryo the creation of which may be brought about with the use of those gametes being used for one or more of the purposes mentioned in paragraph 2(1) above.

(2) An embryo the creation of which was brought about *in vitro* must not be received by any person unless there is an effective consent by each person whose gametes were used to bring about the creation of the embryo to the use for one or more of the purposes mentioned in paragraph 2(1) above of the embryo.

(3) An embryo the creation of which was brought about *in vitro* must not be used for any purpose unless there is an effective consent by each person whose gametes were used to bring about the creation of the embryo to the use for that purpose of the embryo and the embryo is used in accordance with those consents.

(4) Any consent required by this paragraph is in addition to any consent that may be required by paragraph 5 above.

Embryos obtained by lavage, etc.

7.—(1) An embryo taken from a woman must not be used for any purpose unless there is an effective consent by her to the use of the embryo for that purpose and it is used in accordance with the consent.

(2) An embryo taken from a woman must not be received by any person for use for any purpose unless there is an effective consent by her to the use of the embryo for that purpose.

(3) This paragraph does not apply to the use, for the purpose of providing a woman with treatment services, of an embryo taken from her.

Storage of gametes and embryos

8.—(1) A person's gametes must not be kept in storage unless there is an effective consent by that person to their storage and they are stored in accordance with the consent.

(2) An embryo the creation of which was brought about *in vitro* must not be kept in storage unless there is an effective consent, by each person whose gametes were used to bring about the creation of the embryo, to the storage of the embryo and the embryo is stored in accordance with those consents.

(3) An embryo taken from a woman must not be kept in storage unless there is an effective consent by her to its storage and it is stored in accordance with the consent.

Section 49.

SCHEDULE 4
MINOR AND CONSEQUENTIAL AMENDMENTS

Family Law Reform Act 1969 (c. 46.)

1. In section 25 of the Family Law Reform Act 1969 (interpretation), at the end of the definition of "excluded" there is added "to section 27 of the Family Law Reform Act 1987 and to sections 27 to 29 of the Human Fertilisation and Embryology Act 1990".

Social Security Act 1975 (c. 14.)

2. In section 25(1) of the Social Security Act 1975 (widowed mother's allowance), for the words from "or" after paragraph (b) to the end there is substituted "or

(c) if the woman and her late husband were residing together immediately before the time of his death, the woman is pregnant as the result of being artificially inseminated before that time with the semen of some person other than her husband, or as the result of the placing in her before that time of an embryo, of an egg in the process of fertilisation, or of sperm and eggs.".

Social Security (Northern Ireland) Act 1975 (c. 15.)

3. In section 25(1) of the Social Security (Northern Ireland) Act 1975 (widowed mother's allowance), at the end there is inserted "or

(c) if the woman and her late husband were residing together immediately before the time of his death, the woman is pregnant as the result of being artificially inseminated before that time with the semen of some person other than her husband, or as the result of the placing in her before that time of an embryo, of an egg in the process of fertilisation, or of sperm and eggs.".

Adoption Act 1976 (c. 36.)

4. In section 15 of the Adoption Act 1976 (adoption by one person), in subsection (3)(a) (conditions for making an adoption order on application of one

parent), after "found" there is inserted "or, by virtue of section 28 of the Human Fertilisation and Embryology Act 1990, there is no other parent".

Family Law Reform (Northern Ireland) Order 1977 (S.I. 1977/1250 (N.I. 17))

5. In Article 13 of the Family Law Reform (Northern Ireland) Order 1977 (interpretation), at the end of the definition of "excluded" there is added "and to sections 27 to 29 of the Human Fertilisation and Embryology Act 1990".

Adoption (Scotland) Act 1978 (c. 28.)

6. In section 15 of the Adoption (Scotland) Act 1978 (adoption by one person), in subsection (3)(a) (conditions for making an adoption order on application of one parent), after "found" there is inserted "or, by virtue of section 28 of the Human Fertilisation and Embryology Act 1990, there is no other parent".

Adoption (Northern Ireland) Order 1987 (S.I. 1987/2203 (N.I. 22))

7. In Article 15 of the Adoption (Northern Ireland) Order 1987 (adoption by one person), in paragraph (3)(a) (conditions for making an adoption order on the application of one parent), after "found" there is inserted "or, by virtue of section 28 of the Human Fertilisation and Embryology Act 1990, there is no other parent".

Human Organ Transplants Act 1989 (c. 31.)

8. Sections 27 to 29 of this Act do not apply for the purposes of section 2 of the Human Organ Transplants Act 1989 (restrictions on transplants between persons not genetically related).

Human Organ Transplants (Northern Ireland) Order 1989 (S.I. 1989/2408 (N.I. 21))

9. Sections 27 to 29 of this Act do not apply for the purposes of Article 4 of the Human Organ Transplants (Northern Ireland) Order 1989 (restrictions on transplants between persons not genetically related).

Appendix 2
The Abortion Act 1967 (as amended)

1967 Chapter 87. An Act to amend and clarify the law relating to termination of pregnancy by registered medical practitioners. [27 October 1967]

BE IT ENACTED by the Queen's most Excellent Majesty, by and with the advice and consent of the Lords Spiritual and Temporal, and Commons, in this present Parliament assembled, and by the authority of the same, as follows:—

Medical termination of pregnancy.

1.—(1) Subject to the provisions of this section, a person shall not be guilty of an offence under the law relating to abortion when a pregnancy is terminated by a registered medical practitioner if two registered medical practitioners are of the opinion, formed in good faith—

(a) that the pregnancy has not exceeded its twenty-fourth week and that the continuance of the pregnancy would involve risk, greater than if the pregnancy were terminated, of injury to the physical or mental health of the pregnant woman or any existing children of her family; or

(b) that the termination is necessary to prevent grave permanent injury to the physical or mental health of the pregnant woman; or

(c) that the continuance of the pregnancy would involve risk to the life of the pregnant woman, greater than if the pregnancy were terminated; or

(d) that there is a substantial risk that if the child were born it would suffer from such physical or mental abnormalities as to be seriously handicapped.

(2) In determining whether the continuance of a pregnancy would involve such risk of injury to health as is mentioned in paragraph (a) or (b) of subsection (1) of this section, account may be taken of the pregnant woman's actual or reasonably foreseeable environment.

(3) Except as provided by subsection (4) of this section, any treatment for the termination of pregnancy must be carried out in a hospital vested in the Minister of Health or the Secretary of State under the National Health Service Acts, or in a place for the time being approved for the purposes of this section by the said Minister or the Secretary of State.

(3A) The power under subsection (3) of this section to approve a place includes power, in relation to treatment consisting primarily in the use of such medicines as may be specified in the approval and carried out in such manner as may be so specified, to approve a class of places.

(4) Subsection (3) of this section, and so much of subsection (1) as relates to the opinion of two registered medical practitioners, shall not apply to the termination of a pregnancy by a registered medical practitioner in a case where he is of the opinion, formed in good faith, that the termination is immediately necessary to save the life or to prevent grave permanent injury to the physical or mental health of the pregnant woman.

Notification.

2.—(1) The Minister of Health in respect of England and Wales, and the Secretary of State in respect of Scotland, shall by statutory instrument make regulations to provide—

(a) for requiring any such opinion as is referred to in section 1 of this Act to be certified by the practitioners or practitioner concerned in such form and at such time as may be prescribed by the regulations, and for requiring the preservation and disposal of certificates made for the purposes of the regulations;

(b) for requiring any registered medical practitioner who terminates a pregnancy to give notice of the termination and such other information relating to the termination as may be so prescribed;

(c) for prohibiting the disclosure, except to such persons or for such purposes as may be so prescribed, of notices given or information furnished pursuant to the regulations.

(2) The information furnished in pursuance of regulations made by virtue of paragraph (b) of subsection (1) of this section shall be notified solely to the Chief Medical Officers of the Ministry of Health and the Scottish Home and Health Department respectively.

(3) Any person who wilfully contravenes or wilfully fails to comply with the requirements of regulations under subsection (1) of this section shall be liable on summary conviction to a fine not exceeding one hundred pounds.

(4) Any statutory instrument made by virtue of this section shall be subject to annulment in pursuance of a resolution of either House of Parliament.

Application of Act to visiting forces etc.

3.—(1) In relation to the termination of a pregnancy in a case where the following conditions are satisfied, that is to say—

(a) the treatment for termination of the pregnancy was carried out in a hospital controlled by the proper authorities of a body to which this section applies; and

(b) the pregnant woman had at the time of the treatment a relevant association with that body; and

(c) the treatment was carried out by a registered medical practitioner or a person who at the time of the treatment was a member of that body appointed as a medical practitioner for that body by the proper authorities of that body,

this Act shall have effect as if any reference in section 1 to a registered medical practitioner and to a hospital vested in a Minister under the National Health

Service Acts included respectively a reference to such a person as is mentioned in paragraph (c) of this subsection and to a hospital controlled as aforesaid, and as if section 2 were omitted.

(2) The bodies to which this section applies are any force which is a visiting force within the meaning of any of the provisions of Part I of the Visiting Forces Act 1952 and any headquarters within the meaning of the Schedule to the International Headquarters and Defence Organisations Act 1964; and for the purposes of this section—

(a) a woman shall be treated as having a relevant association at any time with a body to which this section applies if at that time—

(i) in the case of such a force as aforesaid, she had a relevant association within the meaning of the said Part I with the force; and

(ii) in the case of such a headquarters as aforesaid, she was a member of the headquarters or a dependant within the meaning of the Schedule aforesaid of such a member; and

(b) any reference to a member of a body to which this section applies shall be construed—

(i) in the case of such a force as aforesaid, as a reference to a member of or of a civilian component of that force within the meaning of the said Part I; and

(ii) in the case of such a headquarters as aforesaid, as a reference to a member of that headquarters within the meaning of the Schedule aforesaid.

Conscientious objection to participation in treatment.

4.—(1) Subject to subsection (2) of this section, no person shall be under any duty, whether by contract or by any statutory or other legal requirement, to participate in any treatment authorised by this Act to which he has a conscientious objection:

Provided that in any legal proceedings the burden of proof of conscientious objection shall rest on the person claiming to rely on it.

(2) Nothing in subsection (1) of this section shall affect any duty to participate in treatment which is necessary to save the life or to prevent grave permanent injury to the physical or mental health of a pregnant woman.

(3) In any proceedings before a court in Scotland, a statement on oath by any person to the effect that he has a conscientious objection to participating in any treatment authorised by this Act shall be sufficient evidence for the purpose of discharging the burden of proof imposed upon him by subsection (1) of this section.

5.—(1) No offence under the Infant Life (Preservation) Act 1929 shall be committed by a registered medical practitioner who terminates a pregnancy in accordance with the provisions of this Act.

(2) For the purposes of the law relating to abortion, anything done with intent to procure a woman's miscarriage (or, in the case of a woman carrying more than one foetus, her miscarriage of any foetus) is unlawfully done unless authorised by section 1 of this Act and, in the case of a woman carrying more than one foetus, anything done with intent to procure her miscarriage of any foetus is authorised by that section if—

(a) the ground for termination of the pregnancy specified in subsection (1)(d) of that section applies in relation to any foetus and the thing is done for the purpose of procuring the miscarriage of the foetus, or

(b) any of the other grounds for termination of the pregnancy specified in that section applies.

Interpretation.

6. In this Act, the following expressions have meanings hereby assigned to them:—

"the law relating to abortion" means sections 58 and 59 of the Offences against the Person Act 1861, and any rule of law relating to the procurement of abortion;

"the National Health Service Acts" means the National Health Service Act 1946 to 1966 or the National Health Service (Scotland) Acts 1947 to 1966.

Short title, commencement and extent.

7.—(1) This Act may be cited as the Abortion Act 1967.

(2) This Act shall come into force on the expiration of the period of six months beginning with the date on which it is passed.

(3) This Act does not extend to Northern Ireland.

Appendix 3
The Congenital Disabilities (Civil Liability) Act 1976 (as amended)

1976 Chapter 28. An Act to make provision as to civil liability in the case of children born disabled in consequence of some person's fault; and to extend the Nuclear Installations Act 1965, so that children so born in consequence of a breach of duty under that Act may claim compensation. [22 July 1976]

BE IT ENACTED by the Queen's most Excellent Majesty, by and with the advice and consent of the Lords Spiritual and Temporal, and Commons, in this present Parliament assembled, and by the authority of the same, as follows:—

Civil liability to child born disabled.
1.—(1) If a child is born disabled as the result of such an occurrence before its birth as is mentioned in subsection (2) below, and a person (other than the child's own mother) is under this section answerable to the child in respect of the occurrence, the child's disabilities are to be regarded as damage resulting from the wrongful act of that person and actionable accordingly at the suit of the child.

(2) An occurrence to which this section applies is one which—

(a) affected either parent of the child in his or her ability to have a normal, healthy child; or

(b) affected the mother during her pregnancy, or affected her or the child in the course of its birth, so that the child is born with disabilities which would not otherwise have been present.

(3) Subject to the following subsections, a person (here referred to as "the defendant") is answerable to the child if he was liable in tort to the parent or would, if sued in due time, have been so; and it is no answer that there could not have been such liability because the parent suffered no actionable injury, if there was a breach of legal duty which, accompanied by injury, would have given rise to the liability.

(4) In the case of an occurrence preceding the time of conception, the defendant is not answerable to the child if at that time either or both of the

parents knew the risk of their child being born disabled (that is to say, the particular risk created by the occurrence); but should it be the child's father who is the defendant, this subsection does not apply if he knew of the risk and the mother did not.

(5) The defendant is not answerable to the child, for anything he did or omitted to do when responsible in a professional capacity for treating or advising the parent, if he took reasonable care having due regard to then received professional opinion applicable to the particular class of case; but this does not mean that he is answerable only because he departed from received opinion.

(6) Liability to the child under this section may be treated as having been excluded or limited by contract made with the parent affected, to the same extent and subject to the same restrictions as liability in the parent's own case; and a contract term which could have been set up by the defendant in an action by the parent, so as to exclude or limit his liability to him or her, operates in the defendant's favour to the same, but no greater, extent in action under this section by the child.

(7) If in the child's action under this section it is shown that the parent affected shared the responsibility for the child being born disabled, the damages are to be reduced to such extent as the court thinks just and equitable having regard to the extent of the parent's responsibility.

Extension of section 1 to cover infertility treatments.

1A.—(1) In any case where—

(a) a child carried by a woman as the result of the placing in her of an embryo or of sperm and eggs or her artificial insemination is born disabled,

(b) the disability results from an act or omission in the course of the selection, or the keeping or use outside the body, of the embryo carried by her or of the gametes used to bring about the creation of the embryo, and

(c) a person is under this section answerable to the child in respect of the act or omission,

the child's disabilities are to be regarded as damage resulting from the wrongful act of that person and actionable accordingly at the suit of the child.

(2) Subject to subsection (3) below and the applied provisions of section 1 of this Act, a person (here referred to as "the defendant") is answerable to the child if he was liable in tort to one or both the parents (here referred to as "the parent or parents concerned") or would, if sued in due time, have been so; and it is no answer that there could not have been such liability because the parent or parents concerned suffered no actionable injury, if there was a breach of legal duty which, accompanied by injury, would have given rise to the liability.

(3) The defendant is not under this section answerable to the child if at the time the embryo, or the sperm and eggs, are placed in the woman or the time of her insemination (as the case may be) either or both of the parents knew the risk of their child being born disabled (that is to say, the particular risk created by the act or omission).

(4) Subsections (5) to (7) of section 1 of this Act apply for the purposes of this section as they apply for the purposes of that but as if references to the parent or the parent affected were references to the parent or parents concerned.

Liability of woman driving when pregnant.

2. A woman driving a motor vehicle when she knows (or ought reasonably to know) herself to be pregnant is to be regarded as being under the same duty to take care for the safety of her unborn child as the law imposes on her with respect to the safety of other people; and if in consequence of her breach of that duty her child is born with disabilities which would not otherwise have been present, those disabilities are to be regarded as damage resulting from her wrongful act and actionable accordingly at the suit of the child.

Disabled birth due to radiation.

3.—(1) Section 1 of this Act does not affect the operation of the Nuclear Installations Act 1965 as to liability for, and compensation in respect of, injury or damage caused by occurrences involving nuclear matter or the emission of ionising radiations.

(2) For the avoidance of doubt anything which—

(a) affects a man in his ability to have a normal, healthy child; or

(b) affects a woman in that ability, or so affects her when she is pregnant that her child is born with disabilities which would not otherwise have been present,

is an injury for the purposes of that Act.

(3) If a child is born disabled as the result of an injury to either of its parents caused in breach of a duty imposed by any of sections 7 to 11 of that Act (nuclear site licensees and others to secure that nuclear incidents do not cause injury to persons, etc.), the child's disabilities are to be regarded under the subsequent provisions of that Act (compensation and other matters) as injuries caused on the same occasion, and by the same breach of duty, as was the injury to the parent.

(4) As respects compensation to the child, section 13(6) of that Act (contributory fault of person injured by radiation) is to be applied as if the reference there to fault were to the fault of the parent.

(5) Compensation is not payable in the child's case if the injury to the parent preceded the time of the child's conception and at that time either or both of the parents knew the risk of their child being born disabled (that it to say, the particular risk created by the injury).

Interpretation and other supplementary provisions.

4.—(1) References in this Act to a child being born disabled or with disabilities are to its being born with any deformity, disease or abnormality, including predisposition (whether or not susceptible of immediate prognosis) to physical or mental defect in the future.

(2) In this Act—

(a) "born" means born alive (the moment of a child's birth being when it first has a life separate from its mother), and "birth" has a corresponding meaning; and

(b) "motor vehicle" means a mechanically propelled vehicle intended or adapted for use on roads.

and references to embryos shall be construed in accordance with section 1 of the Human Fertilisation and Embryology Act 1990.

(3) Liability to a child under section 1, 1A or 2 of this Act is to be regarded—

(a) as respects all its incidents and any matters arising or to arise out of it; and

(b) subject to any contrary context or intention, for the purpose of construing references in enactments and documents to personal or bodily injuries and cognate matters,

as liability for personal injuries sustained by the child immediately after its birth.

(4) No damages shall be recoverable under any of those sections in respect of any loss of expectation of life, nor shall any such loss be taken into account in the compensation payable in respect of a child under the Nuclear Installations Act 1965 as extended by section 3, unless (in either case) the child lives for at least 48 hours.

(4A) In any case where a child carried by a woman as the result of the placing in her of an embryo or of sperm and eggs or her artificial insemination is born disabled, any reference in section 1 of this Act to a parent includes a reference to a person who would be a parent but for sections 27 to 29 of the Human Fertilisation and Embryology Act 1990.

(5) This Act applies in respect of births after (but not before) its passing, and in respect of any such birth it replaces any law in force before its passing, whereby a person could be liable to a child in respect of disabilities with which it might be born; but in section 1(3) of this Act the expression "liable in tort" does not include any reference to liability by virtue of this Act, or to liability by virtue of any such law.

(6) References to the Nuclear Installations Act 1965 are to that Act as amended; and for the purposes of section 28 of that Act (power by Order in Council to extend the Act to territories outside the United Kingdom) section 3 of this Act is to be treated as if it were a provision of that Act.

Crown application.

5. This Act binds the Crown.

Citation and extent.

6.—(1) This Act may be cited as the Congenital Disabilities (Civil Liability) Act 1976.

(2) This Act extends to Northern Ireland but not to Scotland.

Appendix 4
The ILA Guidelines

Guidelines for both Clinical and Research Applications of Human *In Vitro* Fertilisation

Introduction
The purpose of these Guidelines is to set out the principles which the Joint Medical Research Council/Royal College of Obstetricians and Gynaecologists Interim Licensing Authority believes should guide those whose clinical practice or research involves the use of *in vitro* fertilisation with human gametes. They have been based on the recommendations of the 'Committee of Inquiry into Human Fertilisation and Embryology' under the chairmanship of Dame Mary Warnock (the Warnock Committee), the Medical Research Council Statement on 'Research Related to Human Fertilisation and Embryology' (MRC Statement) and the 'Report of the RCOG Ethics Committee on *In Vitro* Fertilisation and Embryo Replacement or Transfer' (the RCOG Ethics Committee Report).

During their discussions the ILA considered it was important to define the term 'pre-embryo' used in these Guidelines. The term 'embryo' has traditionally been used to describe the stage reached in development where organogenesis has started, as shown by the appearance of the primitive streak and the certainty that thereafter one or more individuals are developing rather than a hydatidiform mole, for example. To the collection of dividing cells up to the determination of the primitive streak we use the term 'pre-embryo'.

Background
After many years of medical research the birth of the first child resulting from the technique of *in vitro* fertilisation took place in July 1978.

The Government established in 1982 the Warnock Committee and its Report was published in July 1984.

One of the recommendations made by the Warnock Committee was that urgent action be taken to control work involving *in vitro* fertilisation. Recognising that appropriate legislation would not be enacted immediately the Medical Research Council and the Royal College of Obstetricians and Gynaecologists agreed to set up a Voluntary Licensing Authority for Human *In Vitro* Fertilisation and Embryology (VLA). To emphasise that the Authority was an interim measure until the Government introduced a statutory licensing scheme, the Authority changed its name, in 1989, to the Interim Licensing Authority (ILA).

As its first task the Authority prepared Guidelines which are consistent with the recommendations made by the Warnock Committee together with the MRC Statement and the RCOG Ethics Committee Report.

When preparing these Guidelines the Authority, in addition to referring to reports from various expert committees, was aware of the deep public concern that has been expressed about some aspects of *in vitro* fertilisation and the ethical and moral issues that the application of the technique has raised.

The Authority has agreed that soundly based clinical practice involving *in vitro* fertilisation should proceed and it should be regarded as a developing therapeutic procedure covered by the normal ethics of the doctor/patient relationship.

It has also been agreed that scientifically sound research involving *in vitro* fertilisation — where there is no intent to transfer the pre-embryo to the uterus — should be allowed to proceed if its aims are clearly defined and acceptable.

The Authority will consider research projects on a case by case basis but certain types will not be approved, e.g. modification of the genetic constitution of a pre-embryo: the placing of a human pre-embryo in the uterus of another species for gestation: cloning of pre-embryos by nuclear substitution.

Guidelines

(1) Scientifically sound research involving experiments on the processes and products of *in vitro* fertilisation between gametes is ethically acceptable, subject to certain provisions detailed in sections 2-10 below.

(2) Any application made to the Authority must give reasons why information cannot be obtained from studies of species other than the human.

(3) The aim of the research must be clearly defined and relevant to clinical problems such as the diagnosis and treatment of infertility or of genetic disorders, or for the development of safe and more effective contraceptive measures.

(4) Pre-embryos resulting from or used in research should not be transferred to the uterus, except in the course of clinical research studies designed to enhance the possibility of establishing a successful pregnancy in a particular individual.

(5) Suitable signed consent to research involving human ova and sperm should be obtained in every case from the donors; sperm from sperm banks should not be used unless permission for its use in research has been obtained from the donor. Approval for each project must be obtained from the local ethical committee prior to seeking approval from the ILA.

(6) When human ova have been obtained and fertilised *in vitro* for a therapeutic purpose and are no longer required for that purpose it would be ethical to use them for soundly based research provided that the signed consent of both donors was obtained, subject to the same approval as in the preceding section.

(7) Human ova fertilised with human sperm should not be cultured *in vitro* for more than 14 days excluding any period of storage at low temperature (see Guideline 8) and should not be stored for use in research other than that for which local ethical committee and ILA approval has been obtained.

(8) Where a pre-embryo has been preserved at low temperature, whether donated for research purposes at the time of preservation or subsequently, it may continue to be grown to the equivalent of 14 days' normal development provided that approval has first been obtained from the local ethical committee and the ILA. Storage of individual pre-embryos at low termperature should be reviewed after two years and the maximum storage time should be ten years.

(9) The means of disposal of the pre-embryo must be carefully considered before the start of each project. At the end of a study steps must be taken to stop development of the pre-embryo and the appropriate disposal must be considered in discussion with the local ethical committee and details given to the ILA. The means of disposal will depend on the nature of the particular study that the pre-embryo has been used for. In view of the scarcity of the material, it would be inappropriate to discard any pre-embryo without thorough examination.

(10) Studies on the penetration of animal eggs by human sperm are valuable in providing information on the penetration ability and chromosomal complement of sperm from subfertile men and are considered ethically acceptable provided that development does not proceed beyond the early cleavage stage.

(11) The clinical use of ova stored at low temperatures, involving subsequent *in vitro* fertilisation should not proceed to transfer to the uterus until such time as scientific evidence is available as to the safety of the procedure.

(12) Consideration must be given to ensuring that whilst a woman has the best chance of achieving a pregnancy the risks of a large multiple pregnancy occurring are minimised. For this reason whether IVF or GIFT procedures are used either jointly or separately no more than three eggs or pre-embryos should be transferred in any one cycle, unless there are *exceptional clinical reasons* when up to four may be replaced per cycle.

(13) The following general considerations must be taken into account when establishing clinical facilities where *in vitro* fertilisation or GIFT is carried out:

(a) each centre must have access to an ethical committee, and no procedure should be undertaken without the knowledge and consent of the ethical committee,

(b) detailed records must be kept along the lines recommended in the Warnock Committee Report, and should include details of the children born as a result of *in vitro* fertilisation; the records should be readily available for examination by duly authorised staff and for collation on a national basis for a follow-up study,

(c) where the director either does not have accredited consultant status, or the equivalent, or is a non-clinician full clinical responsibility must be assumed by a Consultant Adviser who takes an active role in overseeing the centre's treatment protocols and emergency procedures; all other medical, nursing and technical staff must have appropriate experience and training,

(d) specialist medical, surgical and nursing facilities appropriate for the specific techniques used for the treatment must be available,

(e) arrangements for emergency treatment must be made,

(f) there must be adequate arrangements, where appropriate, for the transfer of gametes and pre-embryos between clinical facilities and the laboratory,

(g) centres should have appropriate counselling facilities with access to properly trained independent counselling staff,

(h) whenever donor gametes are to be used both donors and recipients should be tested for hepatitis B and HIV antibodies,

(i) donor sperm should be obtained only from a bank where all appropriate screening tests are undertaken including those recommended by the DHSS AIDS Booklet 4 *AIDS and Artificial Insemination — Guidance for Doctors and AI Clinics* (CMO (86) 12),

(j) egg donors should remain anonymous and for this reason donation for clinical purposes from any known person including close relatives should be avoided,

(k) the use of close relatives for IVF surrogacy should be avoided.

(14) The following general considerations must be taken into account when establishing laboratory facilities where *in vitro* fertilisation is carried out:

(a) each centre must have access to an ethical committee,

(b) detailed records must be kept and should be readily available for examination by duly authorised staff,

(c) laboratory staff must have appropriate experience and training in the techniques being used,

(d) laboratory conditions must be of a high standard (e.g. good culture facilities, facilities for microscopic examination, appropriate incubators and training in 'non-touch' techniques),

(e) where gametes and pre-embryos are cultured and stored there must be a very high standard of security and of record keeping and labelling.

(15) The following general conditions must be taken into account when receiving donated oocytes from both those donating for purely altruistic reasons and those receiving free sterilisation or other operative procedures:

(a) Skilled and independent counselling, by somebody other than the medical practitioner involved in the procedure, must be available to the donor to ensure that sufficient information has been given and understood, particularly in relation to discomfort and risk; and that the donor, if she consents, does so with her judgement unimpaired. The counsellor should look for stability of purpose so that neither consent nor withdrawal during treatment would be lightly undertaken.

(b) The donor must know that she is free to withdraw consent to the egg donation at any time without threat of financial penalty and, where appropriate, without impairment of her interest in the successful conduct of the primary operation.

(c) The centre must be prepared to accept, in the event of withdrawal after preparation for egg recovery has begun, the financial loss incurred.

(d) The donor must be informed of the purpose for which her eggs will be used (i.e. research or donation to another woman for clinical purposes) and the centre at which the eggs will be used. Eggs must not be sold.

(e) The donor must be given a copy of the information booklet provided by the ILA. The consent form at the back of the booklet must be signed by the donor and retained in the records of the centre where the donation took place.

(f) The local ethics committee must satisfy itself that the conditions both can and will be met in the centre for which it is responsible.

(16) The following general conditions must also be taken into account when offering free sterilisation (or other related surgery) to women in return for donated oocytes:

(a) Centres wishing to offer free sterilisation to women in consideration of their donating oocytes must apply in writing to the ILA for permission. Each centre's application will be judged independently.

(b) The discussion of egg donation must be entirely separate from decisions concerning the management and clinical care of the patient for whom the sterilisation or other operation may be indicated. Only when those decisions have been made may the question of egg donation be raised.

(c) The fact of egg donation alone should not entitle a patient to transfer to a shorter list or faster lane for sterilisation; such a transfer must have its own clinical justification.

Appendix 5
The RCOG GIFT Guidelines

ROYAL COLLEGE of OBSTETRICIANS & GYNAECOLOGISTS

GUIDELINES ON ASSISTED REPRODUCTION INVOLVING SUPEROVULATION

Introduction

Fellows and Members will wish to be aware of Parliamentary concerns expressed during the passage of the Human Fertilisation and Embryology Bill through Parliament. The unease relates to **triplets and higher order multiple births** resulting from infertility treatment. In these cases there are commonly substantial problems for parents during pregnancy and delivery as well as subsequently. The Minister for Health has now written to the College requesting that consideration be given to issuing College guidelines pointing to the need for—

(a) appropriate counselling about such problems prior to treatment, and

(b) measures which should be taken to seek to avoid these multiple births wherever possible.

The aim should also be to avoid selective foetal reduction being contemplated because infertility treatment has caused a higher order multiple pregnancy.

Hyperstimulation of ovulatory women results in unpredictable numbers of follicles and hence oocytes. Multiple pregnancy occurs in approximately 25% of cases following gonadotrophin induced ovulations.

The Interim Licensing Authority guidelines in relation to IVF and GIFT stipulate that no more than three embryos or three ova should be replaced. In 1988, more multiple pregnancies in the UK resulted from GIFT than IVF. Results in older women (over the age of 39), or when a male contribution to infertility occurs, are poor, so there is a natural temptation to replace more oocytes or embryos which should be resisted. This points to a special need for counselling and monitoring in these circumstances.

Recommendations

1. **Counselling** — prospective parents must be made aware of the problems of multiple pregnancy and the potential risk this carries during the antenatal, intrapartum and neonatal period as well as subsequently.
2. **Gonadotrophins** — for use in ovulation induction; the use of these should always include monitoring of their effect, by means of hormone assays and ultrasound, even when procedures such as IVF or GIFT, etc. are not involved.
3. **GIFT or IVF** — not more than three oocytes in GIFT or three embryos in IVF should be transferred, except under exceptional circumstances where a maximum of four embryos may be replaced.
4. **Male factor** infertility treated by assisted conception should use IVF rather than GIFT initially, to assess fertilisation.
5. **Cryopreservation** — ideally, GIFT and similar procedures should be carried out where IVF is also practised and cryopreservation of embryos is available so that spare eggs may be fertilised and transferred or stored with a view to later treatment if the initial treatment fails.

August 1990

27 Sussex Place, Regent's Park, London NW1 4RG. Tel: 071-262 5425

Appendix 6
ILA Specimen Consent Form

SPECIMEN

Agreement for *In Vitro* Fertilisation

(For use of pre-embryos for research a separate consent form must be used)

Name and address of Centre

We .... (full name of woman)

and .... (full name of man)

of ....

....

....

being unlikely to have a child by other means, have requested the .... Centre, through its medical and scientific staff, to assist the woman to give birth to a child by the man.

1. We had a full discussion with .... on .... and we understand that the methods to be used may include:
   - (i) preparation of the woman by the administration of hormones and other drugs described in the attached schedule;
   - (ii) egg retrieval by means of ....
   - (iii) fertilisation with the man's semen of any eggs from the woman;
   - (iv) maintenance of pre-embryos resulting from such fertilisation until such time as, in the view of the medical and scientific staff, they are ready for replacement in the woman;
   - (v) selection by the medical and scientific staff of the most suitable pre-embryos for such replacement;

(vi) transfer of selected pre-embryos to the woman.

2. We consent to these procedures and to the administration of such drugs and anaesthetics to the woman as may be necessary. We also consent to any further operative measures which may be found to be necessary in the course of the treatment.

3. We understand and accept that there is no certainty that a pregnancy will result from these procedures, since the success rate is uncertain even where an egg is recovered and replacement carried out. We further understand and accept that the medical and scientific staff can give no assurance that pregnancy will result in the delivery of a normal living child.

4.* (a) We request that any pre-embryos which are not replaced should, at the discretion of the medical staff, be preserved by freezing or other methods and stored for a period of not more than two years from the date of fertilisation.

*(b) We understand that if before the period of two years has expired we wish any pre-embryos to be preserved for a further period, the Centre will be prepared, at our request, to consider such further period of preservation on terms to be negotiated.

*(c) We understand that, if we so wish, any suitable pre-embryos so stored may be used for replacement (but only in the above-named woman) and at the discretion of the medical and scientific staff. We further understand that no assurance can be given that any such pre-embryos will survive or be suitable for replacement.

*(d) We agree that no stored pre-embryo shall be removed from the custody of the medical and scientific staff of the Centre without the written consent of both of us (or the survivor), such consent to be given within twenty-eight days before replacement or removal. In the event of both our deaths we request that any stored pre-embryos should be disposed of at the discretion of the Centre, as at section (e).

*(e) We agree that after the period of two years (or such extension as may be agreed) has expired the Hospital or Centre (subject to the general terms of this agreement) may dispose of the stored pre-embryos at its discretion either by:

*(i) donation to another individual determined by the clinician in charge,

*(ii) destroying by approved methods.

5. We accept that decisions as to the suitability and number of pre-embryos for replacement, at any time and whether frozen or not, will be at the discretion of the medical and scientific staff of the Centre, subject to the Guidelines of the ILA.

6. We do not consent to the transfer of any pre-embryos so produced into a woman other than the above-named woman.

7. We have read the information booklet relating to IVF and have understood what is involved in this procedure.

8. We have been given time to consider the contents of this document and we have been given the opportunity to make such further enquiries as we wish before signing.

DATED the .... day of .... 199........

SIGNED .... woman

.... man

.... for the Centre

WITNESS ....

....

....

Agreement for the use of pre-embryos for research

We understand that pre-embryos not used for replacement or storage and any pre-embryos remaining after the agreed period of storage may be used for the advance of medical and scientific knowledge and we welcome such use and consent to it.

We realise that the development of such pre-embryos cannot proceed for long outside the body and the period of survival will be brief.

We have been given at least 24 hours to consider the use of spare pre-embryos for use in an approved research programme and to make such further enquiries as we wish before signing.

DATED the .... day of .... 199........

SIGNED .... woman

.... man

.... for the Centre

WITNESS ....

....

....

---

*Delete as required.

Appendix 7
List of ILA Approved Centres (1990)

ILA APPROVED CENTRES

	Name of Centre	*Director*	*IVF*	*GIFT*	*Licensed Research*	*Date Licensed*
1	Assisted Reproduction Unit, University of **Aberdeen**	Professor A A Templeton	Yes	No	Yes	1986
2	IVF Unit, Royal Maternity Hospital, **Belfast**	Professor W Thompson Dr A I Traub	Yes	Yes	No	1988
3	Department of Obstetrics & Gynaecology, Birmingham Maternity Hospital, **Birmingham**	Mr M Obhrai	Yes	Yes	No	1988
4	AMI Priory Hospital, **Birmingham**	Mr R S Sawers	Yes	Yes	No	1990
5	Department of Obstetrics & Gynaecology, **Bristol** Maternity Hospital	Professor M G R Hull Dr A McDermott	Yes	No	Yes	1985
6	The BUPA Glen Hospital, Durdham Down, **Bristol**	Professor M G R Hull Dr A McDermott	Yes	Yes	Yes	1989
7	Department of Obstetrics & Gynaecology, Southmead General Hospital, **Bristol**	Mr D N Joyce Dr A McDermott	Yes	Yes	No	1985
8	Bourne Hall, Bourn, **Cambridge**	Mr P Brinsden	Yes	Yes	Yes	1986
9	Embryo and Gamete Research Group, The Rosie Maternity Hospital, **Cambridge**	Dr P R Braude	Yes	Yes	Yes	1985

	Name of Centre	*Director*	*IVF*	*GIFT*	*Licensed Research*	*Date Licensed*
10	Fertility Unit, University Hospital of Wales, **Cardiff**	Mrs S Walker	Yes	Yes	Yes	1989
11	Department of Reproductive Medicine, Ninewells Hospital, **Dundee**	Dr J A Mills	Yes	Yes	No	1986
12	Department of Obstetrics & Gynaecology, University of **Edinburgh**	Professor D T Baird	Yes	No	Yes	1985
13	Holly House Hospital, **Essex**	Mr M Ah-Moye	Yes	Yes	No	1990
14	Department of Obstetrics & Gynaecology, Royal Infirmary/Nuffield McAlpin Nursing Home, **Glasgow**	Dr R W S Yates Professor Sir Malcolm Macnaughton	Yes	Yes	Yes	1985
15	Gavin Brown Clinic, Princess Royal Hospital, **Hull**	Mr A G Gordon	Yes	Yes	No	1987
16	Department of Obstetrics & Gynaecology, St James's University Hospital, **Leeds**	Mr D R Bromham	Yes	Yes	Yes	1985
17	Assisted Conception Centre, Fazakerley Hospital, **Liverpool**	Mr P Bousfield	Yes	Yes	No	1989
18	Assisted Conception Unit, Royal **Liverpool** Hospital	Dr C Kingsland	Yes	No	No	1990
19	Assisted Conception Unit, The Women's Hospital, **Liverpool**	Dr J Hewitt	Yes	Yes	No	1989
20	IVF Unit, Blessings Private Clinic, **London**	Dr S E Addo	Yes	Yes	No	1990
21	IVF Unit, Bridge Fertility Centre, London Bridge Hospital, **London**	Mr O Djahanbakhch	Yes	Yes	No	1988
22	The Fertility & IVF Centre, The Churchill Clinic, **London**	Mr R Goswamy	Yes	Yes	No	1988
23	IVF Programme, Cromwell Hospital, **London**	Dr K K Ahuja Professor R W Shaw	Yes	Yes	No	1985

	Name of Centre	*Director*	*IVF*	*GIFT*	*Licensed Research*	*Date Licensed*
24	The Hallam Medical Centre, **London**	Dr B A Mason	Yes	Yes	Yes	1985
25	Institute of Obstetrics & Gynaecology, Hammersmith Hospital, **London**	Professor R M L Winston	Yes	Yes	Yes	1985
26	Fertility & IVF Unit, Humana Hospital Wellington, **London**	Professor I L Craft	Yes	Yes	No	1986
27	Infertility Advisory Centre, **London**	Dr J Glatt	Yes	Yes	No	1987
28	Assisted Conception Unit, King's College Hospital, **London**	Mr J Parsons	Yes	Yes	Yes	1986
29	*In Vitro* Fertilisation Unit, Lister Hospital, **London**	Mr J Studd Mr H Abdalla	Yes	Yes	No	1988
30	MRC Experimental Embryology and Teratology Unit, **London**	Dr D Whittingham	No	No	Yes	1985
31	Fertility Unit, AMI Portland Hospital, **London**	Mr M E Setchell	Yes	Yes	No	1988
32	Academic Department of Obstetrics & Gynaecology, Royal Free Hospital, **London**	Professor R W Shaw	Yes	Yes	Yes	1985
33	IVF Unit, Royal Hospital of St Bartholomew, **London**	Mr M E Setchell Mr R Howell	Yes	Yes	No	1986
34	Royal Masonic Hospital, **London**	Professor R M L Winston	Yes	Yes	No	1990
35	Manchester Fertility Services, BUPA Hospital, **Manchester**	Dr B A Lieberman Dr R W Burslem	Yes	Yes	No	1987
36	Regional IVF Unit, St Mary's Hospital, **Manchester**	Dr B A Lieberman	Yes	Yes	Yes	1985
37	BUPA Hospital, **Norwich**	Mr R Martin	Yes	Yes	No	1987
38	AMI Park Hospital, **Nottingham**	Mr J Webster	Yes	Yes	Yes	1986
39	IVF Unit, John Radcliffe Hospital, **Oxford**	Dr D H Barlow	Yes	No	Yes	1986

	Name of Centre	*Director*	*IVF*	*GIFT*	*Licensed Research*	*Date Licensed*
40	CRC Developmental Tumours Group, University of **Oxford**	Professor C F Graham	No	No	Yes	1987
41	Sheffield Fertility Centre, **Sheffield**	Dr E A Lenton Professor I Cooke	Yes	Yes	No	1989
42	Infertility Advisory Centre, BUPA Parkway Hospital, **Solihull,** West Midlands	Dr J Glatt	Yes	Yes	No	1988
43	Department of Human Reproduction & Obstetrics, Princess Anne Hospital, **Southampton**	Mr G M Masson	Yes	Yes	No	1985
44	IVF Centre, BUPA Hospital, Little Aston, **Sutton Coldfield,** West Midlands	Dr P Bromwich	Yes	No	No	1989
45	Department of Biology, University of **York**	Dr H J Leese	No	No	Yes	1985

The following centres are planning to set up IVF programmes, but have not yet been approved.

Name of Centre	*Director*
Arrowe Park Hospital, **Birkenhead**	Dr M R Darwish
The Grange, Bottisham, **Cambridge**	Dr T Mathews
Chelsfield Park Hospital, **Chelsfield,** Kent	Mr S Jeff
North Devon District Hospital, **Devon**	Mr W P Bradford
Assisted Conception Unit, Esperance Hospital, **Eastbourne**	Mr D Robertson
Cameron Hospital, **Hartlepool**	Mr W G Dawson
The Roding Hospital, **Ilford,** Essex	Mr D Vinker
Allerton Medicare Plc, **Leeds**	Dr M Bark
Guy's Hospital, **London**	Mr M Chapman
Newham General Hospital, **London**	Mr O Djahanbakhch
Welbeck Hospital, **London**	Dr R Ghanadian
Withington Hospital, **Manchester**	Dr S Killick
Princess Mary Maternity Hospital, **Newcastle upon Tyne**	Professor W Dunlop
Royal Victoria Infirmary, **Newcastle upon Tyne**	Professor W Dunlop
The Three Shires Hospital, **Northampton**	Mr W A R Davies
Norfolk & Norwich Hospital, **Norwich**	Mr R Martin
Hope Hospital, **Salford**	Mr G G Mitchell
Cromwell Fertility Centre at The Washington Hospital,	Professor R W Shaw
Tyne and Wear	Dr K K Ahuja
Billinge Maternity Hospital, **Wigan**	Mr C J Chandler
BUPA Murrayfield Hospital, **Wirral**	Mr U Abdalla

CENTRES REGISTERED WITH THE AUTHORITY AS OFFERING GIFT

Name of Centre	*Director*
The Yorkshire Clinic, **Bingley,** West Yorkshire	Mr R Jackson
Arrowe Park Hospital, **Birkenhead**	Mr M R Darwish
Dudley Road Hospital, **Birmingham**	Mr J F Watts
Selly Oak Hospital, **Birmingham**	Dr P G Needham
Princess of Wales Hospital, **Brindgend,** Wales	Dr R P Balfour
Brighton General Hospital, **Brighton**	Mr S Okolo
The Grange, Bottisham, **Cambridge**	Dr T Mathews
Chelsfield Park Hospital, **Chelsfield,** Kent	Mr S Jeff
North Devon District Hospital, **Devon**	Mr W P Bradford
Esperance Hospital, **Eastbourne**	Mr D Robertson
Western General Hospital, **Edinburgh**	Mr T B Hargreave Dr J B Scrimgeour
BUPA Hospital, **Elland,** West Yorkshire	Mr J Campbell
Roding Hospital, **Essex**	Mr G Sadler
Cameron Hospital, **Hartlepool**	Mr W G Dawson
Kettering General and District Hospital, **Kettering,** Northants	Mr M Newman
Allerton Medicare Plc, **Leeds**	Dr M Bark
Clarendon Wing, The General Infirmary, **Leeds**	Mr M Glass
Leicester Royal Infirmary, **Leicester**	Mr R Neuberg
Guy's Hospital, **London**	Mr M Chapman
The London Hospital, Whitechapel, **London**	Professor J G Grudzinskas
Newham General Hospital, **London**	Mr O Djahanbakhch
North Middlesex Hospital, **London**	Mr R Etheridge
St George's Hospital, **London**	Mrs T Varma
Queen Charlotte's and Chelsea Hospital, **London**	Mr D K Edmonds
Luton and Dunstable Hospital, **Luton**	Mr M O Lobb
Withington Hospital, **Manchester**	Dr S Killick
South Cleveland Hospital, **Middlesborough**	Mr P Taylor
Royal Victoria Infirmary, **Newcastle upon Tyne**	Professor W Dunlop
Northampton General Hospital, **Northampton**	Mr W A R Davies
The Three Shires Hospital, **Northampton**	Mr W A R Davies
Norfolk and Norwich Hospital, **Norwich**	Mr R Martin
St Mary's Hospital, **Portsmouth**	Dr I M Golland
Rotherham District General Hospital, **Rotherham**	Dr B C Rosenberg
Hope Hospital, **Salford**	Mr G G Mitchell
Queen Mary's Hospital, **Sidcup,** Kent	Dr S Morcos
Stafford District General Hospital, **Stafford**	Mr A B Duke
Fairfield Independent Hospital, **St Helens**	Mr C J Chandler
North Tees General Hospital, **Stockton-on-Tees**	Mr R Brown
Ryhope Hospital, **Sunderland**	Miss M Dalton
Singleton Hospital, **Swansea,** West Glamorgan	Mr P B Simpkins

Name of Centre	*Director*
Mount Stuart Hospital, **Torquay**	Mr P J Stannard
Hillingdon Hospital, **Uxbridge,** Middlesex	Dr R Bates
Billinge Hospital, **Wigan**	Mr C J Chandler
BUPA Murrayfield Hospital, **Wirral**	Mr U Abdalla
Wrexham Maelor Hospital, **Wrexham,** Clwyd	Mr J D Hamlett

The following centres are planning to set up a GIFT programme:

Monklands District General Hospital, **Airdrie**	Dr D Conway
Heatherwood Hospital, **Ascot,** Berks	Miss J Spring
BUPA Hospital, **Cardiff**	Mr B Turner
James Paget Hospital, **Great Yarmouth**	Mr W B Costley
Northwick Park Hospital, **Harrow,** Middlesex	Mr A M Fisher
The Royal Infirmary, **Huddersfield**	Mr J M Campbell
Welbeck Hospital, **London**	Dr R Ghanadian
Royal Gwent Hospital, **Newport,** Gwent	Mr I Rocker
Cromwell Fertility Centre at The Washington Hospital, **Tyne and Wear**	Professor R W Shaw Dr K K Ahuja

Appendix 8
List of ILA Approved Research Projects (to 1990)

RESEARCH PROJECTS APPROVED BY THE ILA

1985

1. *MRC Experimental Embryology and Teratology Unit, London*
   (a) Culture media and pre-embryo metabolism.
   (b) Storage of human pre-embryos.
   (c) Cell surface changes during egg-sperm interactions.

2. *Royal Free Hospital*
   (a) Studies on ovulation induction and follicular fluid biochemistry.
   (b) Development of technique for cryopreservation of pre-embryos for IVF.

3. *University of York*
Measurement of the uptake of pyruvic acid by single human oocytes and pre-implantation pre-embryos. (Terminated 1988).

4. *Bristol Maternity Hospital/Glen Hospital, Bristol*
   (a) Study of the fertilising ability of oocytes and spermatozoa in relation to defined infertility factors.
   (b) Study of the hormonal preparation of the uterus in women with primary ovarian failure.

5. *The Rosie Maternity Hospital, Cambridge*
   (a) The investigation of factors which contribute to male infertility by fertilisation *in vitro* and donated human oocytes.
   (b) Patterns of enzyme activity (HPRT, APRT, ADA, PNP) and RNA synthesis during the pre–implantation stages of human embryogenesis.
   (c) Effects of temperature changes on the cytoskeleton and fertilisation properties of human oocytes.

6. *University of Edinburgh*
(a) Analysis of karotype of pre-embryo following fertilisation *in vitro*.
(b) An assessment of the effect of varying times at pre-incubation on fertilisation rate of eggs recovered at different times after HCG. (Project completed 1988).
(c) An analysis of the number of follicles, percentage recovery of oocytes and their fertilisation rate following different regimes of superovulation. (Project completed 1988).

1986

1. *Bourn Hall, Cambridge*
(a) Timelapse cinephotography of developing embryos following fertilisation.
(b) Maturation of immature oocytes *in vitro*.
(c) Non-invasive biochemical analysis of human embryos, prior to replacement.
(d) Removal of cumulus cells.
(e) Modifications in the present methods for the cryopreservation of pre-embryos.

2. *John Radcliffe Hospital, Oxford*
(a) Semen characteristics in *in vitro* fertilisation. (Project completed 1988).
(b) Immunological consequences of *in vitro* insemination during *in vitro* fertilisation. (Project completed 1988).

3. *Jessop Hospital, Sheffield*
Hormonal studies to improve IVF treatment. (Terminated 1988).

4. *University of Aberdeen*
The effect of RU486 on the maturation and *in vitro* fertilisation of human oocytes. (Project completed 1987).

1987

1. *St James' University Hospital, Leeds*
Comparison of IVF and GIFT in non-tubal infertility. (Not pursued).

2. *University of Aberdeen*
(a) The effect of two anti-oestrogens of follicle and oocyte maturation. (Project completed 1987).
(b) Follicle maturation and early embryogenesis; a study of chromosome abnormalities.

3. *University of Edinburgh*
(a) Genetic studies of human pre-implantation embryos and oocytes by DNA-DNA *in situ* hybridisation. (Project completed 1989).
(b) Studies of gene expression in human pre-implantation embryos and oocytes. (Project completed 1989).

4. *Hammersmith Hospital*
Pre-implantation diagnosis of Lesch-Nyhan Syndrome.

5. *Royal Free Hospital School of Medicine*
(a) Cryopreservation of human oocytes: a study of the cell membrane permeability co-efficients and their relationship to toxicity and protection during freezing.
(b) An investigation of the activity of genes encoding cell-surface antigens and growth regulatory proteins in the human pre-embryo. (Terminated 1988).

6. *St Mary's Hospital, Manchester*
To compare the outcome of treatment by Gamete Intra Fallopian Transfer (GIFT) to *In Vitro* Fertilisation (IVF) and Embryo Replacement (ER) to couples with unexplained infertility. (Not pursued).

7. *Park Hospital, Nottingham*
(a) The use of micromanipulation techniques in fertilisation.
(b) Micro-injection of spermatozoa into human oocytes.
(c) A study of the existence of viruses in the human oocyte and conceptus.

8. *CRC — University of Oxford*
Derivation of cell lines from the human conceptus to investigate the growth regulation of embryonic and tumour cells for the development of effective pre-implantation diagnosis.

9. *University of York*
Study of the nutrition of single human oocytes and pre-implantation embryos. (In collaboration with Hammersmith Hospital).

10. *King's College Hospital*
(a) The definition of optimal culture conditions for the culture of human pre-implantation embryos *in vitro*.
(b) The identification of criteria for human pre-implantation embryo viability.

1988

1. *Rosie Maternity Hospital, Cambridge*
(a) A study of the factors which induce spontaneous activation of oocytes *in vitro*.
(b) Fertilisation studies using an anti-zona antibody.

2. *Chelsea Hospital for Women*
Study to investigate those couples in whom IVF is unsuccessful due to failure to fertilise.

3. *University of Aberdeen*
A study of the factors affecting the timing and characteristics of the midcycle endogenous LH surge in spontaneous and superovulated cycles.

4. *Bourn Hall, Cambridge*
(a) Pre-implantation diagnosis: sexing of human embryos.
(b) Protocol for zona drilling at Bourne Hall.

5. Optimising biological conditions for IVF — an investigation of the potential of pre-implantation diagnosis.

6. *Hallam Medical Centre*
(a) Surface morphology of arrested human oocytes and embryos observed by scanning electron microscopy.
(b) An investigation of distribution and abundance of intermediate filament proteins in arrested human oocytes.

7. *John Radcliffe Hospital, Oxford*
(a) Transplantation antigen expression on human pre-implantation embryos.
(b) Development of techniques for biopsy of human pre-embryos for pre-natal genetic diagnosis.

8. *University of Edinburgh*
Initiation of x-chromosome inactivation in human embryonic development. (Project completed).

1989

1. *Hammersmith Hospital*
Pre-implantation diagnosis after *in vitro* fertilisation for prevention of x-linked genetic diseases.

2. *Royal Infirmary, Glasgow*
An investigation of the activity of gene encoding cell-surface antigens and growth regulator proteins in the human pre-embryo.

3. *University of Edinburgh*
Development of techniques for pre-implantation diagnosis of human genetic disease.

4. *St James' University Hospital, Leeds*
Role of epidermal growth factor on maturation of oocytes *in vitro*.

5. *King's College Hospital*
(a) Pre-implantation stage diagnosis of sickle cell anaemia and Haemophilia A in the human embryo.
(b) Diagnostic laparoscopy in combination with laparoscopic oocyte collection, as part of the routine investigation and treatment of both infertile donors and recipients.

6. *John Radcliffe Hospital, Oxford*
Partial zona dissection for the alleviation of male infertility.

7. *St Mary's Hospital, Manchester*
(a) The study of the endometrium in *in vitro* fertilisation (IVF) cycles; the effect of superovulation induction regime on endometrial structure around the time of implantation.
(b) Clomiphene challenge test as a screening procedure for IVF patients.

1990

1. *St Mary's Hospital, Manchester*

(a) Cryopreservation of fertilised supernumerary oocytes from GIFT programmes at other hospitals.

(b) The use of biosynthetic human growth hormone (B-hGH) in combination with luteal-phase buserelin and HMG for *in vitro* fertilisation in (a) poor and (b) normal responders.

(c) The use of unfertilised oocytes in a diagnostic test to assess the fertilising capacity of human sperm.

(d) Partial zona dissection (PZD) of human oocytes in the treatment of infertility.

2. *King's College Hospital*

The effect of Lignocaine on human oocytes as assessed by fertilisation, cleavage and parthenogenesis results.

3. *University Hospital of Wales, Cardiff*

Non-invasive investigations of pre-implantation embryos.

Index

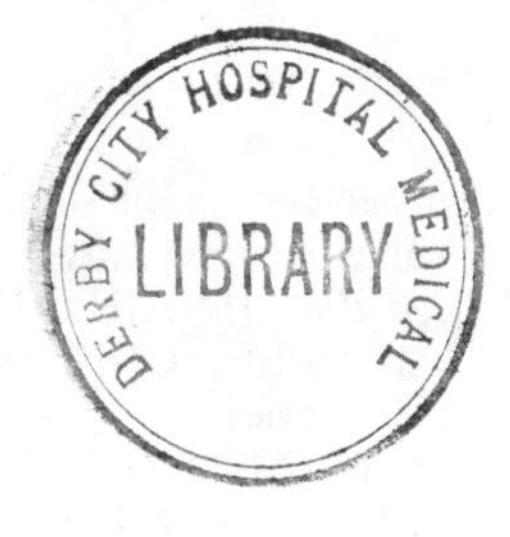